Chronic Obstructive Pulmonary Disease: A Multidisciplinary Approach

Editorial Advisor

JOEL J. HEIDELBAUGH

ELSEVIER

1600 John F. Kennedy Boulevard • Suite 1800 • Philadelphia, Pennsylvania, 19103-2899

http://www.theclinics.com

CLINICS COLLECTIONS
ISSN 2352-7986, ISBN-13: 978-0-323-42822-4

Editor: Patrick Manley (p.manley@elsevier.com)
Developmental Editor: John Vassallo (j.vassallo@elsevier.com)

Clinics Collections (ISSN 2352-7986) is published by Elsevier Inc., 360 Park Avenue South, New York, NY 10010-1710. Business and editorial offices: 1600 John F. Kennedy Boulevard, Suite 1800, Philadelphia, PA 19103-2899. **POSTMASTER:** Send address changes to *Clinics Collections*, Elsevier Health Sciences Division, Subscription Customer Service, 3251 Riverport Lane, Maryland Heights, MO 63043. **Customer Service: Telephone: 1-800-654-2452** (U.S. and Canada); **1-314-447-8871** (outside U.S. and Canada). **Fax: 314-447-8029.** E-mail: **journalscustomerserviceusa@elsevier.com** (for print support); **journalsonlinesupport-usa@elsevier.com** (for online support).

Reprints. For copies of 100 or more of articles in this publication, please contact the Commercial Reprints Department, Elsevier Inc., 360 Park Avenue South, New York, NY 10010-1710. Tel.: 212-633-3874; Fax: 212-633-3820; E-mail: reprints@elsevier.com.

Contributors

EDITORIAL ADVISOR

JOEL J. HEIDELBAUGH, MD, FAAFP, FACG
Clinical Associate Professor, Departments of Family Medicine and Urology; Clerkship Director, University of Michigan Medical School, Ann Arbor; Ypsilanti Health Center, Ypsilanti, Michigan

AUTHORS

ALEXANDER A. BANKIER, MD, PhD
Professor, Department of Radiology, Beth Israel Deaconess Medical Center, Boston, Massachusetts

JEAN BOURBEAU
Montreal Chest Institute, McGill University Health Centre, Montréal, Québec, Canada

DINA BROOKS, PhD, PT
Senior Scientist, Department of Respiratory Medicine, West Park Healthcare Centre; Professor of Physical Therapy, University of Toronto; CIHR Chair in COPD Research, Graduate Department of Rehabilitation Science, Faculty of Medicine, Toronto, Ontario, Canada

PETER CALVERLEY, DSc, FMedSc
Professor, Respiratory Research, Clinical Sciences Department; Professor of Respiratory Medicine, Institute of Ageing & Chronic Diseases, University Hospital Aintree, Liverpool, United Kingdom

GOURAB CHOUDHURY, MBBS, MRCP(UK)
ELEGI and COLT Laboratories, Queens Medical Research Institute, Edinburgh, United Kingdom

ENRIQUE DIAZ-GUZMAN, MD
Division of Pulmonary, Critical Care, and Sleep Medicine, University of Alabama at Birmingham, Birmingham, Alabama

KATHERINE A. DUDLEY, MD
Research and Clinical Fellow, Harvard Combined Program of Pulmonary and Critical Care and Division of Sleep and Circadian Disorders at Brigham and Women's Hospital, Boston, Massachusetts

MARIEKE LEONTINE DUIVERMAN, MD, PhD
Department of Pulmonary Diseases/Home Mechanical Ventilation, University Medical Centre Groningen, Groningen, The Netherlands

VINCENT S. FAN, MD, MPH
Staff Physician, Veterans Affairs Puget Sound Health Care System and Associate Professor of Medicine, Department of Medicine, University of Washington, Seattle, Washington

DELIA E. FREDERICK, MSN, RN
Doctoral Student in Nursing Science, School of Nursing, The University of North Carolina at Greensboro, Oak Street, Franklin, North Carolina

SAMUEL M. GALVAGNO Jr, DO, PhD
Assistant Professor, Department of Anesthesiology, Shock Trauma Center, University of Maryland School of Medicine, Baltimore, Maryland

MARK A. GIEMBYCZ, BSc, PhD
Professor, Tier 1 Canada Research Chair in Pulmonary Pharmacology, Department of Physiology & Pharmacology, Airways Inflammation Research Group, Snyder Institute for Chronic Diseases, University of Calgary, Calgary, Alberta, Canada

ROGER GOLDSTEIN, MB ChB, FRCP
Senior Scientist, Department of Respiratory Medicine, West Park Healthcare Centre; Professor of Medicine and Physical Therapy, University of Toronto; NSA-University of Toronto Chair in Respiratory Rehabilitation Research; Graduate Department of Rehabilitation Science, Faculty of Medicine, Toronto, Ontario, Canada

TREVOR T. HANSEL, FRCPath, PhD
Imperial Clinical Respiratory Research Unit (ICRRU), Biomedical Research Centre (BMRC), Centre for Respiratory Infection (CRI), National Heart and Lung Institute (NHLI), St Mary's Hospital, Imperial College, Paddington, London, United Kingdom

KIRSTEN HARTWICK
Research Assistant, Department of Radiology, Beth Israel Deaconess Medical Center, Boston, Massachusetts

KYLIE HILL, PhD
Associate Professor, School of Physiotherapy and Exercise Science, Faculty of Health Science, Curtin University; Lung Institute of Western Australia, Centre for Asthma, Allergy and Respiratory Research, University of Western Australia; Physiotherapy Department, Royal Perth Hospital, Perth, Western Australia, Australia

ANNE E. HOLLAND, PhD
Associate Professor, Department of Physiotherapy, La Trobe University; Department of Physiotherapy, Alfred Health; Institute for Breathing and Sleep, Melbourne, Victoria, Australia

CARON M. HONG, MD, MSc
Assistant Professor, Department of Anesthesiology, University of Maryland School of Medicine, Baltimore, Maryland

SUZANNE C. LAREAU, RN, MS
Senior Instructor, College of Nursing, University of Colorado, Aurora, Colorado

DIANA E. LITMANOVICH, MD
Assistant Professor, Department of Radiology, Beth Israel Deaconess Medical Center, Boston, Massachusetts

DAVID A. LOMAS, PhD, ScD, FRCP, FMedSci
Professor, University College London, London, United Kingdom

RODERICK MACDONALD, MS
Minneapolis VA Health Care System, Minneapolis, Minnesota

ALEX J. MACKAY, BSc(Hons), MRCP
Clinical Fellow in Respiratory Medicine, Centre for Respiratory Medicine, Royal Free
Campus, University College London, London, United Kingdom

WILLIAM MACNEE, MBChB, MD, FRCP(G), FRCP(E)
ELEGI and COLT Laboratories, Queens Medical Research Institute, Edinburgh,
United Kingdom

ATUL MALHOTRA, MD
Kenneth M. Moser Professor of Medicine, Chief of Pulmonary and Critical Care Medicine,
Director of Sleep Medicine, University of California San Diego, San Diego, California

DAVID M. MANNINO, MD
Division of Pulmonary, Critical Care, and Sleep Medicine, University of Alabama at
Birmingham, Birmingham, Alabama; Department of Preventive Medicine and
Environmental Health, University of Kentucky College of Public Health, Lexington,
Kentucky

STEFAN J. MARCINIAK, PhD, FRCP
Doctor, Division of Respiratory Medicine, Department of Medicine, Addenbrooke's
Hospital; Cambridge Institute for Medical Research (CIMR), University of Cambridge,
Cambridge, United Kingdom

PAULA M. MEEK, RN, PhD
Professor, College of Nursing, University of Colorado, Colorado

ROBERT NEWTON, BSc, PhD
Professor, Alberta Innovates-Health Solutions Senior Scholar, Department of Cell
Biology & Anatomy, Airways Inflammation Research Group, Snyder Institute for Chronic
Diseases, University of Calgary, Calgary, Alberta, Canada

ROBERT L. OWENS, MD
Assistant Professor of Medicine, Divisions of Pulmonary and Critical Care and Sleep and
Circadian Disorders, Brigham and Women's Hospital, Boston, Massachusetts

MILO A. PUHAN, MD, PhD
Professor of Epidemiology and Public Health; Institute of Social and Preventive Medicine,
University of Zurich, Zurich, Switzerland

ROBERTO RABINOVICH, MBBS, MD, PhD
ELEGI and COLT Laboratories, Queens Medical Research Institute, Edinburgh,
United Kingdom

KAMEN RANGELOV, MD
Fellow, Pulmonary and Critical Care Medicine, University at Buffalo, SUNY, Buffalo,
New York

KATHRYN RICE, MD
Minneapolis VA Health Care System, Minneapolis, Minnesota

CLARE L. ROSS, MRCP
Imperial Clinical Respiratory Research Unit (ICRRU), Biomedical Research Centre
(BMRC), Centre for Respiratory Infection (CRI), National Heart and Lung Institute (NHLI),
St Mary's Hospital, Imperial College, Paddington, London, United Kingdom

SUNDEEP SALVI, MD, DNB, PhD, FCCP
Director, Chest Research Foundation, Pune, India

SANJAY SETHI, MD
Professor of Medicine, Division Chief, Pulmonary, Critical Care, and Sleep Medicine, Staff
Physician, VA Western New York Healthcare System, University at Buffalo, The State
University of New York, Buffalo, New York

MARIO SILVA, MD
Research Fellow, Department of Radiology, Beth Israel Deaconess Medical Center,
Boston, Massachusetts; Section of Diagnostic Imaging, Department of Surgical
Sciences, University of Parma, Parma, Italy

RICHA SINGH, BSc(Hons), MRCP
Clinical Fellow in Respiratory Medicine, Centre for Respiratory Medicine, Royal Free
Campus, University College London, London, United Kingdom

JØRGEN VESTBO, DMSc, FRCP
FRCP Professor of Respiratory Medicine, Department of Respiratory Medicine J, Odense
University Hospital, Clinical Institute, University of Southern Denmark, Odense, Denmark;
Respiratory Research Group, Manchester Academic Sciences Centre, University Hospital
South Manchester NHS Foundation Trust, Manchester, United Kingdom

JADWIGA A. WEDZICHA, MD, FRCP
Professor of Respiratory Medicine, Centre for Respiratory Medicine, Royal Free Campus,
University College London, London, United Kingdom

PETER JAN WIJKSTRA, MD, PhD
Department of Pulmonary Diseases/Home Mechanical Ventilation, University Medical
Centre Groningen, Groningen, The Netherlands

TIMOTHY J. WILT, MD, MPH
Minneapolis VA Health Care System, Minneapolis, Minnesota

Contents

syndromes have been poorly studied for a variety of reasons. One difficulty is that each of the underlying disorders in an overlap syndrome occurs along a spectrum of disease severity. Thus, patients with an overlap syndrome are heterogeneous, and the goals of therapy may differ in different patients. However, the importance of overlap syndromes is highlighted by recent data demonstrating increased morbidity and mortality in patients with the overlap of both chronic obstructive pulmonary disease (COPD) and OSA compared with either underlying disorder alone. Unrecognized OSA may also contribute to symptoms of sleepiness/fatigue in patients with chronic lung disease. Clinicians should be mindful of the possibility of overlap syndromes in these patients.

Until now, there has been no conclusive evidence that noninvasive ventilation (NIV) should be provided routinely to stable patients with chronic obstructive pulmonary disease. Nevertheless, patients who are clearly hypercapnic, who receive confirmed effective ventilation by applying higher inspiratory pressures, and have a better compliance, might show clinical benefits. The combination of rehabilitation and nocturnal ventilatory support seems to provide more benefits than rehabilitation alone, so this might be a situation in which chronic NIV is effective.

In this article, the prevalence of depression, anxiety, and cognitive impairment in persons with chronic obstructive pulmonary disease, and the impact of these psychological and cognitive factors on clinical outcomes in COPD is reviewed. Methods for screening and identification of these conditions in COPD are described. The extent to which depression, anxiety or cognitive impairment limit or modify the effectiveness of pulmonary rehabilitation, and whether pulmonary rehabilitation may ameliorate these psychological and cognitive impairments are discussed.

Although primarily a lung disease, chronic obstructive pulmonary disease (COPD) is now recognized to have extrapulmonary effects on distal organs, the so-called systemic effects and comorbidities of COPD. Skeletal muscle dysfunction, nutritional abnormalities including weight loss, cardiovascular complications, metabolic complications, and osteoporosis, among others, are all well-recognized associations in COPD. These extrapulmonary effects add to the burden of mortality and morbidity in COPD and therefore should be actively looked for, assessed, and treated.

Clinical Considerations and Complications

systematic reviews and systematic reviews that have been subsequently reported since the last Cochrane report. The focus of this appraisal was to determine the effectiveness of pulmonary rehabilitation programs versus control therapy in chronic obstructive pulmonary disease patients. This analysis did not evaluate other aspects of the pulmonary rehabilitation intervention.

This article presents evidence that a glucocorticoid, LABA, and phosphodiesterase (PDE) 4 inhibitor in combination can interact in a complex manner to induce a panel of genes that could act collectively to suppress inflammation and improve lung function. The possibility that multivalent ligands may deliver superior efficacy is also being explored. Single molecules that inhibit PDE4 and activate β_2-adrenoceptors at similar concentrations have been described.

Clinical trials with new drugs for chronic obstructive pulmonary disease (COPD) have been performed. Viruses exacerbate COPD and bacteria may play a part in severe COPD; therefore, antibiotic and antiviral approaches have a sound rationale. Antiinflammatory approaches have been studied. Advances in understanding the molecular basis of other processes have resulted in novel drugs to target reactive oxidant species, mucus, proteases, fibrosis, cachexia, and muscle wasting, and accelerated aging. Studies with monoclonal antibodies have been disappointing, highlighting the tendency for infections and malignancies during treatment. Promising future directions are lung regeneration with retinoids and stem cells.

Behavioral change is critical for improving health outcomes in patients with chronic obstructive pulmonary disease. An educational approach alone is insufficient; changes in behavior, especially the acquisition of self-care skills, are also required. There is mounting evidence that embedding collaborative self-management (CSM) within existing health care systems provides an effective model to meet these needs. CSM should be integrated with pulmonary rehabilitation programs, one of the main goals of which is to induce long-term changes in behavior. More research is needed to evaluate the effectiveness of assimilating CSM into primary care, patient-centered medical homes, and palliative care teams.

Despite the well-established benefits of exercise training in people with chronic respiratory disease, there are a group of people in whom it confers minimal gains. Furthermore, there is increasing recognition of the prevalence of comorbid conditions among people with chronic obstructive pulmonary disease and other respiratory diseases, such as musculoskeletal disorders, which make participation in traditional exercise training programs challenging. This article focuses on several adjuncts or strategies that may be implemented by clinicians during exercise training, with the goal of optimizing the proportion of pulmonary rehabilitation participants who achieve significant and meaningful gains on program completion.

Peter Calverley

> The appropriate management of chronic obstructive pulmonary disease (COPD) involves more than taking prescription medicines. The key components have been set out in detail in many treatment guidelines, both national and international. They include the avoidance of identified risk factors, especially tobacco smoking, and the optimization of daily physical activity. This article reviews the key components of the pharmacologic treatment of COPD, both acute and chronic, with an emphasis on those recent studies, which are likely to change practice in the next few years.

Special Considerations

Delia E. Frederick

> This article elicits why critical care nurses need to become aware of the pulmonary issues of older adults. The population of older adults is increasing. Older adults undergo anatomic and physiologic changes of the protective mechanisms of the pulmonary system. These changes alter the rate and effort of breathing. Speech is slowed because of expiratory strength effort. Cognition changes may be the only indication of impaired oxygenation. Bedside nursing care provides protection from pulmonary complications. Health behaviors of smoking cessation, oral hygiene, and exercise promote pulmonary health even in older adults.

Preface

Each year, Elsevier's prestigious *Clinics Review Articles* series publishes more than 250 issues (3000+ articles) encompassing more than 50 medical and surgical disciplines. This curated collection of articles, devoted to Chronic Obstructive Pulmonary Disease, draws from the robust *Clinics* database to provide multidisciplinary teams with practical, clinical advice on comorbidities and complications of this highly prevalent disease.

Featured articles from the *Clinics in Chest Medicine*, *Sleep Medicine Clinics*, *Medical Clinics of North America*, *Radiologic Clinics of North America*, and *Critical Care Nursing Clinics of North America* reflect the wide range of clinicians who manage the patient with chronic obstructive pulmonary disease. This multidisciplinary perspective is essential to successful team-based management.

I hope you share this volume with your colleagues and that it spurs more collaboration, deeper understanding, and safer, more effective care for your patients.

Joel J. Heidelbaugh, MD, FAAFP, FACG
Ypsilanti, MI, USA
June 2015

Clinics Collections 6 (2015) xiii
http://dx.doi.org/10.1016/j.ccol.2015.05.027
2352-7986/15/$ – see front matter © 2015 Published by Elsevier Inc.

COPD: Definition and Phenotypes

Jørgen Vestbo, DMSc, FRCP[a,b,*]

KEYWORDS

- COPD • Definition • Diagnosis • Lung function • Chronic inflammation

KEY POINTS

- The definition of chronic obstructive pulmonary disease (COPD) is pragmatic and highlights the chronicity, the enhanced inflammation, and the importance of exacerbations and comorbidities.
- For the clinical diagnosis of COPD, exposures, symptoms, and airflow limitation are all required.
- Phenotypes are distinct COPD subgroups that deserve attention because they have either specific outcomes or require specific management.
- The frequent exacerbator is an important phenotype with higher future risks and a requirement for preventive treatments.

The definition and phenotypes in chronic obstructive pulmonary disease (COPD) are important topics. Not only should the definition clearly outline the disease but it is also, to a large extent, the conceptual framework on which we build the diagnostic criteria for the disease. *Phenotype* is a more recent term in COPD; however, the notion of COPD consisting of several subgroups is not new at all. In fact, it is often stated that COPD is a syndrome rather than a disease. Snider[1] has dealt with this COPD nosology quite extensively, and this article only deals briefly with these concepts. More space is devoted to the operationalization of the definition, diagnostic criteria, and phenotypes.

This article originally appeared in *Clinics in Chest Medicine*, Volume 35, Issue 1, March 2014.
Disclosure of Interests: J. Vestbo has received honoraria for advising Bioxydyn, Chiesi, GlaxoSmithKline, Novartis, Syntaxin, and Takeda. J. Vestbo has received honoraria for presenting from AstraZeneca, Boehringer-Ingelheim, Chiesi, GlaxoSmithKline, Novartis, and Takeda. J. Vestbo is a member (vice-chair) of the Board of Directors of the Global Initiative for Obstructive Lung Diseases (GOLD), and he is the chair of the GOLD Scientific Committee.
[a] Department of Respiratory Medicine J, Odense University Hospital, Clinical Institute, University of Southern Denmark, Odense, Denmark; [b] Respiratory Research Group, Manchester Academic Sciences Centre, University Hospital South Manchester NHS Foundation Trust, Southmoor Road, M23 9LT Manchester, UK
* Department of Respiratory Medicine J, Odense University Hospital, Sdr Boulevard 29, 5000 Odense C, Denmark.
E-mail address: Jorgen.vestbo@manchester.ac.uk

DEFINITION

Several definitions of COPD exist, and it would be wrong to say that one is clearly superior to another. The first definitions arising from working groups of the major respiratory societies came in 1995 from the American Thoracic Society (ATS)[2] and the European Respiratory Society (ERS).[3] Significant national guidelines have subsequently adopted and modified these definitions. The ATS and ERS definitions are shown in **Box 1**.

Neither of these definitions is particularly precise and can easily include disease entities that are not usually regarded as COPD, such as cystic fibrosis, sarcoidosis, and bronchiectasis. Importantly, neither of these definitions differentiates COPD from chronic asthma with airway remodeling. There are reasons for this; there is a significant overlap, and as acknowledged by the ATS mentioning airway hyperreactivity, one of the hallmarks of asthma, some patients with COPD do have features that make it difficult to separate them from patients with chronic ongoing asthma.

In 2001, the Global Initiative for Chronic Obstructive Lung Diseases (GOLD) was launched; in their seminal document from 2001,[4] COPD is defined as "a disease state characterized by airflow limitation that is not fully reversible. The airflow obstruction is usually both progressive and associated with an abnormal response of the lungs to noxious particles or gases."[4]

This definition differs fundamentally from those of the ATS and ERS in its inclusion of inflammation as well as the disease being a consequence of external stimuli (ie, noxious particles and gases). The GOLD document has been revised twice, in 2006 and 2011. On both occasions, the definition has been changed. In 2006[5] it was changed as follows:

> Chronic obstructive pulmonary disease (COPD) is a preventable and treatable disease with some significant extrapulmonary effects that may contribute to the severity in individual patients. Its pulmonary component is characterized by airflow limitation that is not fully reversible. The airflow limitation is usually progressive and associated with an abnormal inflammatory response of the lung to noxious particles or gases.[5]

The phrase *preventable and treatable* was also included in the definition proposed by the joint ATS/ERS document from 2004 and reflects an attempt to leave previous

---

Box 1
COPD definitions from the ATS and ERS 1995

ATS 1995

"Chronic obstructive pulmonary disease is defined as a disease state characterized by the presence of airflow obstruction caused by chronic bronchitis or emphysema; the airflow obstruction is generally progressive, may be accompanied by airway hyperreactivity, and may be partially reversible."[2]

ERS 1995

"COPD is defined as a disorder characterized by reduced maximum expiratory flow and slow forced emptying of the lungs, features which do not change markedly over several months. Most of the airflow limitation is slowly progressive and irreversible. The airflow limitation is due to varying combinations of airway disease and emphysema; the relative contribution of the two processes is difficult to define *in vivo*."[3]

therapeutic nihilism regarding COPD behind. Importantly, this definition includes extrapulmonary effects as a contributor to severity in individual patients. These extrapulmonary effects were, however, not clearly defined; subsequently, many of these effects were seen as comorbidities. This point is reflected in the most recent GOLD definition[6] and is shown in **Box 2**.

The most recent changes reflect the increased knowledge of the disease that had accumulated since 2006. It has become clear that calling airflow limitation reversible in asthma and irreversible in COPD is too simplistic because patients with COPD can show significant reversibility with bronchodilators. However, airflow is never normalized; the airflow limitation was, thus, described as persistent. Similarly, we have seen that the chronic inflammation in airways and lung parenchyma does not have any specific abnormal characteristics. Rather, it seems that patients with COPD are unable to switch off inflammation; it was, therefore, thought that the phrase *enhanced inflammation* was a better descriptor. Extrapulmonary effects were replaced by comorbidities, and it was thought that the importance of exacerbations for individual patients was sufficient to warrant the inclusion of the term *exacerbations* in the definition.

DIAGNOSTIC CRITERIA

Is the current definition as proposed by GOLD ideal? The many different suggestions for a definition probably illustrates that this is not the case. The most important limitation is probably that it seems difficult to directly translate the definition into diagnostic criteria. In particular, we have no means of easily measuring the enhanced inflammation that we think is the basis for COPD. For this reason, our diagnostic criteria have heavily relied on the physiologic ascertainment of airflow limitation in patients with relevant exposure presenting to a physician.

In the GOLD 2011 revision,[6] the main section on diagnosis states that

A clinical diagnosis of COPD should be considered in any patient who has dyspnea, chronic cough or sputum production, and/or a history of exposure to risk factors for the disease. Spirometry is required to make the diagnosis in this clinical context; the presence of a post-bronchodilator [forced expiratory volume in the first second of expiration/forced vital capacity] $FEV_1/FVC <0.70$ confirms the presence of persistent airflow limitation and thus of COPD.[6]

It is important to note that the aforementioned definition relates to a clinical diagnosis (ie, a doctor making a diagnosis in a patient). Although this is clearly the most important aspect of a diagnosis, the epidemiology of COPD has for decades relied on field measurements of lung function using spirometry and simple questions excluding asthma and sometimes other respiratory disease. It may seem trivial, but this distinction has significant implications, not the least of which is for the discussion on the spirometric criteria for airflow limitation. In epidemiology, there is no proxy for

---

Box 2
COPD definition according to GOLD 2011

"Chronic Obstructive Pulmonary Disease (COPD), a common preventable and treatable disease, is characterized by persistent airflow limitation that is usually progressive and associated with an enhanced chronic inflammatory response in the airways and the lung to noxious particles or gases. Exacerbations and comorbidities contribute to the overall severity in individual patients."[6]

patients going to a doctor; diagnostic criteria in epidemiology, therefore, resemble the criteria that would be used for screening, a tool not advocated by any major respiratory society or body.

However, the devil is often in the details. Importantly, in the 2013 update,[7] the terms *and/or* in the second line have been substituted by the term *and* as shown in **Box 3**.

In simple words, this means that in patients with relevant exposure and respiratory symptoms, a spirometry should be obtained; if airflow limitation (here defined as a postbronchodilator FEV_1/FVC <0.70) is found, this constitutes a diagnosis of COPD unless patients have other respiratory conditions, such as asthma, bronchiectasis, stenosing bronchial tumor, and so forth. Using the aforementioned strategy for COPD case finding will often result in a favorable yield; in Denmark, programs using this approach have resulted in diagnoses in 20% to 30% of those fulfilling the criteria for spirometry.[8]

Unfortunately, most of the debate on diagnostic criteria has focused on the choice of an FEV_1/FVC of less than 0.70 as the defining cutoff for airflow limitation. This cutoff is somewhat arbitrary, and opponents often argue that it has no scientific validity; instead, the lower limit of normal (LLN) is proposed.[9] There is little doubt that in most populations, the fixed 0.70 cutoff will result in more abnormal FEV_1/FVC ratios in the elderly and fewer in patients younger than 50 years.[10] This has led to a heated debate that seems futile because no gold standard exists; therefore, little real evidence exists in this area. In the epidemiologic setting, LLN should be preferred,[11] although great care should be taken when selecting reference values. In the clinical setting, no comparative studies exist. The virtue of the fixed 0.70 cutoff is simplicity and familiarity, and this is the reason why GOLD[7] and the UK National Center for Clinical Excellence have kept this criterion. The LLN is the physiologists' choice because it is anchored in our usual scientific definition of normality. However, this author really does not think it matters in clinical practice, and it seems that far too much energy has been spent on this issue considering the underrecognition, underdiagnosis, and undertreatment of COPD globally.

The probably most critical issue with the current diagnostic criteria is that they do not capture patients with pure emphysema until relatively late in the course of the disease. With an increasing focus on early diagnosis, the lack of sensitivity to a major COPD component – such as emphysema – reliance on simple spirometry for diagnosis may no longer be sufficient.

CONSIDERATIONS FOR FUTURE DIAGNOSTIC CRITERIA

So, because the current diagnostic criteria are far from ideal and the spirometric criteria are frequently the topic of futile debates, it may be worth considering if it is time to rethink diagnosis. When comparing with another chronic illness that in many ways resembles COPD, heart failure, it is clear that others have avoided debate on very specific cutoff values.[12] If we were to transfer similar thinking to COPD as that

---

Box 3
COPD diagnostic criteria according to GOLD 2013

"A clinical diagnosis of COPD should be considered in any patient who has dyspnea, chronic cough or sputum production, and a history of exposure to risk factors for the disease. Spirometry is required to make the diagnosis in this clinical context; the presence of a postbronchodilator FEV_1/FVC <0.70 confirms the presence of persistent airflow limitation and thus of COPD."[7]

of the cardiologists when diagnosing heart failure, future COPD diagnostic criteria could take the shape of 'Symptoms and clinical features compatible with COPD in an individual with relevant exposures, where either physiologic measures or imaging support the presence of functional or structural abnormalities supporting a diagnosis of COPD.'

With the very general definition of COPD and the debated diagnostic criteria, those favoring the use of diagnoses such as emphysema and chronic bronchitis (the splitters) instead of COPD (the lumpers) may wish to go back to the time before the umbrella term *COPD* was launched. But there is little doubt that COPD has come to stay. However, the splitters can comfort themselves in the fact that most COPD researchers and many clinicians find increasing value in splitting COPD into subgroups, into *phenotypes*.

COPD PHENOTYPES

A phenotype is usually considered the physical appearance or biochemical characteristic resulting from an interaction between its genotype and the environment. In COPD, whereby the underlying genes are mainly unknown or poorly characterized, *phenotype* has become almost synonymous with *clinical subgroup*. Several researchers have come up with a consensus definition of phenotypes[13] as shown in **Box 4**. This definition emphasizes that a phenotype has to be a subgroup that impacts on the outcome, that is, that having a particular phenotype means a different prognosis, a higher risk of exacerbation, a better response to a particular therapy, and so forth.

There are a few important issues regarding the concept of phenotypes. One phenotype is unlikely to be unique to one patient. In Snider's[14] original nonproportional Venn diagram, several overlapping subgroups were presented; subsequent studies trying to implement Snider's diagram to patients and populations showed that the overlap was indeed substantial. In addition to belonging to several phenotypes, patients can also have phenotypical traits. Considering emphysema as a phenotype, a patient could have mild emphysema and quite significant airflow limitation; one could speculate if emphysema had any importance in this particular patient. Also, specific combinations of phenotypes could be more important than others. Finally, in asthma, there is a move away from phenotypes toward endotypes,[15] whereby an endotype is basically a phenotype defined by a distinct pathophysiologic mechanism.

SPECIFIC COPD PHENOTYPES

The classic phenotypes of Snider's[14] diagram are asthma, emphysema, and chronic bronchitis. Asthma is likely to be considered a disease entity of its own, or a separate syndrome, despite the significant clinical overlap and the fact that asthma can be regarded as a risk factor for persistent airflow limitation. Features of asthma, such as airway hyperresponsiveness and reversibility, have been associated with a worse prognosis in some studies[16,17]; but particularly reversibility seems to be a very instable phenotype in COPD.[17]

Box 4
Phenotype definition

"A COPD phenotype is a single or combination of disease attributes that describe differences between individuals with COPD as they relate to clinically meaningful outcomes (symptoms, exacerbations, response to therapy, rate of disease progression, or death)."[13]

Emphysema is a significant component of COPD and the extent of emphysema increases with increasing severity of airflow limitation. Emphysema is associated with a significantly increased decline in FEV_1, the hallmark of COPD.[18] Emphysema is a stable phenotype. The same can be said for chronic bronchitis, which in some studies has been associated with excess FEV_1 decline, particularly in younger adults,[19] with hospital admission as well as mortality.

Many other phenotypes are likely to exist as suggested in **Box 5**.

Having frequent exacerbations is a feature that has attracted considerable attention in recent years. Several studies have shown that only some patients with COPD experience exacerbations. But with the analyses of the Evaluation of COPD Longitudinally to Identify Predictive Surrogate Endpoints (ECLIPSE) study,[20] it became evident that having 2 or more exacerbations per year seemed a stable phenotype. This has significant implications. First, exacerbations are associated with a poor prognosis[21] and an excess FEV_1 decline[18,22]; secondly, several treatments are aimed at reducing exacerbations.[7] It can be argued whether 2 annual exacerbations is the right threshold for defining the frequent exacerbator, but at least the current literature seems to support this cutoff.

Another characteristic that has attracted attention lately is the presence of systemic inflammation. Early studies saw systemic inflammation as a feature of COPD; but with larger patient cohorts studied, we have learned more. First, not all patients with COPD have elevated markers of systemic inflammation. The markers most frequently measured have been C-reactive protein (CRP) and fibrinogen, and both are associated with subsequent hospital admission and death.[23] Recent analyses from the ECLIPSE study showed that multiple markers were likely to provide more relevant information than single markers,[24] and an epidemiologic study has shown that the use of 3 biomarkers (CRP, fibrinogen, and white blood cell count) seemed to provide prognostic value regarding incident comorbidities.[25] However, we currently have no treatment aimed at systemic inflammation in COPD.

Several other phenotypes exist and could be discussed. They are all based on our understanding of the disease, and most of them rely on single observational characteristics. Several groups have made an attempt at developing phenotypes based on an unbiased approach, including machine learning. They have been applied in both stable COPD and exacerbations; but, to date, the value of these approaches is difficult to evaluate.

Box 5
Features of suggested phenotypes in COPD

Asthma

Bronchial hyperresponsiveness

Bronchodilator reversibility

Emphysema

Hyperinflation

Cachexia

Chronic bronchitis

Frequent exacerbations

Systemic inflammation

Thus, the whole concept of COPD as a syndrome with specific entities is constantly evolving. The current definition has changed only a little over the last decade. It is likely to change within the coming decade. Whether the concept of phenotypes will evolve and be included in future standards for diagnosis and management remains to be seen.

REFERENCES

1. Snider GL. Definition of chronic obstructive pulmonary disease. In: Calverley PM, MacNee W, Pride NB, et al, editors. Chronic obstructive pulmonary disease. 2nd edition. London: Arnold; 2003. p. 1–10.
2. American Thoracic Society. Standards for the diagnosis and care of patients with chronic obstructive pulmonary disease. Am J Respir Crit Care Med 1995;152: S77–121.
3. Siafakas NM, Vermeire P, Pride NB, et al. Optimal assessment and management of chronic obstructive pulmonary disease (COPD). The European Respiratory Society Task Force. Eur Respir J 1995;8:1398–420.
4. Pauwels RA, Buist AS, Calverley PM, et al. Global strategy for the diagnosis, management, and prevention of chronic obstructive pulmonary disease. NHLBI/WHO Global Initiative for Chronic Obstructive Lung Disease (GOLD) workshop summary. Am J Respir Crit Care Med 2001;163:1256–76.
5. Rabe KF, Hurd S, Anzueto A, et al. Global strategy for the diagnosis, management and prevention of chronic obstructive pulmonary disease, GOLD executive summary. Am J Respir Crit Care Med 2007;176(6):532–55.
6. Vestbo J, Hurd SS, Agusti AG, et al. Global strategy for the diagnosis, management and prevention of chronic obstructive pulmonary disease, GOLD executive summary. Am J Respir Crit Care Med 2013;187:347–65.
7. Available at: http://www.goldcopd.org/uploads/users/files/GOLD_Report_2013_Feb20.pdf. Accessed May 2, 2013.
8. Ulrik CS, Løkke A, Dahl R, et al. Early detection of COPD in general practice. Int J Chron Obstruct Pulmon Dis 2011;6:123–7.
9. Pellegrino R, Brusasco V, Viegi G, et al. Definition of COPD: based on evidence or opinion? Eur Respir J 2008;31:681–2.
10. Vollmer WM, Gislason T, Burney P, et al. Comparison of spirometry criteria for the diagnosis of COPD: results from the BOLD study. Eur Respir J 2009;34:588–97.
11. Bakke PS, Rönmark E, Eagan T, et al. Recommendations for epidemiological studies on COPD. ERS Task Force Report. Eur Respir J 2011;38:1261–77.
12. McMurray JJ, Adamopoulos S, Anker SD, et al. The Task Force for the Diagnosis and Treatment of Acute and Chronic Heart Failure 2012 of the European Society of Cardiology. ESC guidelines for the diagnosis and treatment of acute and chronic heart failure 2012. Eur Heart J 2012;33:1787–847.
13. Han MK, Agusti A, Calverley PM, et al. COPD phenotypes: the future of COPD. Am J Respir Crit Care Med 2010;182:598–604.
14. Snider G. Chronic obstructive pulmonary disease: a definition and implications of structural determinants of airflow obstruction for epidemiology. Am Rev Respir Dis 1989;140(3 Pt 2):S3–8.
15. Lötvall J, Akdis CA, Bacharier LB, et al. Asthma endotypes: a new approach to classification of disease entities within the asthma syndrome. J Allergy Clin Immunol 2011;127:355–60.
16. Scott TW, Sparrow D, editors. Airways responsiveness and atopy in the development of chronic lung disease. New York: Raven Press; 1989.

17. Albert PS, Agusti A, Edwards LD, et al. Bronchodilator responsiveness is not a consistent phenotypic characteristic of COPD. Thorax 2012;67:701–8.
18. Vestbo J, Edwards LD, Scanlon PD, et al, for the ECLIPSE Investigators. Change in forced expiratory volume in 1 second over time in COPD. N Engl J Med 2011; 365:1184–92.
19. Guerra S, Sherrill DL, Venker C, et al. Chronic bronchitis before age 50 years predicts incident airflow limitation and mortality risk. Thorax 2009;64:894–900.
20. Hurst JR, Vestbo J, Anzueto A, et al, for the Evaluation of COPD Longitudinally to Identify Predictive Surrogate Endpoints (ECLIPSE) investigators. Susceptibility to exacerbation in chronic obstructive pulmonary disease. N Engl J Med 2010;363: 1128–38.
21. Soler-Cataluña JJ, Martínez-García MA, Román Sánchez P, et al. Severe acute exacerbations and mortality in patients with chronic obstructive pulmonary disease. Thorax 2005;60:925–31.
22. Celli BR, Thomas NE, Anderson JA, et al. Effect of pharmacotherapy on rate of decline of lung function in COPD: results from the TORCH study. Am J Respir Crit Care Med 2008;178:332–8.
23. Celli BR, Locantore N, Yates J, et al, for the ECLIPSE investigators. Inflammatory biomarkers improve clinical prediction of mortality in chronic obstructive pulmonary disease. Am J Respir Crit Care Med 2012;185:1065–72.
24. Agusti A, Edwards LD, Rennard SI, et al, for the Evaluation of COPD Longitudinally to Identify Predictive Surrogate Endpoints (ECLIPSE) investigators. Persistent systemic inflammation is associated with poor clinical outcomes in COPD: a novel phenotype. PLoS One 2012;7:e37483.
25. Thomsen M, Dahl M, Lange P, et al. Inflammatory biomarkers and comorbidities in chronic obstructive pulmonary disease. Am J Respir Crit Care Med 2012;186: 982–8.

Epidemiology and Prevalence of Chronic Obstructive Pulmonary Disease

Enrique Diaz-Guzman, MD[a], David M. Mannino, MD[a,b,*]

KEYWORDS

• Chronic obstructive pulmonary disease • Prevalence • Trends • Epidemiology

KEY POINTS

• In most studied countries, about 8% to 10% of the adult population has chronic obstructive pulmonary disease, with cigarette smoking as the main risk factor.
• Occupational and environmental exposures are important in the development and progression of chronic obstructive pulmonary disease, particularly in the developing world.
• Recent data suggest that rates of chronic obstructive pulmonary disease morbidity and mortality are starting to decrease in some parts of the world.

INTRODUCTION

Chronic obstructive pulmonary disease (COPD) is a preventable and treatable disease characterized by progressive airflow limitation and represents one of the most prevalent human health disorders in the world.[1] Although mortality associated with cardiovascular disease has been significantly reduced during the last 2 decades, the number of deaths associated with COPD has almost doubled, and COPD is now the fourth leading cause of death globally. More than 15 million people have the disease in the United States[2] and more than 210 million globally.[3] Despite significant public health efforts aimed to better understand and prevent the burden of this disease, the World Health Organization (WHO) has predicted that COPD will become the third most

This article originally appeared in *Clinics in Chest Medicine*, Volume 35, Issue 1, March 2014.
Conflict of Interest Statement: E. Diaz-Guzman reports no conflicts of interest. D.M. Mannino has served as a consultant for Boehringer Ingelheim, GlaxoSmithKline, Astra-Zeneca, Novartis, Merck and Forest and has received research grants from GlaxoSmithKline, Novartis, Boehringer-Ingelheim, Forest and Pfizer.
[a] Division of Pulmonary, Critical Care, and Sleep Medicine, University of Alabama at Birmingham, 625 19th Street, Birmingham, AL 35249, USA; [b] Department of Preventive Medicine and Environmental Health, University of Kentucky College of Public Health, 111 Washington Avenue, Lexington, KY 40536, USA
* Corresponding author.
E-mail address: dmannino@uky.edu

common cause of death in the world by 2030.[4] Moreover, prevalence estimates suggest that up to a quarter of adults 40 years or older have evidence of airflow obstruction.[5] Because of the increase in prevalence, many efforts have been made to measure the epidemiology of COPD at national and international levels. Studies such as the Global Burden of Disease (GBD) and the Global Initiative for Chronic Obstructive Lung Disease (GOLD), have affected our understanding of the burden and impact of chronic respiratory disease.[6,7] This review provides a summary of the most important recent reports addressing the epidemiology of COPD and a description of new COPD guidelines.

DEFINITION OF COPD

The most recent GOLD guidelines define COPD as "a common preventable and treatable disease characterized by persistent airflow limitation that is usually progressive and associated with an enhanced chronic inflammatory response in the airways and the lungs to noxious particles or gases. Exacerbations and comorbidities contribute to the overall severity in individual patients."[7] Although this definition includes the major components of the disease, in practice, COPD consists of different clinical syndromes whose definitions vary according to the presence or absence of symptoms and measures of airflow limitation and reversibility. The following components are frequently considered when defining COPD.

Measures of Airflow Limitation and Reversibility

Airflow limitation, defined as a reduction in velocity of expiratory airflow, consists of a low forced expiratory volume in 1 second (FEV_1) and a low FEV_1 to forced vital capacity (FVC) ratio despite bronchodilator therapy. An FEV_1/FVC ratio of less than 70% continues to be used to identify airflow limitation in patients with COPD.[7,8] The use of lower limit of normal (LLN) values (based on the normal distribution of the population) has been proposed as a more specific tool to diagnose airflow limitation, but current GOLD and American Thoracic Society/European Respiratory Society guidelines continue to recommend the use of a fixed ratio instead of an LLN. Some studies have found that the use of a fixed FEV_1/FVC ratio will result in underestimation of COPD in patients less than 45 years of age (particularly those with mild disease), may overestimate the prevalence of COPD in older adults, and can result in misclassification in some patients.[9] Other studies, however, suggest that the use of a fixed ratio of 0.70 functions reasonably well in classifying most patients.[10]

In addition to airflow limitation, reversibility of airflow obstruction in response to an inhaled bronchodilator or to oral or inhaled corticosteroid is frequently used to identify patients who benefit from bronchodilator therapy.[7,11] Airflow reversibility, defined as an increase in FEV_1 of 200 mL and 12% improvement greater than baseline FEV_1, has been traditionally used to further characterize patients with airflow obstruction. Nevertheless, the degree of reversibility has not been found to increase sensitivity or specificity to diagnose COPD,[12] and current GOLD guidelines do not recommend the use of airflow reversibility as a criterion for the definition of COPD.[7]

Clinical Features and Overlap Syndromes

The characterization of COPD has included the terms *chronic bronchitis* (CB) and *emphysema*. CB is defined as the presence of a chronic productive cough for 3 months in each of 2 consecutive years provided that other medical causes have been excluded.[13] Emphysema is defined as the destruction of alveolar walls and permanent enlargement of the airspaces distal to the terminal bronchioles.[14] Although significant improvements in imaging technologies currently allow of the accurate detection of emphysema in most patients, significant variability in physician diagnosis of emphysema and CB exist, and current GOLD guidelines do not include the use of these terms in the definition of COPD.[7]

Asthma is defined as a "chronic inflammatory disorder of the airways in which many cells and cellular elements play a role. The chronic inflammation causes an associated increase in airway hyper-responsiveness that leads to recurrent episodes of wheezing, breathlessness, chest tightness and coughing, particularly at night or in the early morning. These episodes are usually associated with widespread but variable airflow obstruction that is often reversible either spontaneously or with treatment."[15] Asthma and COPD represent 2 distinct entities with different pathogeneses and risk factors; nevertheless, clinical features of both diseases may overlap, and large population studies have found that a high proportion of patients with respiratory problems are classified with more than one diagnosis (ie, asthma and chronic bronchitis or emphysema).[16,17] Moreover, overlapping diagnoses of asthma and COPD occur more commonly in patients older than 50 years, and its frequency increases with age.[16,18]

RISK FACTORS

The pathophysiology of COPD is complex, and the disease is related to genetic and environmental factors. In addition to smoking tobacco, additional important risk factors have been recognized as important and preventable causes of COPD in industrialized and developing countries. The list of risk factors associated with this condition is extensive and has been previously well described in the literature. Following is a brief description of the most commonly known risk factors in COPD.

Active and Passive Cigarette Smoking

There is overwhelming epidemiologic evidence that confirms that smoking tobacco remains the main risk factor for COPD. Several studies have found increased risk of airway obstruction measured by spirometry[19,20] and increased risk of COPD and hospitalizations for COPD exacerbations.[21] A 25-year follow-up study of the general population in Denmark that included 8045 men and women age 30to 65 years, found that the risk of COPD for continuous smokers was at least 25%.[22] The BOLD (Burden of Obstructive Lung Disease) project analyzed data from 14 different populations older than 40 years and found that pack-years of smoking were associated with increased risk of COPD, including passive cigarette smoke exposure (odds ratio [OR], 1.24, 95% confidence interval [CI], 1.05–1.47 for each 10 pack-year increase).[23] In addition to the risk for COPD, results of a recent study involving 26,851 participants from Sweden found that current smoking is a strong risk factor for any wheeze (including asthmatic wheezing), particularly among young women.[24] Tobacco use remains a major cause of morbidity and mortality, particularly in patients with COPD. A recent study using pooled data from 7 different cohort studies in the United States, analyzed 50-year trends in smoking-related mortality and found that the overall risks associated with smoking plateau compared with the levels seen 2 decades ago, except for a continuing increase in mortality from COPD.[25]

Occupational Risk Factors

Several occupational exposures may increase the risk for COPD. Activities such as farming (exposure to high levels of organic particles such as vegetable dust and bacterial or fungal toxins), textile industry work (exposure to cotton dust), and industrial work (mining, smelting, wood work, building) have been associated with an increased risk for obstructive lung disease.[26] The overall work-related burden of COPD at a population level has been well-characterized. Blanc[27] performed a review of several studies and found a median PAR% (population-attributable risk) for occupationally related COPD of 15% (range 0%–37%) and 15% for occupationally related CB (range 0%–35%). A more recent prospective cohort study by Mehta and colleagues[28] evaluated the incidence of COPD in 4267 Swiss workers exposed to biologic dusts, mineral dusts, gases/fumes, and vapors and found an increased risk (2- to 5-fold) of COPD (stage 2 according to GOLD). The PAR of stage 2 COPD was between 31% and 32% for biologic dusts among smokers and ranged between 43% and 56% for nonsmokers depending on type and level of exposure.

Air Pollution

Environmental exposure to air pollution or inside of the home (particularly among habitants of underdeveloped countries) represents an important risk factor for COPD and other obstructive lung diseases. A multinational study from 3 metropolitan areas in Latin America (ESCALA), recently described that levels of particulate matter are significantly associated with increased mortality from respiratory and cardiovascular causes, including COPD.[29] A more recent population cohort study assessed the risk of COPD associated with residential exposures to traffic-related air pollutants (black carbon, particulate matter <2.5 μm in aerodynamic diameter, nitrogen dioxide, and nitric oxide) and wood smoke. The study found a 7% increased risk of mortality and 15% increased risk of hospitalizations associated with COPD.[30]

Genetic Factors

Genetic factors determining the lung responses to environmental exposures are key for the development of COPD. Nevertheless, the specific genes responsible for this enhanced risk and increase in susceptibility remains poorly understood. The best described genetic factor in COPD is a deficiency in α_1-antitrypsin (PIZZ phenotype), but this abnormality accounts for only 1% to 3% of patients with COPD.[31] Numerous other genes have been studied and implicated in COPD susceptibility, based on different pathogenetic pathways: inflammatory (interleukin-4, -6, -13), tumor necrosis factor, transforming growth factor-β, protease/antiprotease (MMP9, TIMP2, SERPINA3), oxidative stress (glutathione transferase, superoxide dismutase) and others (ACE, ADRB2). A recent review of the literature summarizing possible genetic associations is shown in **Fig. 1**.[32]

PREVALENCE OF COPD

Even though COPD represents one of the most significant health care problems in the world, ascertainment of true prevalence among different countries has been difficult. Estimates of the prevalence of COPD depend on the criteria used. Significant differences in prevalence estimates from well-designed epidemiologic studies have been reported, particularly among studies completed before standardization of an epidemiologic definition of COPD. Furthermore, until recently, few studies were able to provide an estimate of disease prevalence using a standard spirometry-based definition.

Criteria and Impact on Disease Prevalence

In 1997, GOLD recommended spirometry as the gold standard diagnostic test for COPD. Estimations of COPD prevalence before GOLD guidelines were published were plagued with methodologic issues because of lack of quality assurance

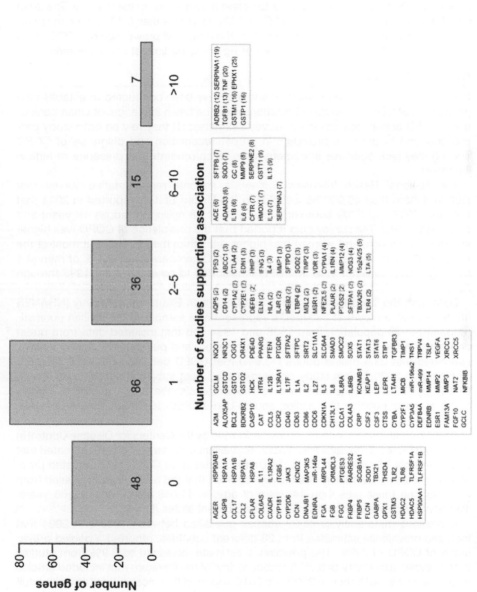

(From Bosse Y. Updates on the COPD gene list. Int J Chron Obstruct Pulmon Dis 2012;7:613.)

Fig. 1. Studies supporting genetic association with COPD.

measures, frequent use of prebronchodilator values (which may result in overestimation of COPD), and inconsistencies in the definition of obstruction being used.[33] In 2002, the Burden of Obstructive Lung Disease (BOLD) project set standards for definition of COPD in epidemiologic studies and recommended the use of a postbronchodilator FEV_1/FVC ratio of less than 0.7 to define the presence of the disease. The 2013 GOLD guidelines continue to use an FEV_1/FVC ratio of less than 0.7 to define the presence of COPD, and studies have found that the observed prevalence of COPD using the GOLD definition is higher than when using the lower limit of normal criteria.[33,34]

Prevalence Estimates

In the United States, several national surveys have been conducted to establish the prevalence of COPD. Two main limitations must be taken into account when considering COPD prevalence based on survey estimates: (1) they rely on both study participants and health care providers in proper recognition and diagnosis of COPD and (2) they lack objective spirometry data to corroborate the presence of airflow limitation.

The National Health Interview Survey, a national representative survey that included more than 40,000 households in the United States, reported in 2011 that between 2007 and 2009 approximately 5.1% (11.8 million) of adults 18 years and older had COPD. The survey also reported that the prevalence of COPD was higher in older age groups, and women had higher rates than men throughout most of the lifespan (6.1% of women [7.4 million] had COPD compared with 4.1% of men [4.4 million]). The prevalence rate of COPD is reported to be stable from 1998 through 2009.[35]

Data from the Third National Health and Nutrition Examination Survey (NHANES III), a national survey that included a representative sample of the civilian noninstitutionalized US population from 1988 and 1994 and that included data from questionnaires in the household, physical examination, and pulmonary function testing, estimated that 23.6 million adults (13.9%) met GOLD definition of COPD (stage 1 or higher) in 2000.[36] This study concluded that most subjects classified as having COPD by GOLD criteria had mild to moderate disease and that approximately 1.4% of the population (2.4 million adults) had an FEV_1 less than 50% of the predicted value.[36]

In 2011, a national telephone survey performed by the Centers for Disease Control in the United States Behavioral Risk Factor Surveillance System (BRFSS), estimated that approximately 15 million adults in the United States have COPD (age-adjusted prevalence of 6.0%). In addition, the survey reported that the prevalence increased from 3.2% among those less than 44 years of age, to 11.6% among those ≥65 years. The prevalence varied significantly across different states (**Fig. 2**).[2]

A previous meta-analysis of 62 studies published between 1990 and 2004 that included prevalence estimates from 28 different countries, reported a pooled prevalence of COPD of 7.6%. The prevalence estimate increased to 8.9% from studies that included spirometry data.[37] A recent review of the literature that included articles in English published between 2000 and 2010, reported that most estimates in the adult population varied widely across countries and populations, with a range from 0.2% in Japan to 37% in the United States. Consistent with previous observations, COPD prevalence was higher among studies using GOLD criteria to define COPD compared with other classification methods.[38] **Table 1** includes a summary of recent studies that have included spirometry data to estimate prevalence of COPD. The table highlights how different definitions and exclusion criteria can result in different estimates of disease prevalence, even when using data from the same study.

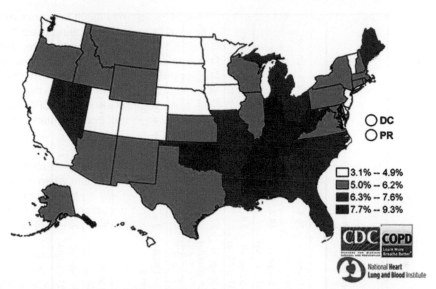

Fig. 2. BRFSS and geographic variation of prevalence estimates in the United States. (*From* Centers for Disease Control and Prevention. Chronic pulmonary obstructive disease among adults - United States 2011. MMWR Morb Mortal Wkly Rep 2012;61(46):938–42.)

Prevalence of COPD and Gender Differences

COPD historically has been considered a disease of male predominance; nevertheless, a significant shift in gender prevalence has been observed over the last few decades. In the United States, data from NHANES studies showed that the prevalence of moderate COPD increased during the last 2 decades in women (50.8–58.2 per 1000), whereas the prevalence decreased in men during the same period (108.1–74.3 per 1000).[39,40] Similarly, the National Health Interview Survey study reported that although the prevalence of COPD has been stable from 1998 through 2009, it has remained higher in women than in men (**Fig. 3**).[35] A similar trend has been observed in other developed countries,[41,42] whereas in developing countries, prevalence of COPD is still higher in men compared with women.[43]

BURDEN OF COPD AND MORTALITY

The GBD study has provided estimates of worldwide global and regional mortality. In 2006, GBD reported that COPD caused the death of at least 3.1 million people, representing the fourth leading cause of mortality in the world.[44] A subsequent report of the GBD that included mortality between 1990 and 2010 shows that COPD is now the third leading cause of mortality in the world, although the number of deaths attributed to COPD decreased from 3.1 million to 2.9 million annually.[45]

In contrast to these optimistic estimates in developed countries, the problem of COPD continues to increase in the rest of the world. Studies estimate that up to 50% of all households in developing countries use coal and biomass as primary sources of energy and therefore are exposed to smoke produced during heating and cooking.[46] The WHO has estimated that approximately 700,000 annual deaths from COPD are caused by solid fuel smoke exposure, although these numbers may severely underestimate the real burden of COPD in underdeveloped countries.[47] Studies calculate that in Latin America, between 30% and 75% of people living in rural areas use

Table 1
Prevalence estimates of COPD

Reference	Study	Dates	Sample	Diagnosis of COPD	Prevalence (%)	Comments
United States						
Celli et al[9]	NHANES III	1988–1994	9838 adults (30–80 y)	GOLD Stage ≥I (2001 criteria)	16.8	Smokers had 21.9% vs never smokers 9.1%
Hnizdo et al[50]	NHANES III	1988–1994	13,824 adults (20–80 y)	GOLD Stage >I (2001 criteria)	14.2	Prevalence by LLN criteria (ATS 1991) of 12.3%
Mannino et al[40]	NHANES III	1991–1994	6600 adults (>25 y) with spirometry data	GOLD Stage >II (2001 criteria)	7.4	Prevalence rates age adjusted to 2000 US population
Vaz Fragoso et al[51]	NHANES III	1988–1994 (followed up until 12/2000)	3502 adults (40–80 y)	GOLD Stage >I (2006 criteria)	27	Mean age 60.7 y. LLN (2008 criteria) prevalence of 13.8%
Multicentric, International (>1 country)						
Cerveri et al[52]	ECRHS (European Community Respiratory Health Survey) involving 25 countries	1991–1993	17,966 adults (20–44 y)	Stage >I (2004 criteria)	3.6	Prevalence for GOLD stage 0 was 11.8%
Buist et al[53]	Burden of Obstructive Lung Disease (BOLD)	—	9425 adults (40 y of age and older)	GOLD Stage >II (2006 criteria)	10.1	11.8% for men and 8.5% for women
Menezes et al[54]	PLATINO Study (5 Latin American countries)	2002–2005	5315 adults (>40 y)	GOLD Stage >0 (2004 criteria)	7.8–19.7	Rates varied significantly across Latin American countries

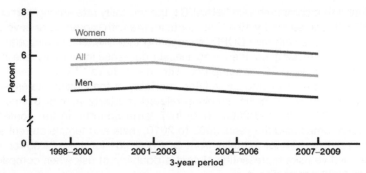

Fig. 3. Prevalence of COPD among adults aged 18 and older: United States, 1998 to 2009. (*From* Akinbami LJ, Liu X. Chronic obstructive pulmonary disease among adults aged 18 and over in the United States, 1998–2009. NCHS Data Brief 2011;(63):1–8.)

biomass fuels for cooking[48] and in India, China, and sub-Saharan Africa, as much as 80%.[49] In 2000, the WHO estimated that approximately 1.6 million deaths in the world were attributed to indoor air pollution. Ten years later, the WHO raised the estimate to 2.0 million deaths annually.

A recent review of the literature that included 58 studies between 2000 and 2010 describes significant variations in mortality rates in the world, with overall mortality rate of 3 to 9 deaths per 100,000 people in Japan to 7 to 111 deaths per 100,000 in the United States. This review found that studies reported an overall increase in COPD mortality rates within the last 30 to 40 years, with a much greater increase in mortality in women compared with men, with some studies suggesting a slight decrease in COPD mortality among men.[38]

In the United States, studies have reported that the age-adjusted mortality rate for COPD doubled from 1970 to 2000.[41] Nevertheless, a recent report by Ford and colleagues[10] that included an analysis from data in the NHANES I and NHANES III

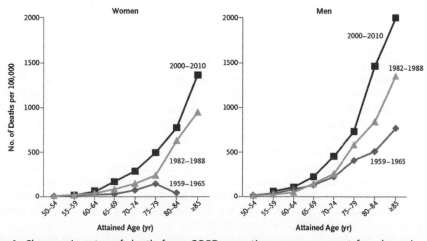

Fig. 4. Changes in rates of death from COPD over time among current female and male smokers in 3 time periods. (*From* Thun MJ, Carter BD, Feskanich D, et al. 50-year trends in smoking-related mortality in the United States. N Engl J Med 2013;368(4):360; with permission.)

studies, found that compared with NHANES I, the mortality rate among participates in the NHANES III decreased by 15.8% for participants with moderate or severe COPD and 25.2% for those with mild COPD, suggesting that overall mortality attributed to COPD may be decreasing, but there was a lesser decrease in mortality rate in women with moderate or severe COPD compared with men (3% vs 17.8%).

A recent assessment of smoking-related mortality in the United States evaluated temporal trends in sex-specific, smoking-related mortality across 3 time periods (1959–1965, 1982–1988, and 2000–2010) in 7 large cohorts. In the contemporary cohort that encompassed the years 2000 to 2010, male and female current smokers had similar relative risks for mortality from COPD (26.61 for men, 22.35 for women), with these relative risks representing almost a doubling of risk when compared with the 1982 to 1988 period (**Fig. 4**).[25]

SUMMARY

Estimating the true prevalence of COPD in the world is a difficult task. Nevertheless, during the last couple of decades, there has been significant progress made in identification and classifications of populations with COPD that currently allow us to determine the impact of this deadly disease in the world. In developed countries, current information estimates a prevalence of 8% to 10% among adults 40 years of age and older, whereas in developing countries, prevalence varies significantly among countries and is difficult to estimate. Recent reports also suggest that prevalence of COPD might have plateaued or even decreased in developed countries, whereas there is overwhelming evidence to suggest that most of the world population is still exposed to biomass fuels and likely will see an increase in prevalence of COPD. Overall, the mortality associated with COPD appears to be improving, except for a trend increase in mortality in women. Further studies will help us better understand these geographic and mortality differences.

REFERENCES

1. Decramer M, Janssens W, Miravitlles M. Chronic obstructive pulmonary disease. Lancet 2012;379(9823):1341–51.
2. Centers for Disease Control and Prevention. Chronic pulmonary obstructive disease among adults - United States 2011. MMWR Morb Mortal Wkly Rep 2012; 61(46):938–42.
3. Bousquet J, Kiley J, Bateman ED, et al. Prioritised research agenda for prevention and control of chronic respiratory diseases. Eur Respir J 2010;36(5):995–1001.
4. WHO. World health statistics. 2008. Available at: http://www.whoint/whosis/whostat/EN_WHS08_Full.pdf. Accessed February 15, 2012.
5. Mannino DM, Buist AS. Global burden of COPD: risk factors, prevalence, and future trends. Lancet 2007;370(9589):765–73.
6. Murray CJ, Lopez AD. Alternative projections of mortality and disability by cause 1990-2020: Global Burden of Disease Study. Lancet 1997;349(9064):1498–504.
7. Global strategy for the diagnosis, management, and prevention of chronic obstructive pulmonary disease. NHLBI/WHO Global Initiative for Chronic Obstructive Lung Disease (GOLD) Workshop summary (Revised 2013). Available at: http://www.goldcopd.org. Accessed February 15, 2013.
8. Celli BR, MacNee W. Standards for the diagnosis and treatment of patients with COPD: a summary of the ATS/ERS position paper. Eur Respir J 2004;23(6):932–46.
9. Celli BR, Halbert RJ, Isonaka S, et al. Population impact of different definitions of airway obstruction. Eur Respir J 2003;22(2):268–73.

10. Ford ES, Mannino DM, Zhao G, et al. Changes in mortality among US adults with COPD in two national cohorts recruited from 1971-1975 and 1988-1994. Chest 2012;141(1):101–10.
11. Dirksen A, Christensen H, Evald T, et al. Bronchodilator and corticosteroid reversibility in ambulatory patients with airways obstruction. Dan Med Bull 1991;38(6): 486–9.
12. Albert P, Agusti A, Edwards L, et al. Bronchodilator responsiveness as a phenotypic characteristic of established chronic obstructive pulmonary disease. Thorax 2012;67(8):701–8.
13. Standards for the diagnosis and care of patients with chronic obstructive pulmonary disease. American Thoracic Society. Am J Respir Crit Care Med 1995; 152(5 Pt 2):S77–121.
14. Snider GL. Chronic obstructive pulmonary disease: a definition and implications of structural determinants of airflow obstruction for epidemiology. Am Rev Respir Dis 1989;140(3 Pt 2):S3–8.
15. Masoli M, Fabian D, Holt S, et al. The global burden of asthma: executive summary of the GINA Dissemination Committee report. Allergy 2004;59(5):469–78.
16. Soriano JB, Davis KJ, Coleman B, et al. The proportional Venn diagram of obstructive lung disease: two approximations from the United States and the United Kingdom. Chest 2003;124(2):474–81.
17. Shaya FT, Dongyi D, Akazawa MO, et al. Burden of concomitant asthma and COPD in a Medicaid population. Chest 2008;134(1):14–9.
18. Gibson PG, Simpson JL. The overlap syndrome of asthma and COPD: what are its features and how important is it? Thorax 2009;64(8):728–35.
19. Gold DR, Wang X, Wypij D, et al. Effects of cigarette smoking on lung function in adolescent boys and girls. N Engl J Med 1996;335(13):931–7.
20. Langhammer A, Johnsen R, Gulsvik A, et al. Sex differences in lung vulnerability to tobacco smoking. Eur Respir J 2003;21(6):1017–23.
21. Prescott E, Bjerg AM, Andersen PK, et al. Gender difference in smoking effects on lung function and risk of hospitalization for COPD: results from a Danish longitudinal population study. Eur Respir J 1997;10(4):822–7.
22. Lokke A, Lange P, Scharling H, et al. Developing COPD: a 25 year follow up study of the general population. Thorax 2006;61(11):935–9.
23. Hooper R, Burney P, Vollmer WM, et al. Risk factors for COPD spirometrically defined from the lower limit of normal in the BOLD project. Eur Respir J 2012; 39(6):1343–53.
24. Bjerg A, Ekerljung L, Eriksson J, et al. Higher Risk of wheeze in female than male smokers. Results from the Swedish GA(2)LEN Study. PLoS One 2013;8(1):e54137.
25. Thun MJ, Carter BD, Feskanich D, et al. 50-year trends in smoking-related mortality in the United States. N Engl J Med 2013;368(4):351–64.
26. Diaz-Guzman E, Aryal S, Mannino DM. Occupational chronic obstructive pulmonary disease: an update. Clin Chest Med 2012;33(4):625–36.
27. Blanc PD. Occupation and COPD: a brief review. J Asthma 2012;49(1):2–4.
28. Mehta AJ, Miedinger D, Keidel D, et al. Occupational exposure to dusts, gases and fumes and incidence of COPD in SAPALDIA. Am J Respir Crit Care Med 2012;185:1292–300.
29. Romieu I, Gouveia N, Cifuentes LA, et al. Multicity study of air pollution and mortality in Latin America (the ESCALA study). Res Rep Health Eff Inst 2012;(171):5–86.
30. Gan WQ, Fitzgerald JM, Carlsten C, et al. Associations of ambient air pollution with chronic obstructive pulmonary disease hospitalization and mortality. Am J Respir Crit Care Med 2013;187:721–7.

31. Stoller JK, Aboussouan LS. Alpha1-antitrypsin deficiency. Lancet 2005;365(9478): 2225–36.
32. Bosse Y. Updates on the COPD gene list. Int J Chron Obstruct Pulmon Dis 2012; 7:607–31.
33. Shirtcliffe P, Weatherall M, Marsh S, et al. COPD prevalence in a random population survey: a matter of definition. Eur Respir J 2007;30(2):232–9.
34. Colak Y, Lokke A, Marott JL, et al. Impact of diagnostic criteria on the prevalence of COPD. Clin Respir J 2013;7:297–303.
35. Akinbami LJ, Liu X. Chronic obstructive pulmonary disease among adults aged 18 and over in the United States, 1998-2009. NCHS Data Brief 2011;(63):1–8.
36. Mannino DM, Gagnon RC, Petty TL, et al. Obstructive lung disease and low lung function in adults in the United States: data from the National Health and Nutrition Examination Survey, 1988–1994. Arch Intern Med 2000;160(11):1683–9.
37. Halbert RJ, Natoli JL, Gano A, et al. Global burden of COPD: systematic review and meta-analysis. Eur Respir J 2006;28(3):523–32.
38. Rycroft CE, Heyes A, Lanza L, et al. Epidemiology of chronic obstructive pulmonary disease: a literature review. Int J Chron Obstruct Pulmon Dis 2012;7:457–94.
39. Camp PG, Goring SM. Gender and the diagnosis, management, and surveillance of chronic obstructive pulmonary disease. Proc Am Thorac Soc 2007;4(8): 686–91.
40. Mannino DM, Homa DM, Akinbami LJ, et al. Chronic obstructive pulmonary disease surveillance–United States, 1971-2000. MMWR Surveill Summ 2002;51(6): 1–16.
41. Gershon AS, Wang C, Wilton AS, et al. Trends in chronic obstructive pulmonary disease prevalence, incidence, and mortality in ontario, Canada, 1996 to 2007: a population-based study. Arch Intern Med 2010;170(6):560–5.
42. Bischoff EW, Schermer TR, Bor H, et al. Trends in COPD prevalence and exacerbation rates in Dutch primary care. Br J Gen Pract 2009;59(569):927–33.
43. Menezes AM, Perez-Padilla R, Jardim JR, et al. Chronic obstructive pulmonary disease in five Latin American cities (the PLATINO study): a prevalence study. Lancet 2005;366(9500):1875–81.
44. Lopez AD, Shibuya K, Rao C, et al. Chronic obstructive pulmonary disease: current burden and future projections. Eur Respir J 2006;27(2):397–412.
45. Lozano R, Naghavi M, Foreman K, et al. Global and regional mortality from 235 causes of death for 20 age groups in 1990 and 2010: a systematic analysis for the Global Burden of Disease Study 2010. Lancet 2012;380(9859):2095–128.
46. Perez-Padilla R, Schilmann A, Riojas-Rodriguez H. Respiratory health effects of indoor air pollution. Int J Tuberc Lung Dis 2010;14(9):1079–86.
47. Zhang J, Smith KR. Indoor air pollution: a global health concern. Br Med Bull 2003;68:209–25.
48. Romieu I, Riojas-Rodriguez H, Marron-Mares AT, et al. Improved biomass stove intervention in rural Mexico: impact on the respiratory health of women. Am J Respir Crit Care Med 2009;180(7):649–56.
49. Desai M, Mehta S, Smith K. Indoor smoke from solid fuels: assessing the environmental burden of disease at national and local levels. Geneva (Switzerland): World Health Organization; 2004.
50. Hnizdo E, Sullivan PA, Bang KM, et al. Association between chronic obstructive pulmonary disease and employment by industry and occupation in the US population: a study of data from the Third National Health and Nutrition Examination Survey. Am J Epidemiol 2002;156(8):738–46.

51. Vaz Fragoso CA, Concato J, McAvay G, et al. The ratio of FEV1 to FVC as a basis for establishing chronic obstructive pulmonary disease. Am J Respir Crit Care Med 2010;181(5):446–51.
52. Cerveri I, Accordini S, Verlato G, et al. Variations in the prevalence across countries of chronic bronchitis and smoking habits in young adults. Eur Respir J 2001; 18(1):85–92.
53. Buist AS, McBurnie MA, Vollmer WM, et al. International variation in the prevalence of COPD (the BOLD Study): a population-based prevalence study. Lancet 2007;370(9589):741–50.
54. Menezes AM, Perez-Padilla R, Hallal PC, et al. Worldwide burden of COPD in high- and low-income countries. Part II. Burden of chronic obstructive lung disease in Latin America: the PLATINO study. Int J Tuberc Lung Dis 2008;12(7): 709–12.

Genetic Susceptibility

Stefan J. Marciniak, PhD, FRCP[a,b,*],
David A. Lomas, PhD, ScD, FRCP, FMedSci[c]

KEYWORDS

- Genetics • COPD • Emphysema • GWAS • SNP

KEY POINTS

- Approximately 20% of the population-attributable risk for chronic obstructive pulmonary disease (COPD) arises from family history.
- Early hypothesis-driven candidate gene approaches identified several genes contributing to risk for COPD, including components of the protease/antiprotease system and of the antioxidant pathway.
- More recent unbiased genome-wide association studies have gone on to reveal unanticipated genetic factors, for example, polymorphisms within the nicotinic acetyla choline receptor.
- The individual risk contributed by most genetic variants that predispose to COPD is small (odds ratios of less than 1.5), but current technological advances have rendered their analysis a tractable and therapeutically important question.

INTRODUCTION

Although most smokers will die of a smoking-related disorder, only 20% suffer from significant chronic obstructive pulmonary disease (COPD). Familial clustering suggests that heritable factors play an important role in the development of this disease.[1,2] In one large series, 18.6% of population-attributable risk for COPD could be accounted for by family history: patients with an affected parent having more severe disease, more frequent exacerbations, and a worse quality of life.[3] Similarly, in twin pairs the risk of developing COPD is higher for monozygotic than for dizygotic twins, with 60% of the individual susceptibility explained by genetic factors.[4] Both the airway and the

This article originally appeared in *Clinics in Chest Medicine*, Volume 35, Issue 1, March 2014.
This work was supported by the Medical Research Council (UK), British Lung Foundation, and Diabetes UK. S.J. Marciniak is an MRC Senior Clinical Fellow (G1002610).
[a] Division of Respiratory Medicine, Department of Medicine, Addenbrooke's Hospital, Cambridge CB2 0QQ, UK; [b] Cambridge Institute for Medical Research (CIMR), University of Cambridge, Wellcome Trust/MRC Building, Hills Road, Cambridge CB2 0XY, UK; [c] University College London, 1st Floor, Maple House, 149 Tottenham Court Road, London W1T 7NF, UK
* Corresponding author. Cambridge Institute for Medical Research (CIMR), University of Cambridge, Wellcome Trust/MRC Building, Hills Road, Cambridge CB2 0XY, UK.
E-mail address: sjm20@cam.ac.uk

emphysema components cluster independently, suggesting that different genetic factors play a role in the development of these 2 components of the disease.[5] Unsurprisingly, for a disorder with a substantial heritable component, race and ethnicity seem to impact on the development of COPD. For example, in the COPDGene Study, 42% of affected African Americans were found to suffer severe early-onset COPD (age <55 years, forced expiratory volume in 1 second [FEV1] <50% predicted) compared with 14% of non-Hispanic whites.[6] In contrast, self-reported Hispanic ethnicity and Native American genetic ancestry have both been reported to be associated with significantly lower risks of developing COPD.[7]

Efforts to identify the genetic determinants of COPD have evolved as the available technologies have changed. The analysis of candidate genes yielded some successes that will be discussed later (in "Candidate Gene Approaches" section), but that approach also led to numerous blind alleys, with initial excitement followed by disappointment as associations proved impossible to reproduce. The analysis of large cohorts of patients in genome-wide association studies (GWAS) using microarray technology to assay up to a million single nucleotide polymorphisms (SNPs) in each case led to the unbiased identification of novel disease-associated loci. This approach is hypothesis-free and so has the potential to open novel avenues of research.

UNBIASED APPROACHES

Until recently, only mutations of the SERPINA1 gene that are responsible for α_1-antitrypsin deficiency were unambiguously linked with the development of COPD. However, this disorder accounts for only 1% to 2% of cases of COPD and so other disease-associated alleles must exist. Recent large multinational GWAS have shed much light on this. In addition to validating the involvement of some candidate genes previously suspected of playing a role in the pathogenesis of COPD, these landmark studies have identified novel pathways that might plausibly lead to novel therapies for COPD.

SNPs in chromosome 15 at the α-nicotinic acetylcholine receptor CHRNA3/5 locus (15q25.1, rs8034191, and rs1051730) were found to reach genome-wide significance and have subsequently been replicated in several independent studies.[8-13] This locus is significantly associated with pack-years of smoking, emphysema (by computed tomography [CT]), and airflow obstruction.[9,14] Notably, the C allele of the rs8034191 SNP was estimated to have a population attributable risk for COPD of 12.2% and has previously been identified in genome-wide association studies of lung cancer, being thought to be important in nicotine addiction.[8] Individuals who carry this SNP may require more cigarettes to satisfy nicotine addiction, may inhale more deeply, and may find it more difficult to withdraw from cigarette smoking. Indeed, it has been reported that the association of the CHRNA3/5 locus is substantially mediated by smoking phenotype,[12] although this finding has been disputed.[14] However, IREB2 is a gene in tight linkage disequilibrium with CHRNA3/5 and has also been identified as a potential determinant of COPD.[9,15,16] This gene encodes an iron regulatory protein localized in epithelia that may plausibly affect oxidative stress responses in smoked-exposed lungs. These candidate genes are not mutually exclusive and it remains possible that both genes within the haplotype contribute to the disease phenotype.[12]

GWAS have also identified a locus at 4q22.1 containing the gene FAM13A to be significantly associated with COPD and lung function in multiple cohorts.[9,17] Although the function of FAM13A is unclear, another gene at 4q31 newly identified and replicated by GWAS as being associated with both COPD and lung function encodes hedgehog interacting protein, which appears to play a role in signaling that modulates lung development or remodeling.[8,18-20] Hedgehog interacting protein is expressed in pulmonary tissues but at lower levels in COPD-affected lungs, and disease-associated SNPs have been identified within the gene's promoter (rs6537296A and rs1542725C) that appear to reduce its transcription.[21] Other loci that have been identified using similar techniques include 2q35, 4q24, 5q33, 6p21, 15q23, and 19q13, although these require validation.[19,22] Other COPD-related phenotypes have also been linked with specific loci, for example, low body mass index in COPD is significantly association with SNP rs8050136 within the first intron of the fat mass and obesity-associated (*FTO*) gene,[23] whereas an SNP in *BICD1* (rs10844154 in 12p11.2) is associated with the presence and severity of emphysema on CT scan.[24]

CANDIDATE GENE APPROACHES
The Extracellular Matrix

Alveolar tissue consists of epithelial cells, capillaries, and extracellular matrix (ECM), the latter comprising a complex network of scaffolding proteins, principally elastin and collagen. The elastin filaments form from tropoelastin monomers that self-assemble into aggregates and then fuse with microfilaments. Multiple covalent cross-links between the lysines in neighboring filaments provide stability. Cutis laxa is a family of autosomal-dominant (OMIM #123700), X-linked (OMIM #304150), and recessive (OMIM #219100, 219200) human diseases characterized by excessively slack connective tissues. Several families with the milder autosomal-dominant form show early-onset pulmonary pathologic abnormality including emphysema,[25] particularly if inherited with the Z allele of α_1-antitrypsin.[26] Two groups independently identified separate mutations within the ELN (elastin) gene that cause mild cutis laxa and early-onset COPD.[27,28] The ELN gene maps to 7q11.23 in man, but as chromosome 7 has not been identified in linkage analysis as a site associated with COPD, it is likely that ELN mutations are a rare cause of this disease.

Elastin fibers bind other proteins including fibulins, which in turn bind multiple ECM components and the basement membrane. The fibulins are a family of 6 proteins, at least 2 of which are mutated in severe autosomal-recessive forms of cutis laxa and whose phenotype often includes early-onset emphysema.[29,30] A novel mutation in the fibulin-4 gene (FBLN4; 11q13) was recently identified in autosomal-recessive cutis laxa with developmental emphysema.[29] The mutation caused an amino acid substitution in an epidermal growth factor–like domain of FBLN-4, leading to very low levels of extracellular protein. In a consanguineous Turkish family, a homozygous mutation in the related fibulin-5 gene (FBLN5; 14q32.1) was also found to cause cutis laxa and emphysema complicated by recurrent pulmonary infections.[30] Once again, the mutation was located within an epidermal growth factor–like domain, suggesting these are critical for fibulins to maintain the integrity of the ECM within the lung. Interestingly, analogous mutations in fibrillin, which bare homology to the fibulins, cause Marfan syndrome. Moreover, mutations of fibrillin (FBN1; 15q21.1) have been described in neonatal Marfan with very early-onset emphysema.[31–33]

Menkes disease (OMIM #309400), characterized by abnormal hair and dysmorphic features, is caused by mutations in an intracellular copper transporter (ATP7A; Xq13.3). The clinical features are due to defective connective tissue synthesis thought to be the result of dysfunction of lysyl oxidase. This copper-dependent enzyme is required for proper cross-linking of both collagen and elastin fibers. A recent case report described a child with Menkes disease and severe bilateral pan-lobular emphysema who died at the age of 14 months.[34] Gene sequencing revealed a splice-site mutation in ATP7A, suggesting that proper ECM cross-linking is vital for stability of the lung parenchyma.

In contrast to animal models of COPD, mutations in collagen have not been identified in humans, but does not appear to be due to an incompatibility of mutated collagen with survival, as numerous collagen mutations have been described that cause other human diseases. Instead, it may reflect a more important role for elastin integrity in emphysema in humans than in mice. However, aberrant collagen synthesis has been implicated in COPD. The signaling molecule TGFβ1 enhances collagen synthesis in vivo, and polymorphisms in its gene (TGFB1; 19q13.1) have been associated with COPD,[35–39] although a recent, large study found no association between TGFB1 polymorphisms and the rate of lung function decline in smokers.[40] Intriguingly, the TGFβ1 gene maps to a locus on chromosome 19, which has high linkage (LOD 3.3) with FEV_1 in smokers.[36,41] However, as is frequently the case with polymorphism studies, the literature is unclear. For example, 2 TGFB1 SNPs, rs1800469 and rs1982073, were found to be independently associated with COPD in 2 studies,[35,38] but in another, they were only significant when analyzed as part of a haplotype (combination of alleles), whereas yet another SNP, rs6957, was significant in its own right.[39] Detailed analysis of the Boston Early-Onset COPD Study data revealed further complexity.[36] Although some alleles of TGFB1 were associated with FEV_1 (rs2241712, rs2241718, rs6957), there was a separate but partially overlapping set of alleles associated with airflow obstruction (rs2241712, rs1800469, rs1982073). TGFβ1 protein is inactive when first secreted owing to the presence of an inhibitory N-terminal propeptide. It is secreted associated with latent TGFβ1 binding proteins (LTBP), which share structural features with fibrillins and are assembled into the ECM. Mice with mutations in LTBP4 develop severe emphysema.[42] Intriguingly, the sole study that has addressed LTBP4 (19q13.1-q13.2) polymorphisms found an association with COPD in man.[38] More recently, genome-wide linkage analysis of pedigrees stratified by emphysema status (on CT scan) identified a region on chromosome 1p (LOD score = 2.99).[43] An intronic SNP in TGFB-receptor-3 at this locus was found to be associated with COPD status, FEV_1, and CT emphysema.

Taken together, these studies provide strong evidence in support of a crucial role for the loss of ECM integrity, in particular, the elastic components, in the development of COPD. It is therefore important to consider the enzymes implicated in degradation of the ECM.

Protease-Antiprotease Balance

The protease antiprotease theory has its roots in the observation that individuals with α_1-antitrypsin are particularly susceptible to COPD and in experimental models of emphysema from the 1960s. This theory suggests that the pathogenesis of COPD and emphysema is the result of an imbalance between enzymes that degrade the ECM within the lung and proteins that oppose this proteolytic activity. Many proteases play important roles in remodeling or inflammation within the lung. It is essential that they be controlled by antiproteases to protect against uncontrolled degradation of the ECM.

The best-understood example of genetically induced emphysema results from mutations in the α_1-antitrypsin gene (SERPINA1; 14q32.1). These mutations increase the protein's propensity to form ordered polymers, which are incapable of inhibiting its target enzyme, neutrophil elastase. This abnormal behavior leads to retention of the protein within hepatocytes as periodic acid Schiff–positive inclusions and results in plasma deficiency of an important protease inhibitor (OMIM #107400). It is now increasingly recognized that mutant α_1-antitrypsin can also form polymers within the interstitium and alveolar spaces of the lung. These polymers are chemotactic for neutrophils and so combine with the deficiency of α_1-antitrypsin to focus and amplify the inflammatory response within the lung.[44] In most Northern European populations the frequency of the most severe Z allele is about 1/2000. Classically, Z α_1-antitrypsin homozygotes carry the Glu342Lys mutation and suffer from early-onset emphysema when compared with normal MM α_1-antitrypsin individuals. The onset and progression of emphysema are markedly accelerated by cigarette smoking. Moreover, it appears that even a single allele of Z α_1-antitrypsin may increase the risk of COPD. In the longitudinal Copenhagen City Heart Study, the MZ α_1-antitrypsin genotype increased the rate of decline of FEV_1 by 19% compared with those who were MM homozygotes, causing a 30% increased risk of obstructive lung function and a 50% increased risk of physician-diagnosed COPD.[45] The authors found that the frequency of the MZ genotype in their Danish population was as high as 5% and so calculated that it would account for 2.4% of cases of COPD. This finding is in contrast to the ZZ genotype, which was causal in only 0.8% of cases. In meta-analysis, heterozygosity for the Z allele carried an odds ratio for COPD of 2.31.[46] In one study, the MZ (but not MS; the S allele has the Glu264Val mutation) α_1-antitrypsin genotype was associated with a rapid decline in FEV_1, which was even more marked if there was also a family history of COPD, suggesting an interaction with additional genetic factors.[47] A further meta-analysis combining 17 studies found a 3-fold increase in COPD in SZ α_1-antitrypsin heterozygotes and a small increase in MS α_1-antitrypsin heterozygotes. Other polymorphisms of the SERPINA1 gene do not appear to be associated with increased risk of developing COPD.[48]

Other pulmonary serine protease inhibitors may also be involved in the pathogenesis of COPD. Following earlier linkage studies demonstrating an association between chromosome 2q and COPD, expression profiling of genes within that locus identified SERPINE2 (2q33-q35) as being up-regulated during murine lung development and in the lungs of individuals with COPD.[49] The authors went on to demonstrate an association between SNPs in SERPINE2 and COPD. SERPINE2 SNPs were found to segregate with COPD in a large multicenter family-based study and to be associated with COPD in a case-control analysis.[50] However, another large study failed to replicate the association with COPD despite having adequate power.[51] The latter study included individuals with COPD with and without emphysema, whereas the studies by Demeo and colleagues[49] included a preponderance of patients with emphysema assessed for lung volume reduction surgery. Nevertheless, although these differences may reflect different COPD phenotypes, they illustrate the need to replicate the findings of genetic association studies in multiple populations before drawing firm conclusions. A recent study of Finish construction workers found that 3 SNPs within SERPINE2 (rs729631, rs975278, and rs6748795) were in tight linkage disequilibrium and so focused solely on one (rs729631),[52] which showed a significant association with panlobular emphysema, as seen with mutants of SERPINA1.

Because mutations of α_1-antitrypsin so clearly lead to emphysema, one might infer that its target, neutrophil elastase, is central to the pathogenesis of disease. However, mutations in this protease have not been shown to be important, despite being studied extensively in other conditions. Instead, most evidence implicates matrix metalloproteases (MMPs) in the pathogenesis of COPD. These MMPs are zinc-dependent endopeptidases involved in the degradation of many ECM components. An SNP of MMP9 (20q11) was associated with COPD in Japanese[53] and Chinese[54] populations; however, a further Japanese study found an association with emphysema distribution rather than COPD per se.[55] Another large study failed to show MMP9 association with COPD, but instead MMP1 (11q22) and MMP12 (11q22) polymorphisms were identified.[56] Further support for a role for MMP9, but not MMP1 polymorphisms, has also been published.[57] Tissue inhibitors of metalloproteinases inhibit the MMPs, but thus far, only one polymorphism in tissue inhibitors of metalloproteinases 2 (17q25) has been associated with COPD.[58] When more than 8000 individuals were analyzed, the minor allele of the promoter of MMP12 (rs2276109 [−82A→G]) showed clear association with FEV_1 in a combined analysis of adult ever-smokers and children with asthma and with a reduced risk of COPD.[59] In a separate study, a haplotype containing this SNP in MMP-12 (rs652438 and rs2276109) was found to be associated with severe COPD (Global Initiative for Chronic Obstructive Lung Disease stages III and IV; 20078883). When expressed in cells in vitro, the COPD-associated A allele of rs652438 was 3-fold more proteolytically active than the G allele, suggesting that it might mediate enhanced ECM degradation.[60]

Reactive Oxygen Species

Cigarette smoke contains vast numbers of free radicals that impose an oxidative stress on the lung. Such stress is thought to induce damage through multiple mechanisms, including direct oxidation of cellular lipids and DNA, and through inactivation of key proteins such as α_1-antitrypsin. For this reason, much work has gone into assessing the role of endogenous antioxidant enzymes in protecting against smoke-induced lung damage.

Many toxins in cigarette smoke are subject to first-pass metabolism in the liver. Among the many enzymes involved, microsomal epoxide hydrolase (EPHX1; 1q42.1) has been intensely studied in the context of COPD. Several EPHX1 SNPs have been described that affect its activity. One of these leads to a 40% loss of in vitro activity (rs1051740 Tyr113His, the "slow" allele), whereas another increases activity by 25% (rs2234922 His139Arg, the "fast" allele). In 1997, the "slow" variant of EPHX1 was found to increase the risk of emphysema by a staggering odds ratio of 5.0 and of COPD by an odds ratio of 4.1.[61] Since then, numerous studies have attempted to reproduce this effect with varying success.[38,62–73] Recently, analysis of randomly selected white Danish individuals participating in the Copenhagen City Heart Study (n = 10,038) and the Copenhagen General Population Study (n = 37,022) for the rs1051740 and rs2234922 variants in the EPHX1 gene combined with a meta-analysis of 19 previous studies indicates that genetically reduced EPHX1 activity is not a major risk factor for COPD or asthma in the Danish population.[74]

Glutathione S-transferase (GST) comprises a large family of enzymes capable of catalyzing the conjugation of reduced glutathione to endogenous and xenobiotic electrophilic compounds. The GSTs are important in the detoxification of many compounds and are highly polymorphic. These polymorphisms have been linked to susceptibility to toxins and carcinogens. SNPs in GSTP1 have been associated with COPD,[75] the distribution of emphysema,[76] and more rapid decline in lung function.[77] However, the data should be interpreted with caution because one-third of the cohorts[77] have been used in multiple analyses[68] and there was a lack of Hardy-Weinberg equilibrium for GSTP1 in their population, suggesting either a systematic defect in genotyping or an unidentified bias in the selection of subjects. Moreover, no convincing association was found in other studies.[70,78] The null mutation of GSTM1 (1p13.1) has also been associated with COPD,[63] but others have failed to reproduce this finding.[71]

Heme-oxygenase catalyses the first step in heme degradation. Heme-oxygenase 1 (HMOX1; 22q13.1) is the inducible isoform that can be up-regulated by a wide range of stresses. Bile pigments generated by heme cleavage are thought to have antioxidant properties; thus, HMOX1 induction is protective during cellular oxidant injury and over-expression of HMOX1 in lung tissue protects against hyperoxia. The HMOX1 gene 5′-flanking region contains stretches of group-specific component (GC) repeats that are highly polymorphic in length. An early report found a higher proportion of long repeats in patients with COPD and also demonstrated that long repeats were associated with impaired promoter activity.[79] Attempts to reproduce this effect have had varied success.[64,77,80,81] Although HMOX1 GC-repeat length has not convincingly been shown to be associated with developing COPD, there are some data to support an association between the long allele and increased severity of disease,[81,82] although a recent study of smokers in the NHLBI Lung Health Study found no association between 5 HMOX1 SNPs and the decline of lung function.[83] Moreover, that study failed to detect evidence that the promoter polymorphisms affected regulation of the HMOX1 gene.

Superoxide dismutase (SOD) is an important antioxidant enzyme that catalyses the conversion of superoxide to oxygen and hydrogen peroxide. The extracellular isoform (SOD3; 4p15) is abundant in lung parenchyma. In the cross-sectional Copenhagen Heart Study, the R213G allele that results in higher plasma levels was associated with significantly less COPD in smokers.[84] A second study found similar results for the SOD3 isoenzyme, but not for other forms of SOD.[85]

While biologically very plausible, current genetic evidence fails to provide clear support for the involvement of detoxifying enzymes in the pathogenesis of COPD. Because the potential list of candidates to detoxify cigarette smoke remains long, it would be preferable if future studies were to take an unbiased approach to target identification rather than studying small numbers of candidate genes.

Inflammation

Tumor necrosis factor-α (TNF; 6p21) is a multifunctional cytokine whose levels are elevated in bronchoalveolar lavage, induced sputa, and biopsies from patients with COPD. It is a plausible candidate gene for susceptibility to inflammatory disease, especially as well-studied promoter polymorphisms clearly alter expression levels. Consequently, considerable effort has been invested into determining whether the promoter polymorphism in TNFα also predisposes smokers to COPD. Much interest was generated when an early study revealed an association (with a staggering odds ratio of greater than 10) between allele 2 and "bronchitis" in Taiwanese men.[86] This study is difficult to interpret as one-third of the men were "never smokers". Despite some supportive evidence,[87] many subsequent studies appeared to find little evidence that TNF polymorphisms are associated with, or modify, the progression of COPD.[68,73,88–97]

GC (4q12), also known as vitamin D binding globulin, is a multifunctional protein that enhances the neutrophil and monocyte chemotactic activity of complement component 5a. It is a highly polymorphic protein with more than 124 forms, although 3, Gc*1F, Gc*1S, and Gc2, make up the majority. Kueppers and colleagues[98] found Gc2 homozygotes to be protected from COPD. Others have seen this protective effect,[99,100] whereas Gc*1F homozygosity has been found to be associated with COPD.[101,102] However, a much larger recent study has failed to reproduce these associations.[103]

SUMMARY

Although environmental exposure to smoke remains the preeminent risk factor for developing COPD, the evidence that heredity plays a major role in an individual's risk is clear. The combination of GWAS and carefully conducted candidate gene approaches is helping to tease out those genetic variants responsible for the familial clustering of this disease, offering both the personalization of individual risk stratification and, more excitingly, the hope for rational therapeutic interventions based on a better understanding of the underlying molecular pathologic abnormality. The confusion surrounding many of the early (and some current) studies lies almost entirely with study power. Apart from the notable exception of SERPINA1, the contribution of individual genetic variants to risk of disease will prove to be small; for this reason, large stratified cohorts of well-phenotyped individuals are likely to prove invaluable. A recent large systematic review of all case control candidate genetic studies in COPD before 2008 concluded that although most such studies were underpowered to detect small genetic effects (OR 1.2–1.5), 4 genetic variants (or the 27 for which adequate data were available) remained significantly associated with COPD: the GSTM1 null variant (OR 1.45), rs1800470 in TGFB1 (0.73), rs1800629 in TNFα (OR 1.19), and rs1799896 in SOD3 (OR 1.97).[104] Such findings, combined with the hypothesis generating observations from GWAS, will direct COPD research for the next decade.

REFERENCES

1. Silverman EK, Chapman HA, Drazen JM, et al. Genetic epidemiology of severe, early-onset chronic obstructive pulmonary disease. Risk to relatives for airflow obstruction and chronic bronchitis. Am J Respir Crit Care Med 1998;157(6 Pt 1): 1770–8.
2. McCloskey SC, Patel BD, Hinchliffe SJ, et al. Siblings of patients with severe chronic obstructive pulmonary disease have a significant risk of airflow obstruction. Am J Respir Crit Care Med 2001;164(8 Pt 1):1419–24.
3. Hersh CP, Hokanson JE, Lynch DA, et al. Family history is a risk factor for COPD. Chest 2011;140(2):343–50.
4. Ingebrigtsen T, Thomsen SF, Vestbo J, et al. Genetic influences on chronic obstructive pulmonary disease - a twin study. Respir Med 2010;104(12):1890–5.
5. Patel BD, Coxson HO, Pillai SG, et al. Airway wall thickening and emphysema show independent familial aggregation in chronic obstructive pulmonary disease. Am J Respir Crit Care Med 2008;178(5):500–5.
6. Foreman MG, Zhang L, Murphy J, et al. Early-onset chronic obstructive pulmonary disease is associated with female sex, maternal factors, and African American race in the COPDGene Study. Am J Respir Crit Care Med 2011;184(4):414–20.
7. Bruse S, Sood A, Petersen H, et al. New Mexican Hispanic smokers have lower odds of chronic obstructive pulmonary disease and less decline in lung function than non-Hispanic whites. Am J Respir Crit Care Med 2011;184(11):1254–60.
8. Pillai SG, Ge D, Zhu G, et al. A genome-wide association study in chronic obstructive pulmonary disease (COPD): identification of two major susceptibility loci. PLoS Genet 2009;5(3):e1000421.
9. Pillai SG, Kong X, Edwards LD, et al. Loci identified by genome-wide association studies influence different disease-related phenotypes in chronic obstructive pulmonary disease. Am J Respir Crit Care Med 2010;182(12):1498–505.
10. Kaur-Knudsen D, Nordestgaard BG, Bojesen SE. CHRNA3 genotype, nicotine dependence, lung function and disease in the general population. Eur Respir J 2012;40(6):1538–44.
11. Hardin M, Zielinski J, Wan ES, et al. CHRNA3/5, IREB2, and ADCY2 are associated with severe chronic obstructive pulmonary disease in Poland. Am J Respir Crit Care Med 2012;47(2):203–8.
12. Siedlinski M, Tingley D, Lipman PJ, et al. Dissecting direct and indirect genetic effects on chronic obstructive pulmonary disease (COPD) susceptibility. Hum Genet 2013;132:431–41.

13. Wilk JB, Shrine NR, Loehr LR, et al. Genome-wide association studies identify CHRNA5/3 and HTR4 in the development of airflow obstruction. Am J Respir Crit Care Med 2012;186(7):622–32.

14. Lambrechts D, Buysschaert I, Zanen P, et al. The 15q24/25 susceptibility variant for lung cancer and chronic obstructive pulmonary disease is associated with emphysema. Am J Respir Crit Care Med 2010;181(5):486–93.

15. DeMeo DL, Mariani T, Bhattacharya S, et al. Integration of genomic and genetic approaches implicates IREB2 as a COPD susceptibility gene. Am J Hum Genet 2009;85(4):493–502.

16. Chappell SL, Daly L, Lotya J, et al. The role of IREB2 and transforming growth factor beta-1 genetic variants in COPD: a replication case-control study. BMC Med Genet 2011;12:24.

17. Cho MH, Boutaoui N, Klanderman BJ, et al. Variants in FAM13A are associated with chronic obstructive pulmonary disease. Nat Genet 2010;42(3):200–2.

18. Wilk JB, Chen TH, Gottlieb DJ, et al. A genome-wide association study of pulmonary function measures in the Framingham Heart Study. PLoS Genet 2009;5(3): e1000429.

19. Repapi E, Sayers I, Wain LV, et al. Genome-wide association study identifies five loci associated with lung function. Nat Genet 2010;42(1):36–44.

20. Van Durme YM, Eijgelsheim M, Joos GF, et al. Hedgehog-interacting protein is a COPD susceptibility gene: the Rotterdam Study. Eur Respir J 2010;36(1):89–95.

21. Zhou X, Baron RM, Hardin M, et al. Identification of a chronic obstructive pulmonary disease genetic determinant that regulates HHIP. Hum Mol Genet 2012; 21(6):1325–35.

22. Cho MH, Castaldi PJ, Wan ES, et al. A genome-wide association study of COPD identifies a susceptibility locus on chromosome 19q13. Hum Mol Genet 2012; 21(4):947–57.

23. Wan ES, Cho MH, Boutaoui N, et al. Genome-wide association analysis of body mass in chronic obstructive pulmonary disease. Am J Respir Cell Mol Biol 2011; 45(2):304–10.

24. Kong X, Cho MH, Anderson W, et al. Genome-wide association study identifies BICD1 as a susceptibility gene for emphysema. Am J Respir Crit Care Med 2011;183(1):43–9.

25. Callewaert B, Renard M, Hucthagowder V, et al. New insights into the pathogenesis of autosomal-dominant cutis laxa with report of five ELN mutations. Hum Mutat 2011;32(4):445–55.

26. Corbett E, Glaisyer H, Chan C, et al. Congenital cutis laxa with a dominant inheritance and early onset emphysema. Thorax 1994;49(8):836–7.

27. Urban Z, Gao J, Pope FM, et al. Autosomal dominant cutis laxa with severe lung disease: synthesis and matrix deposition of mutant tropoelastin. J Invest Dermatol 2005;124(6):1193–9.

28. Kelleher CM, Silverman EK, Broekelmann T, et al. A functional mutation in the terminal exon of elastin in severe, early-onset chronic obstructive pulmonary disease. Am J Respir Cell Mol Biol 2005;33(4):355–62.

29. Hucthagowder V, Sausgruber N, Kim KH, et al. Fibulin-4: a novel gene for an autosomal recessive cutis laxa syndrome. Am J Hum Genet 2006;78(6):1075–80.

30. Loeys B, Van Maldergem L, Mortier G, et al. Homozygosity for a missense mutation in fibulin-5 (FBLN5) results in a severe form of cutis laxa. Hum Mol Genet 2002;11(18):2113–8.

31. Revencu N, Quenum G, Detaille T, et al. Congenital diaphragmatic eventration and bilateral uretero-hydronephrosis in a patient with neonatal Marfan syndrome

caused by a mutation in exon 25 of the FBN1 gene and review of the literature. Eur J Pediatr 2004;163(1):33–7.

32. Shinawi M, Boileau C, Brik R, et al. Splicing mutation in the fibrillin-1 gene associated with neonatal Marfan syndrome and severe pulmonary emphysema with tracheobronchomalacia. Pediatr Pulmonol 2005;39(4):374–8.

33. Tekin M, Cengiz FB, Ayberkin E, et al. Familial neonatal Marfan syndrome due to parental mosaicism of a missense mutation in the FBN1 gene. Am J Med GenetA 2007;143(8):875–80.

34. Grange DK, Kaler SG, Albers GM, et al. Severe bilateral panlobular emphysema and pulmonary arterial hypoplasia: unusual manifestations of Menkes disease. Am J Med GenetA 2005;139(2):151–5.

35. Wu L, Chau J, Young RP, et al. Transforming growth factor-beta1 genotype and susceptibility to chronic obstructive pulmonary disease. Thorax 2004;59(2): 126–9.

36. Celedon JC, Lange C, Raby BA, et al. The transforming growth factor-beta1 (TGFB1) gene is associated with chronic obstructive pulmonary disease (COPD). Hum Mol Genet 2004;13(15):1649–56.

37. Su ZG, Wen FQ, Feng YL, et al. Transforming growth factor-beta1 gene polymorphisms associated with chronic obstructive pulmonary disease in Chinese population. Acta Pharmacol Sin 2005;26(6):714–20.

38. Hersh CP, Demeo DL, Lazarus R, et al. Genetic association analysis of functional impairment in chronic obstructive pulmonary disease. Am J Respir Crit Care Med 2006;173(9):977–84.

39. van Diemen CC, Postma DS, Vonk JM, et al. Decorin and TGF-beta1 polymorphisms and development of COPD in a general population. Respir Res 2006; 7:89.

40. Ogawa E, Ruan J, Connett JE, et al. Transforming growth factor-beta1 polymorphisms, airway responsiveness and lung function decline in smokers. Respir Med 2007;101(5):938–43.

41. Silverman EK, Palmer LJ, Mosley JD, et al. Genomewide linkage analysis of quantitative spirometric phenotypes in severe early-onset chronic obstructive pulmonary disease. Am J Hum Genet 2002;70(5):1229–39.

42. Sterner-Kock A, Thorey IS, Koli K, et al. Disruption of the gene encoding the latent transforming growth factor-beta binding protein 4 (LTBP-4) causes abnormal lung development, cardiomyopathy, and colorectal cancer. Genes Dev 2002;16(17):2264–73.

43. Hersh CP, Hansel NN, Barnes KC, et al. Transforming growth factor-beta receptor-3 is associated with pulmonary emphysema. Am J Respir Cell Mol Biol 2009; 41(3):324–31.

44. Gooptu B, Lomas DA. Polymers and inflammation: disease mechanisms of the serpinopathies. J Exp Med 2008;205(7):1529–34.

45. Dahl M, Tybjaerg-Hansen A, Lange P, et al. Change in lung function and morbidity from chronic obstructive pulmonary disease in alpha1-antitrypsin MZ heterozygotes: a longitudinal study of the general population. Ann Intern Med 2002;136(4):270–9.

46. Hersh CP, Dahl M, Ly NP, et al. Chronic obstructive pulmonary disease in alpha1-antitrypsin PI MZ heterozygotes: a meta-analysis. Thorax 2004;59(10): 843–9.

47. Sandford AJ, Weir TD, Spinelli JJ, et al. Z and S mutations of the alpha1-antitrypsin gene and the risk of chronic obstructive pulmonary disease. Am J Respir Cell Mol Biol 1999;20(2):287–91.

48. Quint JK, Donaldson GC, Kumari M, et al. SERPINA1 11478G→A variant, serum alpha1-antitrypsin, exacerbation frequency and FEV1 decline in COPD. Thorax 2011;66(5):418–24.
49. Demeo DL, Mariani TJ, Lange C, et al. The SERPINE2 gene is associated with chronic obstructive pulmonary disease. Am J Hum Genet 2006;78(2):253–64.
50. Zhu G, Warren L, Aponte J, et al. The SERPINE2 gene is associated with chronic obstructive pulmonary disease in two large populations. Am J Respir Crit Care Med 2007;176(2):167–73.
51. Chappell S, Daly L, Morgan K, et al. The SERPINE2 gene and chronic obstructive pulmonary disease. Am J Hum Genet 2006;79(1):184–6.
52. Kukkonen MK, Tiili E, Hamalainen S, et al. SERPINE2 haplotype as a risk factor for panlobular type of emphysema. BMC Med Genet 2011;12:157.
53. Minematsu N, Nakamura H, Tateno H, et al. Genetic polymorphism in matrix metalloproteinase-9 and pulmonary emphysema. Biochem Biophys Res Commun 2001;289(1):116–9.
54. Zhou M, Huang SG, Wan HY, et al. Genetic polymorphism in matrix metalloproteinase-9 and the susceptibility to chronic obstructive pulmonary disease in Han population of south China. Chin Med J (Engl) 2004;117(10):1481–4.
55. Ito I, Nagai S, Handa T, et al. Matrix metalloproteinase-9 promoter polymorphism associated with upper lung dominant emphysema. Am J Respir Crit Care Med 2005;172(11):1378–82.
56. Joos L, He JQ, Shepherdson MB, et al. The role of matrix metalloproteinase polymorphisms in the rate of decline in lung function. Hum Mol Genet 2002; 11(5):569–76.
57. Tesfaigzi Y, Myers OB, Stidley CA, et al. Genotypes in matrix metalloproteinase 9 are a risk factor for COPD. Int J Chron Obstruct Pulmon Dis 2006;1(3):267–78.
58. Hirano K, Sakamoto T, Uchida Y, et al. Tissue inhibitor of metalloproteinases-2 gene polymorphisms in chronic obstructive pulmonary disease. Eur Respir J 2001;18(5):748–52.
59. Hunninghake GM, Cho MH, Tesfaigzi Y, et al. MMP12, lung function, and COPD in high-risk populations. N Engl J Med 2009;361(27):2599–608.
60. Haq I, Lowrey GE, Kalsheker N, et al. Matrix metalloproteinase-12 (MMP-12) SNP affects MMP activity, lung macrophage infiltration and protects against emphysema in COPD. Thorax 2011;66(11):970–6.
61. Smith CA, Harrison DJ. Association between polymorphism in gene for microsomal epoxide hydrolase and susceptibility to emphysema. Lancet 1997; 350(9078):630–3.
62. Korytina GF, Ianbaeva DG, Viktorova TV. Role of polymorphic variants of cytochrome P450 genes (CYP1A1, CYP2E1) and microsomal epoxide hydrolase (mEPHX) in pathogenesis of cystic fibrosis and chronic respiratory tract diseases. Mol Biol (Mosk) 2003;37(5):784–92 [in Russian].
63. Cheng SL, Yu CJ, Chen CJ, et al. Genetic polymorphism of epoxide hydrolase and glutathione S-transferase in COPD. Eur Respir J 2004;23(6):818–24.
64. Fu WP, Sun C, Dai LM, et al. Relationship between COPD and polymorphisms of HOX-1 and mEPH in a Chinese population. Oncol Rep 2007;17(2):483–8.
65. Hersh CP, Demeo DL, Lange C, et al. Attempted replication of reported chronic obstructive pulmonary disease candidate gene associations. Am J Respir Cell Mol Biol 2005;33(1):71–8.
66. Matheson MC, Raven J, Walters EH, et al. Microsomal epoxide hydrolase is not associated with COPD in a community-based sample. Hum Biol 2006;78(6): 705–17.

67. Park JY, Chen L, Wadhwa N, et al. Polymorphisms for microsomal epoxide hydrolase and genetic susceptibility to COPD. Int J Mol Med 2005;15(3):443–8.
68. Sandford AJ, Chagani T, Weir TD, et al. Susceptibility genes for rapid decline of lung function in the lung health study. Am J Respir Crit Care Med 2001;163(2):469–73.
69. Takeyabu K, Yamaguchi E, Suzuki I, et al. Gene polymorphism for microsomal epoxide hydrolase and susceptibility to emphysema in a Japanese population. Eur Respir J 2000;15(5):891–4.
70. Xiao D, Wang C, Du MJ, et al. Relationship between polymorphisms of genes encoding microsomal epoxide hydrolase and glutathione S-transferase P1 and chronic obstructive pulmonary disease. Chin Med J (Engl) 2004;117(5):661–7.
71. Yim JJ, Park GY, Lee CT, et al. Genetic susceptibility to chronic obstructive pulmonary disease in Koreans: combined analysis of polymorphic genotypes for microsomal epoxide hydrolase and glutathione S-transferase M1 and T1. Thorax 2000;55(2):121–5.
72. Yoshikawa M, Hiyama K, Ishioka S, et al. Microsomal epoxide hydrolase genotypes and chronic obstructive pulmonary disease in Japanese. Int J Mol Med 2000;5(1):49–53.
73. Brogger J, Steen VM, Eiken HG, et al. Genetic association between COPD and polymorphisms in TNF, ADRB2 and EPHX1. Eur Respir J 2006;27(4):682–8.
74. Lee J, Nordestgaard BG, Dahl M. EPHX1 polymorphisms, COPD and asthma in 47,000 individuals and in meta-analysis. Eur Respir J 2011;37(1):18–25.
75. Ishii T, Matsuse T, Teramoto S, et al. Glutathione S-transferase P1 (GSTP1) polymorphism in patients with chronic obstructive pulmonary disease. Thorax 1999;54(8):693–6.
76. DeMeo DL, Hersh CP, Hoffman EA, et al. Genetic determinants of emphysema distribution in the national emphysema treatment trial. Am J Respir Crit Care Med 2007;176(1):42–8.
77. He JQ, Ruan J, Connett JE, et al. Antioxidant gene polymorphisms and susceptibility to a rapid decline in lung function in smokers. Am J Respir Crit Care Med 2002;166(3):323–8.
78. Rodriguez F, de la Roza C, Jardi R, et al. Glutathione S-transferase P1 and lung function in patients with alpha1-antitrypsin deficiency and COPD. Chest 2005;127(5):1537–43.
79. Yamada N, Yamaya M, Okinaga S, et al. Microsatellite polymorphism in the heme oxygenase-1 gene promoter is associated with susceptibility to emphysema. Am J Hum Genet 2000;66(1):187–95.
80. Nakayama K, Kikuchi A, Yasuda H, et al. Heme oxygenase-1 gene promoter polymorphism and decline in lung function in Japanese men. Thorax 2006;61(10):921.
81. Budhi A, Hiyama K, Isobe T, et al. Genetic susceptibility for emphysematous changes of the lung in Japanese. Int J Mol Med 2003;11(3):321–9.
82. Fu WP, Zhao ZH, Fang LZ, et al. Heme oxygenase-1 polymorphism associated with severity of chronic obstructive pulmonary disease. Chin Med J (Engl) 2007;120(1):12–6.
83. Tanaka G, Aminuddin F, Akhabir L, et al. Effect of heme oxygenase-1 polymorphisms on lung function and gene expression. BMC Med Genet 2011;12:117.
84. Juul K, Tybjaerg-Hansen A, Marklund S, et al. Genetically increased antioxidative protection and decreased chronic obstructive pulmonary disease. Am J Respir Crit Care Med 2006;173(8):858–64.

85. Young RP, Hopkins R, Black PN, et al. Functional variants of antioxidant genes in smokers with COPD and in those with normal lung function. Thorax 2006;61(5): 394-9.
86. Huang SL, Su CH, Chang SC. Tumor necrosis factor-alpha gene polymorphism in chronic bronchitis. Am J Respir Crit Care Med 1997;156(5):1436-9.
87. Cordoba-Lanus E, Baz-Davila R, de-Torres JP, et al. TNFA-863 polymorphism is associated with a reduced risk of chronic obstructive pulmonary disease: a replication study. BMC Med Genet 2011;12:132.
88. Higham MA, Pride NB, Alikhan A, et al. Tumour necrosis factor-alpha gene promoter polymorphism in chronic obstructive pulmonary disease. Eur Respir J 2000;15(2):281-4.
89. Ishii T, Matsuse T, Teramoto S, et al. Neither IL-1beta, IL-1 receptor antagonist, nor TNF-alpha polymorphisms are associated with susceptibility to COPD. Respir Med 2000;94(9):847-51.
90. Ferrarotti I, Zorzetto M, Beccaria M, et al. Tumour necrosis factor family genes in a phenotype of COPD associated with emphysema. Eur Respir J 2003;21(3):444-9.
91. Patuzzo C, Gile LS, Zorzetto M, et al. Tumor necrosis factor gene complex in COPD and disseminated bronchiectasis. Chest 2000;117(5):1353-8.
92. Seifart C, Plagens A, Dempfle A, et al. TNF-alpha, TNF-beta, IL-6, and IL-10 polymorphisms in patients with lung cancer. Dis Markers 2005;21(3):157-65.
93. Chierakul N, Wongwisutikul P, Vejbaesya S, et al. Tumor necrosis factor-alpha gene promoter polymorphism is not associated with smoking-related COPD in Thailand. Respirology 2005;10(1):36-9.
94. Hegab AE, Sakamoto T, Saitoh W, et al. Polymorphisms of TNFalpha, IL1beta, and IL1RN genes in chronic obstructive pulmonary disease. Biochem Biophys Res Commun 2005;329(4):1246-52.
95. Tanaka G, Sandford AJ, Burkett K, et al. Tumour necrosis factor and lymphotoxin A polymorphisms and lung function in smokers. Eur Respir J 2007;29(1):34-41.
96. Ruse CE, Hill MC, Tobin M, et al. Tumour necrosis factor gene complex polymorphisms in chronic obstructive pulmonary disease. Respir Med 2007;101(2): 340-4.
97. Papatheodorou A, Latsi P, Vrettou C, et al. Development of a novel microarray methodology for the study of SNPs in the promoter region of the TNF-alpha gene: their association with obstructive pulmonary disease in Greek patients. Clin Biochem 2007;40(12):843-50.
98. Kueppers F, Miller RD, Gordon H, et al. Familial prevalence of chronic obstructive pulmonary disease in a matched pair study. Am J Med 1977;63(3):336-42.
99. Horne SL, Cockcroft DW, Dosman JA. Possible protective effect against chronic obstructive airways disease by the GC2 allele. Hum Hered 1990;40(3):173-6.
100. Schellenberg D, Pare PD, Weir TD, et al. Vitamin D binding protein variants and the risk of COPD. Am J Respir Crit Care Med 1998;157(3 Pt 1):957-61.
101. Ishii T, Keicho N, Teramoto S, et al. Association of Gc-globulin variation with susceptibility to COPD and diffuse panbronchiolitis. Eur Respir J 2001;18(5):753-7.
102. Ito I, Nagai S, Hoshino Y, et al. Risk and severity of COPD is associated with the group-specific component of serum globulin 1F allele. Chest 2004;125(1): 63-70.
103. Kasuga I, Pare PD, Ruan J, et al. Lack of association of group specific component haplotypes with lung function in smokers. Thorax 2003;58(9):790-3.
104. Castaldi PJ, Cho MH, Cohn M, et al. The COPD genetic association compendium: a comprehensive online database of COPD genetic associations. Hum Mol Genet 2010;19(3):526-34.

Pulmonary Overlap Syndromes, with a Focus on COPD and ILD

Katherine A. Dudley, MD[a], Robert L. Owens, MD[b],*,
Atul Malhotra, MD[c]

KEYWORDS

- Overlap syndrome • Sleep • Chronic obstructive pulmonary disease
- Idiopathic pulmonary fibrosis • Obstructive sleep apnea

KEY POINTS

- Overlap syndrome refers to the coexistence of chronic lung disease and obstructive sleep apnea (OSA) in the same patient. To date, overlap syndromes have been poorly studied for a variety of reasons.
- One difficulty is that each of the underlying disorders in an overlap syndrome occurs along a spectrum of disease severity. Thus, patients with an overlap syndrome are heterogeneous, and the goals of therapy may differ in different patients.
- However, the importance of overlap syndromes is highlighted by recent data demonstrating increased morbidity and mortality in patients with the overlap of both chronic obstructive pulmonary disease (COPD) and OSA compared with either underlying disorder alone.
- Unrecognized OSA may also contribute to symptoms of sleepiness/fatigue in patients with chronic lung disease. Clinicians should be mindful of the possibility of overlap syndromes in these patients.

First described in the 1980s by pulmonologist David Flenley,[1] *overlap* syndromes (OVSs) refer to the coexistence of chronic lung disease and obstructive sleep apnea (OSA). Although it could refer to any of the lung diseases and OSA, *the* OVS is usually reserved for the coexistence of OSA and chronic obstructive pulmonary disease (COPD), which Flenley thought to have unique adverse health consequences distinct from either condition alone. Given the high prevalence of each disorder alone, OVS is also likely to be common and clinically relevant. However, although OVS has been

This article originally appeared in *Sleep Medicine Clinics*, Volume 9, Issue 3, September 2014.
[a] Harvard Combined Program of Pulmonary and Critical Care and Division of Sleep and Circadian Disorders at Brigham and Women's Hospital, 221 Longwood Avenue, Boston, MA 02115, USA; [b] Divisions of Pulmonary and Critical Care and Sleep and Circadian Disorders, Brigham and Women's Hospital, 221 Longwood Avenue, Boston, MA 02115, USA; [c] University of California, San Diego, San Diego, CA
* Corresponding author.
E-mail address: rowens@partners.org

described in the literature for nearly 30 years, the lack of standard diagnostic criteria for the syndrome has limited rigorous discussion of diagnosis, prevalence, pathophysiology, treatment, and outcomes. These challenges are explored in more detail later and throughout this review. Importantly, several recent studies suggest that OVS does, as Flenley thought, have worse outcomes than either disease in isolation. These findings have highlighted the urgent need for further study of both *the* OVS and all overlaps between OSA and chronic lung disease.

CLINICAL AND RESEARCH CHALLENGES OF THE OVS

OVSs are poorly understood for many reasons. Using *the* OVS as a prototype:

1. The diagnosis of OVS is nebulous, as both OSA and COPD are heterogeneous disorders. COPD and OSA both have wide ranges of severity, in terms of both objective measurements of disease (eg, forced expiratory volume in 1 second [FEV_1], and apnea-hypopnea index [AHI]) and patient-reported symptoms (eg, dyspnea and daytime tiredness). OVS is defined by the presence of both conditions regardless of the relative burden of one or the other. Therefore, patients with OVS may represent a very heterogeneous population, falling into one of many potential categories: mild COPD with mild OSA, mild COPD with severe OSA, severe COPD with mild OSA, severe COPD with severe OSA, and so forth. Prognosis and treatment, therefore, could be considerably different depending on the relative impact of each condition. Although it is a minor point, there is not a single *International Classification of Diseases, Ninth Revision* code for OVS, which impedes even epidemiologic research.

2. The diagnosis of OSA in the setting of hypoxemic lung disease is uncertain. The definition of OSA includes hypopneas and reductions in airflow with associated desaturation, which is more likely to occur in those with chronic lung disease. The AHI, used to grade OSA severity, does not differentiate between apneas and hypopneas. Thus, a patient with severe COPD might have the same AHI consistent with severe OSA (based on a large number of hypopneas) as another patient with a very collapsible upper airway without lung disease (who predominantly has apneas). In addition, a 10-minute prolonged desaturation caused by hypoventilation may be scored as a single hypopnea because the event duration has minimal effect on the definitions used. More rigorous definitions of OSA might be useful, such as the apnea index or scoring based on airflow alone and arousals independent of oxygen desaturation.

3. The interactions of COPD and OSA are not understood. Thus, it is unknown at a pathophysiologic level whether each disorder might predispose to the other disease. As discussed earlier, the baseline hypoxemia of COPD likely predisposes to a diagnosis of OSA. But other links are possible; for example, the changes in lung volumes that occur with COPD might impact upper airway collapsibility. How COPD and OSA interact to cause the increased morbidity and mortality attributable to OVS is not known. Is it simply from more prolonged hypoxemia or hypercapnia than either disorder alone? Or are poor outcomes caused by the indirect effects of the disorders, such as cardiovascular disease?

4. Thus, the goals of therapy in OVS are poorly defined. For a patient with severe OSA with many apneas, the goal of therapy may be to support patency of the upper airway and eliminate apneic events. For a patient with evidence of hypoventilation, the goal may be to improve nocturnal gas exchange and hypercarbia. Maybe the best approach would be intensive modification of cardiovascular risk factors (eg, blood pressure, cholesterol modification). These uncertainties contribute to the confusion as to the ideal therapy to use.

5. The optimal treatment of OVS is unknown. Few large clinical trials have been undertaken, and no large studies have compared long-term outcomes between randomized therapies. Although continuous positive airway pressure (CPAP) is the most commonly applied therapy, some groups have used bilevel positive airway pressure, which provides a higher pressure during inspiration than during expiration. Bilevel may have benefits over CPAP for some patients, particularly among patients with severe COPD whereby it may aid with nocturnal ventilation and resting of respiratory muscles. Finally, the role of oxygen therapy, another treatment used clinically, has not been fully explored in this population. The role of medical therapy aimed at limiting cardiovascular events has also not been explored.
6. An additional under-recognized consideration is that sleep is poor in chronic lung diseases, independent of upper airway collapse. Many studies have highlighted the high prevalence of sleep complaints among patients with chronic lung diseases. There are many reasons behind this finding, ranging from cough interfering with sleep, increased anxiety and insomnia, side effects of medications (eg, chronic glucocorticoids, beta agonists), and frequent arousals. Although treatment of OVS with CPAP may improve upper airway patency, CPAP will not address many of the nonrespiratory problems that plague sleep in this population. Thus, CPAP adherence may be challenged in ways that are unique compared with those without chronic lung disease.

These points are illustrated as the authors discuss what is known about OVSs, focusing on OSA and idiopathic pulmonary fibrosis (IPF), perhaps the most common of the interstitial lung diseases (ILDs).

COPD AND OSA

Throughout this section, *OVS* refers exclusively to those with COPD and OSA.

COPD

COPD is a progressive lung disease characterized by irreversible airway obstruction (FEV_1/forced vital capacity [FVC]<70%). This disease can involve the small airways, pulmonary parenchyma, or both. COPD results from an inflammatory response that can result in chronic sputum production (chronic bronchitis) as well as the destruction of alveolar walls distal to the terminal bronchioles, leading to enlargement of the airspaces (emphysema). Although tobacco use is strongly associated with the development of COPD, it is not the only risk factor. In developing countries, exposure to indoor air pollution plays a critical role, in particular as a result of fuels burned for cooking and heating. Occupational causes are also well described, such as irritants and fumes. Estimates are now that most COPD worldwide is non–smoking related, emphasizing caution about labeling the disease as self-inflicted. COPD may present as dyspnea, wheezing, cough, sputum production, poor exercise tolerance, hypoxic and/or hypercarbic respiratory failure, and right heart failure (cor pulmonale). There are Global Initiative for Chronic Obstructive Lung Disease (GOLD)–defined stages of disease severity based on pulmonary function testing (the FEV_1) and symptoms. In the United States, more than 5% of the population (at least 13.7 million people) is burdened by COPD,[2,3] which is a leading cause of morbidity. Worldwide, about 10% of the population is affected.[4] Although medications may improve symptomatic control of the disease and slow progression, the health-related consequences of COPD remain high.[3] As of 2011, COPD was the third leading cause of death in the United States.[5] Annual expenditures for the disease are approaching $40 billion when direct and indirect costs are considered.[6]

Although COPD is often considered a respiratory condition, the impact on other organ systems and overall health is increasingly well recognized. The most recent GOLD definition of the disease highlights COPD as a systemic process with "significant extrapulmonary effects that may contribute to the severity in individual patients."[7] Indeed, depression, skeletal-muscle myopathy, anemia, and osteoporosis are all common in COPD. Similarly, as is discussed later, sleep disturbance and its consequences could be thought of as one of these extrapulmonary manifestations. COPD is also associated with adverse cardiac outcomes, which may be of particularly importance when thinking about the overlap with OSA, which also has cardiovascular consequences.[8–12] Even after consideration of shared risk factors, such as cigarette smoking, COPD is associated with higher rates of coronary artery disease, congestive heart failure, and arrhythmias.[13,14] Additional mechanisms by which COPD may play a role in cardiovascular disease include increased oxidative stress, inflammation, and increased platelet activation.

Of particular interest in the current discussion, COPD is a heterogeneous disorder, with variable amounts of airway and parenchymal disease. Most patients have a predominance of one phenotype, though there is usually some overlap. In the past, patients with chronic bronchitis were described as *blue bloaters*, referring to hypoxemia, polycythemia, and cor pulmonale that often accompanies patients with this form of COPD. *Pink puffers* were those with an emphysematous phenotype of COPD, often with muscle wasting and hyperinflation but without oxygen desaturation. The GOLD criteria are designed to be inclusive to maximize disease recognition and prompt treatment and, therefore, do not highlight these distinctions. However, there may be critical differences in the pathophysiology among different phenotypes that are important when considering OVS.

Sleep and COPD

More than three-quarters of patients with COPD report bothersome nocturnal symptoms, such as dyspnea.[15,16] Patients who report cough and wheeze during the day are more likely to have sleep disturbances than those who do not.[17] Patients report trouble falling asleep, frequent awakening, difficultly returning to sleep, and nonrestorative sleep. In a survey of patients with COPD, more than 60% had experienced at least one sleep symptom in the preceding 28 days.[15] Rates of clinical insomnia are high among patients with COPD, present in more than one-fourth.[18] As compared with controls, COPD confers an increased risk of insomnia nearly twice that of non-COPD patients.[19] These sleep disturbances are chronic, persisting over many years.[20]

Sleep complaints increase with more severe disease. Although mild obstructive lung disease is associated with preserved sleep quality,[21] a more severe obstructive disease is associated with increased sleep complaints.[22] Severe disease negatively impacts several objective sleep parameters, such as total sleep time, sleep efficiency, rapid eye movement (REM) sleep,[23] as well as sleep-onset latency, arousals, and sleep-stage transitions.[24–27]

The mechanisms behind the sleep disturbances are likely multifactorial. Symptoms such as cough and wheezing may play a role as noted earlier.[28,29] Recent work has also highlighted nonrespiratory factors that also perturb sleep among patients with COPD.[30] For example, restless leg syndrome has been found in up to one-third of patients with COPD, and periodic limb movements are associated with worse insomnia.[31] As a result of all of these factors, the use of medications to aid sleep is common, especially sedative hypnotics, which are used by 25% of patients with COPD.[17] Although data are sparse, these medications could theoretically worsen hypoxemia/hypercapnia, though this may not be true for all patients.[32–35]

Changes in Respiration During Sleep with COPD and Nocturnal Oxygen Desaturation

Nocturnal oxygen desaturation (NOD) in chronic lung disease is the result of the normal changes that occur in ventilation with sleep. Put another way, sleep is a stress test for those patients with chronic lung disease that leads to nocturnal hypoxemia and hypercapnia. Understanding the normal changes in respiration that occur with sleep is key to understanding NOD.

Normal Changes in Respiration During Sleep

Sleep is divided into different stages based on electroencephalography waveforms, muscle tone, eye movement, and breathing pattern, with the main distinction being between non-REM sleep and REM sleep. The main respiratory changes that occur during sleep are a decrease in ventilation (largely a decrease in tidal volume without a compensatory increase in respiratory rate) and decreased accessory muscle activity. The changes in respiration are most pronounced in REM sleep, which is notable for skeletal muscle atonia (with the exception of certain muscles, including the diaphragm); in addition to decreased ventilation, the breathing pattern becomes very irregular (especially during bursts of REMs). The decrease in respiratory drive reflects both a decrease in metabolic rate, which results in less carbon dioxide (CO_2) production and, thus, requirement for elimination, and an increase in the CO_2 set point.[36] The reduction in minute ventilation is further pronounced during REM, when ventilation may be 40% less compared with wakefulness.[37,38] In addition to the decrease in the respiratory set point, there is decreased responsiveness to hypercapnia and hypoxia compared with wakefulness.[39–41] Finally, upper airway resistance increases during sleep, even in those without OSA.[42] An overview of the changes is outlined in **Fig. 1**.

Sleep and Breathing with COPD

All of the aforementioned changes are physiologic changes that occur from wakefulness to sleep. However, in the presence of lung disease, the consequences may be

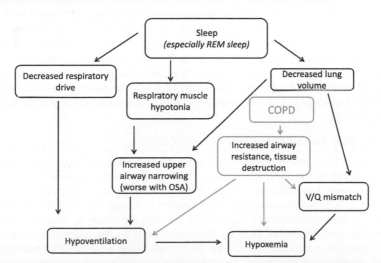

Fig. 1. The normal physiologic changes that occur with sleep. With sleep onset, respiratory drive is decreased, and there is respiratory muscle hypotonia and a decrease in lung volumes. Even without OSA, the result is hypoventilation compared with wakefulness. Particularly with OSA and COPD, there are further pathophysiologic changes that lead to greater hypoventilation and hypoxemia.

dramatic and lead to oxygen desaturation. First, these patients may already have borderline hypoxemia, which puts them on the steep part of the oxygen hemoglobin binding curve; that is, small changes in Pao_2 lead to a decrease in oxygen saturation. Second, patients with COPD have increased minute ventilation for a variety of reasons and frequently rely on accessory muscles to aid ventilation. As a result, ventilation can decrease dramatically during sleep and particularly in REM sleep when muscle activity decreases. Furthermore, patients with COPD may have chest hyperinflation, which stretches the diaphragm and impairs contractile function.[43]

NOD is perhaps the most common sleep abnormality attributed to COPD, occurring in anywhere from one-quarter to three-quarters of patients with an awake oxygen saturation greater than 90% to 95%.[44-46] During sleep, desaturations are frequent among patients with an FEV_1/FVC less than 65%[21]; increasing severity of obstructive disease is associated with more severe desaturations during sleep. Among those with severe obstructive lung disease ($FEV_1<30\%$), a 20% decrease of oxygen saturation can be seen during non-REM sleep and an impressive decline of 40% during REM.[37] There is substantial variation in reported NOD rates, in part caused by the heterogeneous nature of COPD as well as the definition of NOD, which may be based either on nadir levels or the duration of low oxygen tension.

COPD and OSA: the OVS

OSA is a common disorder, characterized by partial or complete collapse of the upper airway during sleep, resulting in intermittent hypoxia and arousals. The repetitive nature of these breathing events results in fragmented and nonrestorative sleep. Among middle-aged men (50–70 years old), the prevalence of moderate to severe OSA is predicted to be as high as 17% and slightly lower but still concerning at 9% among middle-aged women.[47] OSA is associated with an increased risk of serious neurocognitive and cardiovascular consequences, including hypertension, congestive heart failure, and stroke.[48-51] CPAP is the gold standard treatment of OSA and consists of a mask worn during sleep connected to a machine that delivers pressurized air, thereby splinting open the airway during sleep. Although CPAP is efficacious in treating OSA in almost all cases, its effectiveness is limited by patient adherence. Although adherence rates may be improved through intensive support and behavioral therapy, the real-world nonadherence rates may approach 50%. In the context of OVS, these facts illustrate the potentially large number of patients with OSA at risk for OVS, that both OSA and COPD have substantial cardiovascular morbidity and mortality, and that positive airway pressure is unlikely to be accepted by many patients.

Diagnosing OSA Among Those Patients with COPD

OSA is diagnosed through polysomnography, with apneas and hypopneas recorded during sleep. The tendency toward oxygen desaturation described earlier in those patients with chronic lung disease impacts the diagnosis of OSA. Although the designation of apneas is straightforward and independent of oxygen desaturation, hypopneas are based on flow limitation of at least 30% and require either an accompanying 3% or greater oxygen desaturation or an arousal. Based on the sigmoidal shape of the oxygen-hemoglobin desaturation curve, any small change in Pao_2 that occurs during sleep will be reflected as a larger (and therefore scorable as a hypopnea) change in oxygen saturation. Put another way, 2 patients with the same upper airway tendency to collapse, but one healthy and the other with chronic lung disease, might have very different apnea-hypopnea indices. A similar observation that makes the same point is that the AHI improves with descent from altitude, largely because of a decrease in the number of hypopneas.[52] Nevertheless, there are no current alternative scoring criteria or guidelines for OSA diagnosis in the setting of chronic lung disease.

Among patients with COPD, there are clues to suggest OSA beyond the classic symptoms of snoring, witnessed apneas, and daytime sleepiness. For example, headaches with the initiation of nocturnal supplemental oxygen suggest coexistent OSA (caused by increased hypercapnia). Hypercapnia, despite relatively preserved pulmonary function tests, may also signal the presence of sleep-disordered breathing and prompt evaluation. Indeed, based on findings from one cohort, FEV_1 was severely decreased among patients with COPD only with hypercapnia but only moderately reduced in patients who had both COPD and OSA. Despite this difference in pulmonary function tests, daytime $Paco_2$ was higher among those with OVS compared with COPD only.[53,54] Additionally, obesity is more common among hypercarbic patients with COPD who have OSA as compared with COPD only.[54] For comparison, the characteristics of COPD alone, OSA alone, and OVS from one cohort are outlined in **Table 1**.

The American Thoracic Society/European Respiratory Society's guidelines also highlight the role of referring for overnight testing among those with mild COPD and evidence of pulmonary hypertension. Although only 16% of patients with OSA have been observed to have pulmonary hypertension, this number jumps to 86% for those with OVS.[55] This is an intriguing finding, given that traditional markers of OSA severity and nocturnal hypoxia in COPD are not predictive of pulmonary hypertension. However, time spent with oxygen saturation less than 90% is high among patients with OVS, even without a severe obstructive pattern on spirometry.

Prevalence and Epidemiology of OVS

In general, small studies from the early 1990s suggested that severe COPD was a risk factor for OSA.[56] For example, one early study found greater than 80% prevalence of OSA among patients with COPD and excessive daytime sleepiness referred for evaluation.[12] In certain populations, too, such as Veterans Administration patients, the

Table 1
Characteristics and physiologic measures of patients with COPD only, OSA only, and OVS

	COPD Group (n = 32)	Overlap Group (n = 29)	Pure OSA Group (n = 152)
Age (y)	60.1 ± 10.4	57.2 ± 9.5	48.9 ± 12.9
Weight (kg)	87.6 ± 17.5	102.2 ± 20.6	106.8 ± 28.8
BMI (kg/m^2)	31 ± 7	36 ± 6	39 ± 10
FVC (% predicted)	60 ± 19	72 ± 17	89 ± 21
FEV_1 (% predicted)	47 ± 16	63 ± 16	89 ± 20
FEV_1/FVC (%)	59 ± 9	67 ± 5	87 ± 9
P_{ao2} (mm Hg)	69 ± 10	70 ± 11	79 ± 12
P_{aco2} (mm Hg)	40 ± 5	45 ± 5	39 ± 4
AHI (events/h)	6 ± 5	40 ± 20	42 ± 23
Time S_{pO2} <90% (%)	16 ± 28	48 ± 28	30 ± 28

Overlap refers to both COPD and OSA.
Abbreviations: BMI, body mass index; S_{pO2}, oxygen saturation.
Values are mean $\pm$ SD.
Adapted from Resta O, Foschino Barbaro MP, Brindicci C, et al. Hypercapnia in overlap syndrome: possible determinant factors. Sleep Breath 2002;6(1):14; with permission.

coexistence of OSA and COPD was high (29%) among patients who had polysomnogram and spirometry data available.[57]

More recently, larger epidemiology studies including a more broad range of subjects, such as the Sleep Heart Health Study and Multinational Monitoring of Trends and Determinants in Cardiovascular Disease, have not demonstrated an increased risk of OSA among those with obstructive lung disease, at least among those with mild obstructive lung disease.[21,58] In these large cohorts, the prevalence of OSA was 11% to 14%, which was similar in those with or without obstructive lung disease.[21,58] Thus, it seems likely that there is little connection among those with mild COPD; whether more severe COPD can contribute to OSA is not clear.

Although the answer is not yet known, proposed mechanisms of OSA risk in severe COPD include the following: fluid shifts in those with cor pulmonale from lower extremity edema to the neck,[59] a generalized myopathy from COPD alone that affects the upper airway muscles,[60] or a steroid-induced myopathy from systemic or inhaled corticosteroids. All of these changes would increase upper airway collapsibility.

Clinical Consequences of OSA and COPD

The large aforementioned cohort studies did highlight that among those with obstructive lung disease and OSA, the nocturnal desaturations and sleep disturbances are greater (both oxygen saturation nadir and duration of hypoxemia) than would be expected for either disease alone.[21] Whether causal or not, more recent reports have suggested an increased mortality in OVS compared with COPD and OSA alone and have increased awareness about OVSs. First, Marin and colleagues[61] found decreased survival among patients with OVS compared with either COPD or OSA alone (**Fig. 2**). There were differences in death from any cause and cardiovascular causes when patients with OVS using CPAP were compared with those not on CPAP. No differences were seen between COPD only and patients with OVS using CPAP.[61] That patients with OVS using CPAP have reduced mortality compared with OVS without CPAP has now also been reported in other cohorts[62-64] Jaoude and colleagues[64] found that CPAP only improved outcomes from OVS in those patients who were also hypercapnic. Further exploring the observed therapeutic benefit of CPAP,

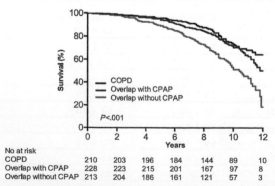

Fig. 2. Kaplan-Meier survival curves for patients with COPD. Patients with OVS on CPAP, and patients with OVS not on CPAP. Treatment with CPAP seems to prevent against the excess mortality in patients with OVS. Importantly, these data are observational. (*Adapted from* Marin JM, Soriano JB, Carrizo SJ, et al. Outcomes in patients with chronic obstructive pulmonary disease and obstructive sleep apnea: the overlap syndrome. Am J Respir Crit Care Med 2010;182(3):328; with permission.)

Stanchina and colleagues[63] found that greater time on CPAP was associated with reduced mortality in patients with OVS.

Although the improvement with CPAP seems dramatic, these are not randomized data; these were cohort studies in which subjects chose to adhere to or abandon CPAP therapy. Patients who did not adhere to CPAP may have been those with more COPD/less OSA; had more respiratory symptoms, such as dyspnea or sputum that limit CPAP use; or were less likely to adhere to other medication therapy, which is also important for limiting poor outcomes (eg, statin therapy). Nevertheless, these findings highlight the need to focus more resources on the care and understanding of these patients.

It is assumed, but not known, that the worse outcomes in OVS are caused by excess cardiovascular events. As discussed earlier, both COPD and OSA increase cardiovascular risk. Some data support this potential mechanism, suggesting that OSA can augment vascular changes among patients with COPD, such as arterial stiffness.[65] Sharma and colleagues[66] found that patients with OSA have more extensive remodeling of the right ventricle seen on cardiac magnetic resonance compared with those with COPD alone; the extent of right ventricle remodeling was correlated with the oxygen desaturation index.

Treatment of OVS

Treatment of OVS may be thought of as addressing the underlying COPD, OSA, or both. Although the specific goals of treatment remain poorly defined, most clinicians strive to eliminate sleep-disordered breathing and eliminate NOD. What to target for ideal oxygen saturation, however, remains unclear, as does the impact of normalizing hypercarbia. The most commonly applied therapy is CPAP.

Before CPAP is applied, however, it is critical to consider the use of therapies that target the underlying COPD, such as bronchodilators and antiinflammatories. Therapies aimed at COPD alone can improve nocturnal oxygen saturation as well as decrease symptoms. Ipratropium and tiotropium, cholinergic bronchodilators, long-acting beta-agonists, and oral steroids all have data to support improvements in oxygen saturation during sleep.[67–70] Some of these agents, such as ipratropium, have also been shown to improve sleep quality and increase REM and total sleep time, although, surprisingly, tiotropium did not.[67,68,70] Although the mechanism of these improvements has yet to be teased out, these studies suggest that optimizing COPD treatment can play a key role in the degree of nocturnal oxygen saturation. The impact on upper airway patency is unknown; some have hypothesized that (inhaled) steroids might predispose the upper airway to myopathy and increased collapsibility. However, at least in asthmatic patients receiving high-dose inhaled corticosteroids, there was no increase in collapsibility.[71]

Nocturnal oxygen is a mainstay of therapy for hypoxemia in COPD with demonstrated mortality benefits.[72,73] Among patients with OSA, nocturnal oxygen therapy alone may improve hypoxemia; however, arousals, sleep architecture, and daytime symptoms, such as sleepiness, are not impacted,[74] pointing to the potential impact of sleep fragmentation caused by arousals triggered by airway obstruction, which is not addressed by oxygen therapy. Thus, supplemental oxygen alone for OSA seems unlikely to be of benefit.

CPAP and Lung Function in COPD

There are a few studies that have assessed treatment with CPAP in patients with OVS. Small studies have demonstrated improvements in daytime oxygen saturation and degree of hypercarbia with nocturnal CPAP use.[75,76] Improvements in FEV_1, echocardiogram estimates of mean pulmonary artery pressure, Pao_2, and $Paco_2$ have been documented.[75,77,78] Other studies have found a decline in lung function among patients with OVS who were adherent to CPAP therapy.[79] Differences in study design, and subject characteristics make it difficult to generalize or reconcile the findings from these studies. It has been hypothesized that improvements in gas exchange may reflect improvement in daytime lung function, although the mechanism remains unclear and controversial. The prevention of repetitive upper airway collapse in an animal model seemed to improve lower airway resistance.[80] Off-loading of respiratory muscles during sleep through CPAP may also be important, contributing to decreased oxygen consumption, CO_2 production, and reducing sleep hypoventilation. After CPAP initiation, fewer COPD-related hospital admissions are seen in some populations.[63,81]

As discussed earlier, recent papers suggest that the treatment of OVS with CPAP is associated with reduced mortality. First, in the Brazilian cohort, 5-year survival with CPAP was 71%, as compared with 26% among patients using oxygen alone.[62] This cohort included more than 600 patients who required long-term oxygen therapy for hypoxemic COPD and had at least moderate OSA. Patients with OSA were prescribed CPAP, and those who were nonadherent to CPAP continued to use oxygen for COPD. Similarly, the findings from a Spanish cohort of patients with OVS also suggested a benefit, lowering the mortality risk to that of COPD alone.[61] The striking improvement in both cohorts supports a beneficial role of CPAP as well as highlighting the very poor outcomes in those with OVS. Again, patients in both studies were not randomized but were self-selected based on adherence to CPAP (or were not able to afford CPAP therapy). That is, these are observational studies comparing patients with OVS who are and are not adherent to CPAP. Although these studies do not elicit the mechanism for the reduced mortality, if caused by CPAP, this may be through the reduction in cardiac risk factors. Indeed, CRP levels, a nonspecific marker of inflammation, were significantly reduced in patients with OVS using CPAP as compared with pretreatment.[82]

Noninvasive ventilation (NIV), such as bilevel positive airway pressure, is an attractive treatment modality in this population. Even in the absence of OSA, nocturnal NIV is often applied for patients with more severe COPD to off-load respiratory muscles, supplement ventilation, decrease hypercapnia, and reduce hypoxemia. Studies in this area have generally been small, nonrandomized, and in patients with stable disease. Taken together, these studies did not demonstrate any improvements in lung function, gas, exchange, sleep efficiency, or mortality according to a 2003 meta-analysis.[83] Since that time, however, 2 areas of investigation deserve to be highlighted. Among patients with OVS with stable hypercapnic COPD (patients with OSA were excluded), one moderately large randomized trial demonstrated a mortality benefit with NIV use, though NIV was accompanied by a decrease in quality of life.[84] A mortality benefit compared with historical controls has also been seen using very high ventilation settings.[85] These investigators argue that so-called high-intensity noninvasive positive pressure ventilation (with very high driving pressures, for example, inspiratory pressures of 28 cm of H_2O and respiratory rate of more than 20 breaths per minute) among patients with COPD does not seem to impact sleep quality and may have some benefits, such as improvement in gas exchange and lung function.[86–88]

Weight loss is beneficial among patients with OSA and obesity.[89] Among patients with COPD alone, however, weight loss is often a concerning finding, stemming from pulmonary cachexia, infection, malignancy, or deconditioning. The role of weight loss among patients with OVS has not been examined; however, it is probably safe for obese patients with OVS to target weight loss.[90] Although purely speculative, given the high rates of cardiovascular disease in OSA and COPD, it may also make sense to consider cardioprotective therapies (eg, aspirin, statin) as the primary prevention in patients with OVS.

Based on all of the aforementioned information, the authors propose the diagnostic and treatment algorithm in **Fig. 3**.

OSA AND ILD, WITH EMPHASIS ON IPF
ILD/IPF Background

ILD may refer to several heterogeneous conditions, such as IPF; sarcoidosis; autoimmune-related pulmonary disorders, such as systemic sclerosis and hypersensitivity pneumonitis; or secondary to an environmental or drug exposure, such as amiodarone. The common features of the ILDs are (1) that these are distinct from obstructive lung diseases (such as COPD) and demonstrate restrictive physiology and (2) that the anatomic basis of the disease is usually the interstitium (the alveolar epithelium, pulmonary capillary endothelium, basement membrane, perivascular, and perilymphatic tissues). The focus of the authors' discussion is primarily among patients with IPF.

IPF is a restrictive lung disease of unknown cause. It is characterized by chronic, progressive lung fibrosis of unknown cause.[91] It is an irreversible process, with an

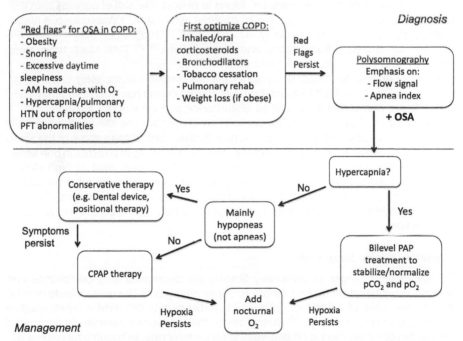

Fig. 3. Management algorithm for patients with COPD. Patients with COPD should be assessed for any red flags that might suggest the presence of concurrent OSA. If present, COPD should be optimized before undergoing polysomnography. Attention should be paid to the flow signal and apnea index when assessing the severity of OSA. If hypercapnia is present, patients can begin on bilevel positive airway pressure (PAP). If flow limitation is present without significant apneas, conservative therapy, such as a mandibular advancement device, weight loss, and positional therapy, should be considered. If apneas predominate, CPAP should be started. Supplemental oxygen should be added if hypoxemia persists. HTN, hypertension; PFT, pulmonary function tests.

unpredictable course. Progression can vary markedly on an individual basis, from slow chronic decline to a rapid acceleration of disease; acute exacerbations may also punctuate the disease course. Prognosis is generally very poor, and there are no known effective medical treatments. Despite ongoing research, the cause of the disease remains poorly understood. Histologically, IPF correlates with the pattern of usual interstitial pneumonitis; the terms are sometimes used synonymously.

As compared with COPD, IPF is a rare condition, affecting approximately 14 to 28 per 100,000 people in the United States.[92] It is more common in older individuals and mens.[93] The relatively low prevalence of IPF means that, as compared with COPD, the prevalence of coexisting OSA and IPF (or any ILD) is presumably also rare. However, OSA and IPF might be worth studying if (1) IPF predisposes to OSA, (2) symptoms traditionally ascribed to IPF (eg, fatigue) are actually caused by OSA and can be successfully treated with OSA treatment, and (3) treatment of OSA in these patients improves outcomes.

Sleep in IPF

Poor sleep is common among patients with IPF. Global measures of sleep quality and excessive daytime sleepiness are significantly different as compared with controls, with patients with IPF complaining of poor sleep and excessive daytime sleepiness.[94] Insomnia is also a frequent occurrence, found in almost one-half of patients with IPF, which may contribute to the high rates of daytime symptoms.[95] When sleep is objectively assessed by polysomnography, as compared with controls, patients with IPF have increased sleep fragmentation and stage I sleep.[96–98] Total sleep time, sleep efficiency, and REM sleep are all reduced.[96–98]

The mechanisms for these sleep abnormalities remain incompletely understood, though are likely to be multifactorial. Disruption from cough has been frequently cited as one factor that contributes to sleep disturbance and the inability to sleep.[95,99–101] The effect of medications, such as corticosteroids, which are still used empirically given the lack of other treatment options, may further contribute to some of the sleep abnormalities reported by patients with IPF. Nearly two-thirds of patients in one series were on prednisone,[94] which may interfere with sleep when used at high doses. Patients with IPF are often additionally burdened by depression and other mood disorders, which are often characterized by sleep disturbances and changes in energy level; the medications used to treat these disorders may also impact sleep and daytime function.

Respiration During Sleep in IPF

The pathologic changes in pulmonary fibrosis are decreased lung compliance and increased ventilation/perfusion mismatch. These changes will increase minute ventilation and the work of breathing. As a result, patients with IPF exhibit rapid, shallow breathing during wakefulness.[98] During sleep, the tachypnea persists; as compared with normal controls, there is no decrease in respiratory rate, although tidal volume decreases.[98] Thus, similar to COPD as discussed earlier, among patients with ILD, sleep may serve as a stressor to the respiratory system. Oxygen desaturation is frequently more profound than during wakefulness. The importance of evaluating nighttime respiratory patterns has been recently highlighted, as it may have prognostic value in assessing mortality in ILD.[102] Specifically, among patients with newly diagnosed IPF, the degree of nocturnal desaturation was greater than seen during exercise and was predictive of survival,[103–105] possibly mediated through worsening pulmonary artery hypertension.[103]

ILD and Sleep-Disordered Breathing

The prevalence of sleep-disordered breathing is reported to be extraordinarily high among patients with ILD. Symptoms such as fatigue, commonly reported in patients with IPF, may be attributable to this.[98] In published series, the incidence of OSA ranges from more than two-thirds to nearly 90%.[106–108] **Fig. 4** outlines the symptoms that are commonly reported in IPF and how they may overlap with OSA. The nature of OSA in these populations remains incompletely characterized, such as whether events are caused by airway collapse and flow limitation or oxygen desaturations. Among patients with IPF, AHI is not strongly correlated with the body mass index, again suggesting that other mechanisms, aside from obesity, may be contributing to the diagnosis of OSA in this population.[108] Indeed, as compared with controls, patients with IPF spend more time with an oxygen saturation less than 90%, even when the AHI is similar. These observations raise the possibility that the lower baseline oxygen saturation and increased tendency toward desaturation are overestimating the collapsibility of the upper airway. The 2009 study by Lancaster and colleagues[108] is helpful in this regard. First, their subjects with mild OSA had a mean AHI of 10.7 events per hour, of which less than 1 event per hour was apnea. Additionally, approximately half of the hypopneas were scored based on a 3% oxygen desaturation (rather than arousal). In those with moderate to severe OSA, the average AHI was 39.4 events per hour. But again, the apnea index was only 7.1 events per hour; nearly half of all hypopneas were scored based on oxygen desaturation.

In support of a mechanistic link between IPF and OSA, some investigators have invoked so-called tracheal traction, the link between lung volumes and the upper airway.[109,110] Briefly, in patients without lung disease, a decrease in lung volumes leads to increased upper airway resistance, increased collapsibility, and worse OSA severity.[111,112] However, whether this relationship still holds when compliance of the lung is altered is not clear; no formal measurement of airway resistance or collapsibility has been made in patients with IPF to test this hypothesis. Again, in the study by Lancaster and colleagues,[108] total lung capacity did not seem to predict OSA.

Treatment

There are no proven therapies that target the underlying disease process in IPF. Oxygen therapy is widely used as supportive care. Studies suggest that oxygen therapy can be associated with improvements in exercise performance.[113,114] However, no studies have demonstrated a mortality benefit[115] or improvement in exertional dyspnea,[116] as rapid shallow breathing persists despite addressing hypoxemia.

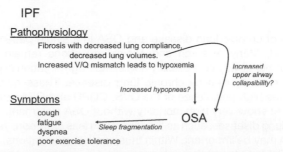

Fig. 4. Links between IPF and OSA. Many symptoms and findings among by patients with IPF overlap with those of OSA, including daytime fatigue, poor sleep, and nocturnal hypoxia. Similarly, the pathophysiologic changes of IPF may contribute to OSA.

Treatment with CPAP among patients with IPF with at least moderate OSA results in gains in sleep-related quality-of-life measures, though adherence to CPAP may be challenging in light of chronic cough and other barriers.[117] There are no studies that have explored the impact of CPAP on outcomes in IPF, such as disease progression or mortality. Taken together, OSA may be common in IPF; treatment with CPAP may improve OSA symptoms.

Other OVS: Beyond COPD and IPF

From the earlier discussion, it is clear that there are many research and clinical questions that remain for OVS, even for *the* OVS, which is relatively common. Even less is known about the prevalence, consequences, and best management of OSA among other chronic lung diseases. However, there are some pearls that the sleep physician should know regarding other lung diseases.

Sarcoidosis is a chronic condition of unknown cause characterized by the formation of granulomas in many organs, most commonly the lung. Lung disease may range from mild to severe and fibrosing in nature. Steroids are often given in more severe disease. Fatigue and excessive daytime sleepiness are more common among patients with sarcoid as compared with controls.[118–120] Consideration of OSA among these patients is, therefore, important, particularly among those with abnormal lung function.[118] There remains a population of patients, however, with hypersomnolence unrelated to OSA. Relevant for sleep medicine physicians, fatigue improves with stimulant therapy (armodafinil).[121] This improvement may serve as a paradigm for patients with chronic lung disease and fatigue to receive empiric therapy.

Although most of the data are in pediatric populations, OSA seems to be more common among patients with sickle cell anemia as compared with controls.[122–124] OSA among patients with sickle cell disease is accompanied by more severe nocturnal desaturations and hypercarbia.[123] Although larger studies are needed to better describe the relationship, OSA, through nocturnal hypoxia, may serve as a trigger for vasoocclusive sickle events.[125] This relationship highlights the potential importance of recognizing and treating OSA among those with sickle cell disease.

Cystic fibrosis (CF) is a systemic disease characterized by abnormal chloride channel function. Obstructive lung disease, bronchiectasis, and repeated pulmonary infections caused by tenacious sputum are common among patients with CF. Sleep apnea is common (in up to 70% of children with CF).[126] OSA presents at an early age as compared with controls, as young as preschool age.[126] NOD is also common among patients with CF, particularly those with awake oxygen saturation less than 94%.[127]

SUMMARY

The combination of chronic lung disease and OSA in a single patient is still, as yet, poorly understood. Many research and clinical questions remain, including how best to quantify upper airway collapsibility and sleep fragmentation in patients already at risk for hypoxemia caused by chronic lung disease. These questions must be answered given the high prevalence of the OVS, COPD and OSA, and observational cohort studies that show very high mortality without OSA treatment.

Other chronic lung diseases, such as IPF, are much less common; yet diagnosis and treatment of OSA may be important. Within these patient populations, there are few or no therapies available to target the underlying disease and its consequences. Recognition and treatment of OSA, therefore, could offer key benefits, such as improvements in quality of life or fatigue level.

REFERENCES

1. Flenley DC. Sleep in chronic obstructive lung disease. Clin Chest Med 1985; 6(4):651–61.
2. Pauwels RA, Buist AS, Calverley PM, et al, GOLD Scientific Committee. Global strategy for the diagnosis, management, and prevention of chronic obstructive pulmonary disease. NHLBI/WHO Global Initiative for Chronic Obstructive Lung Disease (GOLD) workshop summary. Am J Respir Crit Care Med 2001;163(5): 1256–76.
3. Ford ES, Croft JB, Mannino DM, et al. COPD surveillance–United States, 1999-2011. Chest 2013;144(1):284–305.
4. Buist AS, McBurnie MA, Vollmer WM, et al. International variation in the prevalence of COPD (the BOLD study): a population-based prevalence study. Lancet 2007;370(9589):741–50.
5. Hoyert DL, Xu J. Deaths: preliminary data for 2011. Natl Vital Stat Rep 2012; 61(6):1–65 Hyattsville, MD: National Center for Health Statistics. 2012.
6. Foster TS, Miller JD, Marton JP, et al. Assessment of the economic burden of COPD in the U.S.: a review and synthesis of the literature. COPD 2006;3(4): 211–8.
7. Rabe KF, Hurd S, Anzueto A, et al. Global strategy for the diagnosis, management, and prevention of chronic obstructive pulmonary disease: GOLD executive summary. Am J Respir Crit Care Med 2007;176(6):532–55.
8. Shepard JW Jr, Schweitzer PK, Keller CA, et al. Myocardial stress. Exercise versus sleep in patients with COPD. Chest 1984;86(3):366–74.
9. Fletcher EC, Luckett RA, Miller T, et al. Exercise hemodynamics and gas exchange in patients with chronic obstruction pulmonary disease, sleep desaturation, and a daytime PaO2 above 60 mm hg. Am Rev Respir Dis 1989;140(5): 1237–45.
10. Fletcher EC, Luckett RA, Miller T, et al. Pulmonary vascular hemodynamics in chronic lung disease patients with and without oxyhemoglobin desaturation during sleep. Chest 1989;95(4):757–64.
11. Boysen PG, Block AJ, Wynne JW, et al. Nocturnal pulmonary hypertension in patients with chronic obstructive pulmonary disease. Chest 1979;76(5):536–42.
12. Guilleminault C, Cummiskey J, Motta J. Chronic obstructive airflow disease and sleep studies. Am Rev Respir Dis 1980;122(3):397–406.
13. Cheong TH, Magder S, Shapiro S, et al. Cardiac arrhythmias during exercise in severe chronic obstructive pulmonary disease. Chest 1990;97(4):793–7.
14. Slutsky R, Hooper W, Ackerman W, et al. Evaluation of left ventricular function in chronic pulmonary disease by exercise gated equilibrium radionuclide angiography. Am Heart J 1981;101(4):414–20.
15. Price D, Small M, Milligan G, et al. Impact of night-time symptoms in COPD: a real-world study in five European countries. Int J Chron Obstruct Pulmon Dis 2013;8:595–603.
16. Agusti A, Hedner J, Marin JM, et al. Night-time symptoms: a forgotten dimension of COPD. Eur Respir Rev 2011;20(121):183–94.
17. Klink ME, Dodge R, Quan SF. The relation of sleep complaints to respiratory symptoms in a general population. Chest 1994;105(1):151–4.
18. Budhiraja P, Budhiraja R, Goodwin JL, et al. Incidence of restless legs syndrome and its correlates. J Clin Sleep Med 2012;8(2):119–24.
19. Budhiraja R, Roth T, Hudgel DW, et al. Prevalence and polysomnographic correlates of insomnia comorbid with medical disorders. Sleep 2011;34(7):859–67.

20. Dodge R, Cline MG, Quan SF. The natural history of insomnia and its relationship to respiratory symptoms. Arch Intern Med 1995;155(16):1797–800.
21. Sanders MH, Newman AB, Haggerty CL, et al. Sleep and sleep-disordered breathing in adults with predominantly mild obstructive airway disease. Am J Respir Crit Care Med 2003;167(1):7–14.
22. Krachman S, Minai OA, Scharf SM. Sleep abnormalities and treatment in emphysema. Proc Am Thorac Soc 2008;5(4):536–42.
23. Valipour A, Lavie P, Lothaller H, et al. Sleep profile and symptoms of sleep disorders in patients with stable mild to moderate chronic obstructive pulmonary disease. Sleep Med 2011;12(4):367–72.
24. McSharry DG, Ryan S, Calverley P, et al. Sleep quality in chronic obstructive pulmonary disease. Respirology 2012;17(7):1119–24.
25. Manni R, Cerveri I, Bruschi C, et al. Sleep and oxyhemoglobin desaturation patterns in chronic obstructive pulmonary diseases. Eur Neurol 1988;28(5): 275–8.
26. Fleetham J, West P, Mezon B, et al. Sleep, arousals, and oxygen desaturation in chronic obstructive pulmonary disease. the effect of oxygen therapy. Am Rev Respir Dis 1982;126(3):429–33.
27. Brezinova V, Catterall JR, Douglas NJ, et al. Night sleep of patients with chronic ventilatory failure and age matched controls: number and duration of the EEG episodes of intervening wakefulness and drowsiness. Sleep 1982;5(2):123–30.
28. Kwon JS, Wolfe LF, Lu BS, et al. Hyperinflation is associated with lower sleep efficiency in COPD with co-existent obstructive sleep apnea. COPD 2009; 6(6):441–5.
29. Krachman SL, Chatila W, Martin UJ, et al. Physiologic correlates of sleep quality in severe emphysema. COPD 2011;8(3):182–8.
30. Hynninen MJ, Pallesen S, Hardie J, et al. Insomnia symptoms, objectively measured sleep, and disease severity in chronic obstructive pulmonary disease outpatients. Sleep Med 2013;14(12):1328–33.
31. Lo Coco D, Mattaliano A, Lo Coco A, et al. Increased frequency of restless legs syndrome in chronic obstructive pulmonary disease patients. Sleep Med 2009; 10(5):572–6.
32. Timms RM, Dawson A, Hajdukovic RM, et al. Effect of triazolam on sleep and arterial oxygen saturation in patients with chronic obstructive pulmonary disease. Arch Intern Med 1988;148(10):2159–63.
33. Steens RD, Pouliot Z, Millar TW, et al. Effects of zolpidem and triazolam on sleep and respiration in mild to moderate chronic obstructive pulmonary disease. Sleep 1993;16(4):318–26.
34. Stege G, Heijdra YF, van den Elshout FJ, et al. Temazepam 10mg does not affect breathing and gas exchange in patients with severe normocapnic COPD. Respir Med 2010;104(4):518–24.
35. Ekstrom MP, Bornefalk-Hermansson A, Abernethy AP, et al. Safety of benzodiazepines and opioids in very severe respiratory disease: national prospective study. BMJ 2014;348:g445.
36. Douglas NJ, White DP, Pickett CK, et al. Respiration during sleep in normal man. Thorax 1982;37(11):840–4.
37. Becker HF, Piper AJ, Flynn WE, et al. Breathing during sleep in patients with nocturnal desaturation. Am J Respir Crit Care Med 1999;159(1):112–8.
38. Catterall JR, Douglas NJ, Calverley PM, et al. Transient hypoxemia during sleep in chronic obstructive pulmonary disease is not a sleep apnea syndrome. Am Rev Respir Dis 1983;128(1):24–9.

39. Douglas NJ, White DP, Weil JV, et al. Hypoxic ventilatory response decreases during sleep in normal men. Am Rev Respir Dis 1982;125(3):286–9.
40. Douglas NJ, White DP, Weil JV, et al. Hypercapnic ventilatory response in sleeping adults. Am Rev Respir Dis 1982;126(5):758–62.
41. Douglas NJ. Control of ventilation during sleep. Clin Chest Med 1985;6(4):563–75.
42. Hudgel DW, Martin RJ, Johnson B, et al. Mechanics of the respiratory system and breathing pattern during sleep in normal humans. J Appl Physiol Respir Environ Exerc Physiol 1984;56(1):133–7.
43. Ottenheijm CA, Heunks LM, Sieck GC, et al. Diaphragm dysfunction in chronic obstructive pulmonary disease. Am J Respir Crit Care Med 2005;172(2):200–5.
44. Chaouat A, Weitzenblum E, Kessler R, et al. Sleep-related O2 desaturation and daytime pulmonary haemodynamics in COPD patients with mild hypoxaemia. Eur Respir J 1997;10(8):1730–5.
45. Fletcher EC, Miller J, Divine GW, et al. Nocturnal oxyhemoglobin desaturation in COPD patients with arterial oxygen tensions above 60 mm hg. Chest 1987; 92(4):604–8.
46. Lewis CA, Fergusson W, Eaton T, et al. Isolated nocturnal desaturation in COPD: prevalence and impact on quality of life and sleep. Thorax 2009,64(2):133–8.
47. Peppard PE, Young T, Barnet JH, et al. Increased prevalence of sleep-disordered breathing in adults. Am J Epidemiol 2013;177(9):1006–14.
48. Yaggi HK, Concato J, Kernan WN, et al. Obstructive sleep apnea as a risk factor for stroke and death. N Engl J Med 2005;353(19):2034–41.
49. Kendzerska I, Mollayeva T, Gorchon AS, et al. Untreated obstructive sleep apnea and the risk for serious long-term adverse outcomes: a systematic review. Sleep Med Rev 2014;18(1):49–59.
50. Shahar E, Whitney CW, Redline S, et al. Sleep-disordered breathing and cardiovascular disease: cross-sectional results of the sleep heart health study. Am J Respir Crit Care Med 2001;163(1):19–25.
51. Findley LJ, Barth JT, Powers DC, et al. Cognitive impairment in patients with obstructive sleep apnea and associated hypoxemia. Chest 1986;90(5):686–90.
52. Patz D, Spoon M, Corbin R, et al. The effect of altitude descent on obstructive sleep apnea. Chest 2006;130(6):1744–50.
53. Sharma B, Feinsilver S, Owens RL, et al. Obstructive airway disease and obstructive sleep apnea: effect of pulmonary function. Lung 2011;189(1):37–41.
54. Resta O, Foschino Barbaro MP, Brindicci C, et al. Hypercapnia in overlap syndrome: possible determinant factors. Sleep Breath 2002;6(1):11–8.
55. Hawrylkiewicz I, Palasiewicz G, Plywaczewski R, et al. Pulmonary hypertension in patients with pure obstructive sleep apnea. Pol Arch Med Wewn 2004;111(4): 449–54.
56. Chaouat A, Weitzenblum E, Krieger J, et al. Association of chronic obstructive pulmonary disease and sleep apnea syndrome. Am J Respir Crit Care Med 1995;151(1):82–6.
57. Lopez-Acevedo MN, Torres-Palacios A, Elena Ocasio-Tascon M, et al. Overlap syndrome: an indication for sleep studies?: a pilot study. Sleep Breath 2009; 13(4):409–13.
58. Bednarek M, Plywaczewski R, Jonczak L, et al. There is no relationship between chronic obstructive pulmonary disease and obstructive sleep apnea syndrome: a population study. Respiration 2005;72(2):142–9.
59. White LH, Motwani S, Kasai T, et al. Effect of rostral fluid shift on pharyngeal resistance in men with and without obstructive sleep apnea. Respir Physiol Neurobiol 2014;192:17–22.

60. Agusti AG, Noguera A, Sauleda J, et al. Systemic effects of chronic obstructive pulmonary disease. Eur Respir J 2003;21(2):347–60.
61. Marin JM, Soriano JB, Carrizo SJ, et al. Outcomes in patients with chronic obstructive pulmonary disease and obstructive sleep apnea: the overlap syndrome. Am J Respir Crit Care Med 2010;182(3):325–31.
62. Machado MC, Vollmer WM, Togeiro SM, et al. CPAP and survival in moderate-to-severe obstructive sleep apnoea syndrome and hypoxaemic COPD. Eur Respir J 2010;35(1):132–7.
63. Stanchina ML, Welicky LM, Donat W, et al. Impact of CPAP use and age on mortality in patients with combined COPD and obstructive sleep apnea: the overlap syndrome. J Clin Sleep Med 2013;9(8):767–72.
64. Jaoude P, Kufel T, El-Solh AA. Survival benefit of CPAP favors hypercapnic patients with the overlap syndrome. Lung 2014;192(2):251–8.
65. Shiina K, Tomiyama H, Takata Y, et al. Overlap syndrome: additive effects of COPD on the cardiovascular damages in patients with OSA. Respir Med 2012;106(9): 1335–41.
66. Sharma B, Neilan TG, Kwong RY, et al. Evaluation of right ventricular remodeling using cardiac magnetic resonance imaging in co-existent chronic obstructive pulmonary disease and obstructive sleep apnea. COPD 2013;10(1):4–10.
67. Martin RJ, Bartelson BL, Smith P, et al. Effect of ipratropium bromide treatment on oxygen saturation and sleep quality in COPD. Chest 1999;115(5):1338–45.
68. McNicholas WT, Calverley PM, Lee A, et al, Tiotropium Sleep Study in COPD Investigators. Long-acting inhaled anticholinergic therapy improves sleeping oxygen saturation in COPD. Eur Respir J 2004;23(6):825–31.
69. Ryan S, Doherty LS, Rock C, et al. Effects of salmeterol on sleeping oxygen saturation in chronic obstructive pulmonary disease. Respiration 2010;79(6):475–81.
70. Sposato B, Mariotta S, Palmiero G, et al. Oral corticosteroids can improve nocturnal isolated hypoxemia in stable COPD patients with diurnal PaO2 > 60 mm Hg. Eur Rev Med Pharmacol Sci 2007;11(6):365–72.
71. Teodorescu M, Xie A, Sorkness CA, et al. Effects of inhaled fluticasone on upper airway during sleep and wakefulness in asthma: a pilot study. J Clin Sleep Med 2014;10(2):183–93.
72. Continuous or nocturnal oxygen therapy in hypoxemic chronic obstructive lung disease: a clinical trial. Nocturnal oxygen therapy trial group. Ann Intern Med 1980;93(3):391–8.
73. Long term domiciliary oxygen therapy in chronic hypoxic cor pulmonale complicating chronic bronchitis and emphysema. Report of the medical research council working party. Lancet 1981;1(8222):681–6.
74. Loredo JS, Ancoli-Israel S, Kim EJ, et al. Effect of continuous positive airway pressure versus supplemental oxygen on sleep quality in obstructive sleep apnea: a placebo-CPAP-controlled study. Sleep 2006;29(4):564–71.
75. Mansfield D, Naughton MT. Effects of continuous positive airway pressure on lung function in patients with chronic obstructive pulmonary disease and sleep disordered breathing. Respirology 1999;4(4):365–70.
76. Sforza E, Krieger J, Weitzenblum E, et al. Long-term effects of treatment with nasal continuous positive airway pressure on daytime lung function and pulmonary hemodynamics in patients with obstructive sleep apnea. Am Rev Respir Dis 1990;141(4 Pt 1):866–70.
77. de Miguel J, Cabello J, Sanchez-Alarcos JM, et al. Long-term effects of treatment with nasal continuous positive airway pressure on lung function in patients with overlap syndrome. Sleep Breath 2002;6(1):3–10.

78. Toraldo DM, De Nuccio F, Nicolardi G. Fixed-pressure nCPAP in patients with obstructive sleep apnea (OSA) syndrome and chronic obstructive pulmonary disease (COPD): a 24-month follow-up study. Sleep Breath 2010;14(2):115–23.
79. O'Brien A, Whitman K. Lack of benefit of continuous positive airway pressure on lung function in patients with overlap syndrome. Lung 2005;183(6):389–404.
80. Nadel JA, Widdicombe JG. Reflex effects of upper airway irritation on total lung resistance and blood pressure. J Appl Physiol 1962;17:861–5.
81. Peker Y, Hedner J, Johansson A, et al. Reduced hospitalization with cardiovascular and pulmonary disease in obstructive sleep apnea patients on nasal CPAP treatment. Sleep 1997;20(8):645–53.
82. Nural S, Gunay E, Halici B, et al. Inflammatory processes and effects of continuous positive airway pressure (CPAP) in overlap syndrome. Inflammation 2013; 36(1):66–74.
83. Wijkstra PJ, Lacasse Y, Guyatt GH, et al. A meta-analysis of nocturnal noninvasive positive pressure ventilation in patients with stable COPD. Chest 2003; 124(1):337–43.
84. McEvoy RD, Pierce RJ, Hillman D, et al. Nocturnal non-invasive nasal ventilation in stable hypercapnic COPD: a randomised controlled trial. Thorax 2009;64(7): 561–6.
85. Windisch W, Haenel M, Storre JH, et al. High-intensity non-invasive positive pressure ventilation for stable hypercapnic COPD. Int J Med Sci 2009;6(2):72–6.
86. Dreher M, Ekkernkamp E, Walterspacher S, et al. Noninvasive ventilation in COPD: impact of inspiratory pressure levels on sleep quality. Chest 2011;140(4):939–45.
87. Windisch W, Kostic S, Dreher M, et al. Outcome of patients with stable COPD receiving controlled noninvasive positive pressure ventilation aimed at a maximal reduction of pa(CO2). Chest 2005;128(2):657–62.
88. Windisch W, Dreher M, Storre JH, et al. Nocturnal non-invasive positive pressure ventilation: physiological effects on spontaneous breathing. Respir Physiol Neurobiol 2006;150(2–3):251–60.
89. Poulain M, Doucet M, Major GC, et al. The effect of obesity on chronic respiratory diseases: pathophysiology and therapeutic strategies. CMAJ 2006;174(9): 1293–9.
90. Sood A, Petersen H, Meek P, et al. Spirometry and health status worsen with weight gain in obese smokers but improve in normal-weight smokers. Am J Respir Crit Care Med 2014;189(3):274–81.
91. Raghu G. Idiopathic pulmonary fibrosis: guidelines for diagnosis and clinical management have advanced from consensus-based in 2000 to evidence-based in 2011. Eur Respir J 2011;37(4):743–6.
92. Nalysnyk L, Cid-Ruzafa J, Rotella P, et al. Incidence and prevalence of idiopathic pulmonary fibrosis: review of the literature. Eur Respir Rev 2012;21(126):355–61.
93. Raghu G, Weycker D, Edelsberg J, et al. Incidence and prevalence of idiopathic pulmonary fibrosis. Am J Respir Crit Care Med 2006;174(7):810–6.
94. Krishnan V, McCormack MC, Mathai SC, et al. Sleep quality and health-related quality of life in idiopathic pulmonary fibrosis. Chest 2008;134(4):693–8.
95. Bajwah S, Higginson IJ, Ross JR, et al. The palliative care needs for fibrotic interstitial lung disease: a qualitative study of patients, informal caregivers and health professionals. Palliat Med 2013;27(9):869–76.
96. Perez-Padilla R, West P, Lertzman M, et al. Breathing during sleep in patients with interstitial lung disease. Am Rev Respir Dis 1985;132(2):224–9.
97. Bye PT, Issa F, Berthon-Jones M, et al. Studies of oxygenation during sleep in patients with interstitial lung disease. Am Rev Respir Dis 1984;129(1):27–32.

98. Mermigkis C, Stagaki E, Amfilochiou A, et al. Sleep quality and associated day-time consequences in patients with idiopathic pulmonary fibrosis. Med Princ Pract 2009;18(1):10–5.

99. Swigris JJ, Stewart AL, Gould MK, et al. Patients' perspectives on how idiopathic pulmonary fibrosis affects the quality of their lives. Health Qual Life Outcomes 2005;3:61.

100. Mermigkis C, Mermigkis D, Varouchakis G, et al. CPAP treatment in patients with idiopathic pulmonary fibrosis and obstructive sleep apnea–therapeutic difficulties and dilemmas. Sleep Breath 2012;16(1):1–3.

101. Rasche K, Orth M. Sleep and breathing in idiopathic pulmonary fibrosis. J Physiol Pharmacol 2009;60(Suppl 5):13–4.

102. Corte TJ, Wort SJ, Talbot S, et al. Elevated nocturnal desaturation index predicts mortality in interstitial lung disease. Sarcoidosis Vasc Diffuse Lung Dis 2012; 29(1):41–50.

103. Kolilekas L, Manali E, Vlami KA, et al. Sleep oxygen desaturation predicts survival in idiopathic pulmonary fibrosis. J Clin Sleep Med 2013;9(6):593–601.

104. Lettieri CJ, Nathan SD, Browning RF, et al. The distance-saturation product predicts mortality in idiopathic pulmonary fibrosis. Respir Med 2006;100(10):1734–41.

105. Triantafillidou C, Manali E, Lyberopoulos P, et al. The role of cardiopulmonary exercise test in IPF prognosis. Pulm Med 2013;2013:514817.

106. Pihtili A, Bingol Z, Kiyan E, et al. Obstructive sleep apnea is common in patients with interstitial lung disease. Sleep Breath 2013;17(4):1281–8.

107. Mermigkis C, Stagaki E, Tryfon S, et al. How common is sleep-disordered breathing in patients with idiopathic pulmonary fibrosis? Sleep Breath 2010; 14(4):387–90.

108. Lancaster LH, Mason WR, Parnell JA, et al. Obstructive sleep apnea is common in idiopathic pulmonary fibrosis. Chest 2009;136(3):772–8.

109. Van de Graaff WB. Thoracic influence on upper airway patency. J Appl Physiol (1985) 1988;65(5):2124–31.

110. Ruhle KH. Commentary on how common is sleep-disordered breathing in patients with idiopathic pulmonary fibrosis? Mermigkis C. et al. Sleep Breath 2010;14(4):289.

111. Heinzer RC, Stanchina ML, Malhotra A, et al. Effect of increased lung volume on sleep disordered breathing in patients with sleep apnoea. Thorax 2006;61(5): 435–9.

112. Owens RL, Malhotra A, Eckert DJ, et al. The influence of end-expiratory lung volume on measurements of pharyngeal collapsibility. J Appl Physiol (1985) 2010; 108(2):445–51.

113. Harris-Eze AO, Sridhar G, Clemens RE, et al. Oxygen improves maximal exercise performance in interstitial lung disease. Am J Respir Crit Care Med 1994; 150(6 Pt 1):1616–22.

114. Harris-Eze AO, Sridhar G, Clemens RE, et al. Role of hypoxemia and pulmonary mechanics in exercise limitation in interstitial lung disease. Am J Respir Crit Care Med 1996;154(4 Pt 1):994–1001.

115. Crockett AJ, Cranston JM, Antic N. Domiciliary oxygen for interstitial lung disease. Cochrane Database Syst Rev 2001;(3):CD002883.

116. Nishiyama O, Miyajima H, Fukai Y, et al. Effect of ambulatory oxygen on exertional dyspnea in IPF patients without resting hypoxemia. Respir Med 2013; 107(8):1241–6.

117. Mermigkis C, Bouloukaki I, Antoniou KM, et al. CPAP therapy in patients with idiopathic pulmonary fibrosis and obstructive sleep apnea: does it offer a better quality of life and sleep? Sleep Breath 2013;17(4):1137–43.

118. Patterson KC, Huang F, Oldham JM, et al. Excessive daytime sleepiness and obstructive sleep apnea in patients with sarcoidosis. Chest 2013;143(6):1562–8.
119. De Vries J, Rothkrantz-Kos S, van Dieijen-Visser MP, et al. The relationship between fatigue and clinical parameters in pulmonary sarcoidosis. Sarcoidosis Vasc Diffuse Lung Dis 2004;21(2):127–36.
120. Drent M, Lower EE, De Vries J. Sarcoidosis-associated fatigue. Eur Respir J 2012;40(1):255–63.
121. Lower EE, Malhotra A, Surdulescu V, et al. Armodafinil for sarcoidosis-associated fatigue: a double-blind, placebo-controlled, crossover trial. J Pain Symptom Manage 2013;45(2):159–69.
122. Salles C, Ramos RT, Daltro C, et al. Prevalence of obstructive sleep apnea in children and adolescents with sickle cell anemia. J Bras Pneumol 2009;35(11): 1075–83.
123. Kaleyias J, Mostofi N, Grant M, et al. Severity of obstructive sleep apnea in children with sickle cell disease. J Pediatr Hematol Oncol 2008;30(9):659–65.
124. Samuels MP, Stebbens VA, Davies SC, et al. Sleep related upper airway obstruction and hypoxaemia in sickle cell disease. Arch Dis Child 1992;67(7): 925–9.
125. Okoli K, Irani F, Horvath W. Pathophysiologic considerations for the interactions between obstructive sleep apnea and sickle hemoglobinopathies. Med Hypotheses 2009;72(5):578–80.
126. Spicuzza L, Sciuto C, Leonardi S, et al. Early occurrence of obstructive sleep apnea in infants and children with cystic fibrosis. Arch Pediatr Adolesc Med 2012;166(12):1165–9.
127. Perin C, Fagondes SC, Casarotto FC, et al. Sleep findings and predictors of sleep desaturation in adult cystic fibrosis patients. Sleep Breath 2012;16(4): 1041–8.

Ventilatory Support During Sleep in Patients with Chronic Obstructive Pulmonary Disease

Peter Jan Wijkstra, MD, PhD*,
Marieke Leontine Duiverman, MD, PhD

KEYWORDS

- Chronic obstructive pulmonary disease • Noninvasive ventilation
- Chronic respiratory failure • Monitoring • Adequate ventilation

KEY POINTS

- There is no conclusive evidence that chronic noninvasive ventilation (NIV) should be provided routinely to stable patients with chronic obstructive pulmonary disease.
- Level of baseline $Paco_2$, height of inspiratory pressures, and compliance seem to be important components in providing effective ventilatory support.
- The combination of rehabilitation and nocturnal ventilatory support seems to provide more benefits than rehabilitation alone.
- The option of providing chronic NIV after acute respiratory failure has to be investigated.

INTRODUCTION

Chronic ventilatory support is a well-accepted and effective therapy in patients with chronic respiratory failure due to thoracic cage abnormalities or in patients with neuromuscular disease. This is in contrast with patients with chronic obstructive pulmonary disease (COPD), where despite several positive uncontrolled trials, the evidence to start it routinely is lacking. This article will first discuss the different rationales why chronic nocturnal noninvasive ventilation (NIV) might be effective in these patients. It will then discuss the benefits of chronic NIV in stable disease, in combination with rehabilitation, and after acute respiratory failure. Thereafter the authors will elaborate on different issues that might be important in making NIV more effective in patients with COPD.

This article originally appeared in *Sleep Medicine Clinics*, Volume 9, Issue 3, September 2014.
Conflict of Interest: P.J. Wijkstra reports grants and fees from Philips/Respironics, RESMED, VIVISOL, Medicq TEFA, Emdamed, Air Liquide and Goedegebeure.
Department of Pulmonary Diseases/Home Mechanical Ventilation, University Medical Centre Groningen, Post-Box 30.001, Groningen 9700 RB, The Netherlands
* Corresponding author.
E-mail address: p.j.wijkstra@int.azg.nl

Clinics Collections 6 (2015) 59–71
http://dx.doi.org/10.1016/j.ccol.2015.05.032

RATIONALE FOR VENTILATORY SUPPORT DURING SLEEP IN STABLE COPD

During sleep, ventilation is decreased due to several factors such as increased upper airway resistance, a decrease in the reticular activating system and metabolic rate, and a decreased chemosensitivity. During rapid eye movement (REM) sleep, breathing becomes more variable; upper airway resistance increases even further, and a generalized muscle hypotonia of the respiratory muscles leads to a decreased contribution of the intercostal muscles relative to the diaphragm.[1]

In COPD, respiratory failure during sleep occurs frequently, and various mechanisms are thought to contribute. First, it seems apparent that in patients with daytime respiratory failure, physiologic changes during sleep exacerbate this problem. Second, as during the daytime reliance on intercostal and accessory respiratory muscles is greater in COPD compared with healthy subjects, the generalized muscle atonia occurring in REM sleep leads to loss of this contribution and more reliance on a diaphragm that is in a mechanically disadvantageous position that it simply cannot deliver enough power to keep ventilation at a sufficient level. Third, a blunted chemoresponsiveness during sleep might lead to less frequent arousals, during which ventilation has the opportunity to increase. Fourth, functional residual capacity decreases during sleep, leading to increased ventilation–perfusion mismatching, with more pronounced effects in COPD, especially on oxygen levels.[2]

It seems logical to counterbalance these detrimental effects during sleep in COPD with noninvasive positive pressure ventilation. It has been shown that nocturnal hypoventilation is reversed by nocturnal NIV.[3] However, it is intriguing to find that a therapy applied during the night remains effective during the day. In addition to its effect on reversing nocturnal hypoventilation, three other possible mechanisms for improvement have been proposed.[4] NIV provides rest to (fatigued) respiratory muscles; NIV increases ventilatory sensitivity to carbon dioxide during spontaneous breathing, and NIV improves pulmonary mechanics.

Reversal of Nocturnal Hypoventilation

Reversal of nocturnal hypoventilation leads to improvements in arterial blood gases during sleep, and ideally this improvement can (at least partially) be sustained during the day.

It has been suggested that improved blood gases improve muscle function by improving the internal milieu; however, studies on the effects of hypercapnia/acidemia on peripheral and respiratory muscle contractibility, strength, and endurance are controversial.[5–7]

Second, despite decreased chemosensitivity during sleep (especially REM sleep) in COPD, profound hypercapnia may provoke arousals. By reversing hypoventilation, arousals may occur less frequently, leading to improvement in sleep quality. However, sleep quality is affected by several other factors.

Interestingly, it has been shown that after cessation of NIV at awakening, arterial carbon dioxide level ($Paco_2$) decreases even further during the first hours of subsequent spontaneous breathing, an effect more pronounced after patients have been using NIV for a longer period.[8] This suggests that there are additional mechanisms on top of just relying on improvements attained during the night.

Improving Respiratory Muscle Function

In patients with severe COPD, the respiratory muscles have an unfavorable position due to hyperinflation, and therefore the diaphragm is thought to be susceptible to fatigue. This hypothesis is derived from findings in several studies. On the 1 hand, studies have consistently shown that both central neural drive and respiratory muscle work/energy expenditure are increased in severe COPD.[9,10] On the other hand, NIV might reduce respiratory muscle drive[11] and respiratory muscle work load,[12] while capacity is increased, making the respiratory muscles less susceptible to fatigue.

There are also some arguments against the effects of NIV on fatigued muscles. First, it has been shown that the respiratory muscles of hypercapnic COPD patients work hard but are not fatigued; they seem to act as wise fighters, thereby deliberately keeping respiratory muscle work below the fatigue threshold at the expense of decreased tidal volumes and thus alveolar hypoventilation.[13] Second, most studies on NIV in COPD have not shown any effects on maximal respiratory muscle pressures independent from changes in lung volumes,[14] arguing against the hypothesis that if the muscles are rested, they should gain (reserve) capacity. As a consequence, instead of resting fatigued respiratory muscles, NIV might, among other things, lead to a decrease in respiratory muscle work through the induction of a more favorable breathing pattern, a pattern that can be maintained during the day.

Improving Central Drive

Prolonged hypercapnia might lead to a progressive resetting to a higher sensitivity threshold of the central chemoreceptors. After NIV treatment, the threshold might be reset downwards again, although this process has been suggested to occur progressively over several years.[15] In hypercapnic COPD patients, there is a lack of strong evidence that resetting of the CO_2 sensitivity plays a role.[9] However, from the wise fighter concept, it does not seem to be beneficial to increase CO_2 sensitivity, as increased ventilation means an increased load on the already heavily loaded system. Only when a simultaneous reduction in load (eg, by improved pulmonary mechanics) occurs, increased chemosensitivity during sleep and awake states leads to improved ventilation without the occurrence of respiratory muscle fatigue or failure.

Reducing the Load Against Which the Respiratory Muscle Pump Has to Function

Improvement in breathing patterns and pulmonary mechanics seems to be an important part of the improvement in gas exchange, as it was found consistently in most recent studies, especially those using higher pressures.[11,16–18] The mechanical load in severe COPD is high mainly due to a high airway resistance, leading to hyperinflation. Several studies have shown that NIV can reduce hyperinflation, and this reduction is associated with improvements in gas exchange.

A reduction in hyperinflation occurs when a reduction in airway resistance is achieved. A reduction in hypercapnia, causing less retention of salt and water, might lead to a decrease in airway resistance because of less airway edema and/or less airway inflammation.[19] Second, less airway inflammation might be important. Improved sputum expectoration, improved ventilation of peripheral regions, but also less airway edema probably exhibits a positive effect on airway inflammation. Less airway edema might lead to less airway wall remodeling by reducing inflammation when muscle fibers become less overstretched. Third, a reduction in hyperinflation is hypothesized to be a consequence of a slower and deeper breathing pattern, which is facilitated by improved respiratory muscle function that can be preserved from NIV to spontaneous breathing. Furthermore, when patients on NIV have fewer exacerbations, this might prevent any further increase in hyperinflation over time.

Finally, NIV might lead to (small) airway recruitment, probably to less small airway closure. In this respect, by improving ventilation in peripheral lung regions, NIV reduces ventilation–perfusion mismatching, thereby also improving arterial oxygen pressure.[20]

In conclusion, although several theories exist, there are currently no studies on NIV or nasal intermittent positive pressure ventilation (NIPPV) that have provided definitive evidence that the benefits found in gas exchange are related to improvements in respiratory muscle function or altered chemosensitivity. Reversal of nocturnal hypoventilation seems apparent; however, this mechanism does not explain the entire picture, and, furthermore, the effects on sleep efficiency are incompletely explained. The relationship between improved gas exchange and less hyperinflation needs further investigation.

VENTILATORY SUPPORT DURING SLEEP IN STABLE PATIENTS WITH COPD

In the last couple of decades, several trials have investigated the benefits of nocturnal NIV in stable patients with COPD. While in 2000 the opinion was that NIV was not effective in these patients,[21,22] due to new clinical trials there seems to be a shift in this opinion as recently discussed by Schönhofer.[23] This section, will discuss short- and long-term studies investigating the benefits of nocturnal NIV separately and will finish by referring to a recent published meta-analysis.

Uncontrolled Trials

In the past, several uncontrolled trials investigating the effects of NIV showed some encouraging results. A French study showed that 6 months of nocturnal NIV in 14 patients with a mean baseline $Paco_2$ of 7.8 kPa (58.5 mm Hg) significantly improved quality of life.[24] In addition to an improved quality of life, a significant improvement in arterial blood gases was found. In the study by Sivasothy,[25] 26 patients with severe COPD and hypercapnia ($Paco_2$ 8.6 kPa or 64.5 mm Hg) were also ventilated by a volume ventilator during the night. After 18 months, both gas exchange and quality of life improved significantly. A long-term study by Jones showed that after 24 months of pressure ventilation there were significant improvements in arterial blood gases and a reduction in hospital admissions and general practitioner visits.[26] In the last decade, several German studies were published investigating the benefits of high-intensity NIV. Windisch studied the benefits of controlled NIV with mean breathing frequency of 21 breaths per minute and mean inspiratory positive airway pressures of 28 cm H_2O in 73 COPD patients (mean forced expiratory volume in 1 second [FEV_1] 30% predicted). They found significant improvements in blood gas tensions, lung function, and hematocrit after 2 months. In this study, the 2- and 5-year survival rates of all patients were 82% and 58%, respectively.[17] In a randomized controlled crossover trial, the same group compared 6 weeks of high-intensity NIV (using controlled ventilation with mean inspiratory pressures of around 29 cm H_2O) with low-intensity NIV (using assisted ventilation with mean inspiratory pressures of 15 cm H_2O) in 17 patients with severe stable hypercapnic COPD.[17,27] They found a significant reduction in nocturnal $Paco_2$ in favor of high-intensity NIV, which was not unexpected, as high-intensity NIV was targeted in reducing nocturnal $Paco_2$. An important finding was that daily use of NIV was increased in high-intensity NIV compared with low-intensity NIV, meaning that patients tolerated high pressures better than low pressures. In addition, only high-intensity NIV resulted in significant improvements in exercise-related dyspnea, FEV_1, vital capacity, and health-related quality of life. Despite these positive outcomes, the overall opinion is that there is a need for randomized controlled trials (RCTs) evaluating the role of high-intensity NIV in stable hypercapnic COPD patients.

Short-Term RCTs of NIV in COPD

There have been 6 RCTs of NIPPV up to a duration of 3 months that have been published.[3,28–32] Strumpf and colleagues[28] did not find significant changes in any of the measured variables apart from neuropsychological function. Important in this respect is that only 7 of the 19 patients completed the study, and most patients were not hypercapnic. Gay and colleagues[29] investigated the effects of NIPPV in hypercapnic patients and showed that NIPPV did not lead to an improvement in clinical parameters compared with sham ventilation. Still, only a small number of patients completed the study. The study of Meecham Jones and colleagues[3] was the only one to show clear benefits of nocturnal NIPPV in patients with COPD. Three months of NIPPV combined with oxygen were better than oxygen alone for gas exchange, sleep efficiency, and health status. They also showed that patients with an increased level of hypoventilation during the night showed the most benefit in reducing daytime $Paco_2$. Lin and colleagues[30] investigated the effects of only 2 weeks of NIPPV and showed only a positive effect of NIPPV and oxygen on the nighttime oxygenation. The fact that the patients had only 2 weeks of acclimatization on NIPPV might be the reason for this negative study. Renston and colleagues[12] investigated the effects of daytime NIPPV (ie, 2 hours per day) for 5 consecutive days. Although they did not find significant changes in gas exchange, the NIPPV group showed a significant decrease in the level of dyspnea and an improved exercise capacity. A study from Diaz and colleagues[16] investigated the effects of NIPPV during the daytime for 3 hours, 5 days a week for 3 weeks. Although this was a very short-term application of NIV, they found significant improvements in gas exchange, dyspnea, and walking distance. As conflicting results still exist in this field, recently an update of a meta-analysis of individual data from RCTs was published comparing NIV with conventional management of patients with COPD and stable respiratory failure.[31,32] Only studies investigating nocturnal NIPPV applied via a nasal or facemask for at least 4 hours each day for 3 weeks were included. Six RCTs were found that fulfilled the previously mentioned criteria (**Table 1**),[3,29,30,33-35] including the 3-month data of the study of Casanova and colleagues[33] as well. This meta-analysis showed that 3 months of NIPPV in patients with stable COPD did not improve lung function, gas exchange, sleep efficiency, or 6-minute walking distance.

Long-Term RCTs of NIV in COPD

Casanova and colleagues[33] were the first to investigate the effects of long-term NIPPV. This study had a duration of 12 months and randomized 52 patients to either NIPPV plus standard care or to standard care alone. Important issues were that the level of bilevel positive airway preparation (PAP) was only modest (inspiratory positive airway pressure [IPAP] 12–14 cm H_2O), and its effect was not monitored during the night. Therefore, it is not certain that effective ventilation was provided. Notwithstanding these limitations, the study did show some positive effects. The number of hospital admissions was lower after 3 months (5% vs 15%). However, this was not the case after 6 months. Although modest improvements were found in dyspnea and neuropsychological function, no significant changes in arterial blood gases and respiratory muscle strength were found after 12 months. Another long-term study compared the combination of NIPPV and long-term oxygen therapy (LTOT) with LTOT alone for a period of 2 years.[34] Patients with a $Paco_2$ greater than 6.6 kPa (49.5 mm Hg) were included. In this study, 90 patients were randomized, and 47 patients completed the study. The level of NIV was again modest (IPAP of 14 ± 3 cm H_2O). Patients did use the ventilator a considerable number of hours (9 ± 2 h). Compared with the 1-year period before the study, total hospital admissions increased by 27% in the LTOT group, while it decreased by 45% in the NIV group. Intensive care unit ICU admissions decreased in the NIV group by 75%, while in the LTOT group they increased by 20%. However, the outcomes were not statistically

Table 1
Characteristics of studies included in meta-analysis

Trial	Study Design (Compared to Treatment)	IPAP/Expiratory Positive Airway Pressure	Study Population	Outcomes
Short term				
Casanova et al,[33] 2000	Parallel group (LTOT)	12/4	52 randomized patients, 36 completers $Paco_2$ 51 mm Hg, FEV_1 0.84 L	Blood gasses, lung function, PImax/PEmax, dyspnea after 3 mo Exacerbation rate, hospital admissions, intubations, and mortality after 12 mo
Clini et al,[34] 2002	Parallel group (LTOT)	14.4/3.8	90 randomized patients, 78 completers $Paco_2$ 56 mm Hg, FEV_1 0.75 L	Blood gasses and hospitalizations after 3 mo
Gay et al,[29] 1996	Parallel group (sham)	10/2	13 randomized patients, 10 completers $Paco_2$ 52 mm Hg, FEV_1 0.68 L	Blood gasses, 6 MWD, lung function, PImax/ PEmax and sleep study
Meecham Jones et al,[3] 1995	Cross-over (LTOT)	18/2	18 randomized patients, 14 completers. $Paco_2$ 56 mm Hg, FEV_1 0.84 L	Blood gasses, 6 MWD, health-related quality of life, lung function, and sleep study
Sin et al,[35] 2007	Parallel group (sham)	20/4	23 randomized patients, 17 completers $Paco_2$ 43 mm Hg, FEV_1 0.88 L	Blood gasses, 6 MWD, lung function, HRV + natriuretic peptide measurements
Strumpf et al,[28] 1991	Cross-over (standard care)	15/2	19 randomized patients, 7 completers $Paco_2$ 46 mm Hg, FEV_1 0.54 L	Blood gasses, walking test, lung function, PImax/PEmax, sleep study, dyspnea
Long term				
Clini et al,[34] 2002	Parallelgroup (LTOT)	14.6/3.9	90 randomized patients, 57 completers. $Paco_2$ 56 mm Hg, FEV_1 0.75 L	Blood gasses, 6MWD, HRQL, lung function, PImax, sleep study, dyspnea, hospitalizations, mortality
McEvoy et al,[36] 2009	Parallelgroup (LTOT)	12.8/5.1	144 randomized patients, 81 completers. $Paco_2$ 54 mm Hg, FEV_1 0.65 L	Blood gasses, HRQL, lung function, sleep study (only in NIPPV group), hospitalization rates, survival

Abbreviations: HRV, heart rate variability; PEmax, maximal expiratory pressure; PImax, maximal inspiratory pressure; 6 MWD, 6-minute walking distance.
From Struik FM, Lacasse Y, Goldstein RS, et al. Nocturnal noninvasive positive pressure ventilation in stable COPD: a systematic review and individual patient data meta-analysis. Respir Med 2014;108:332; with permission.

significantly different between both groups. After 2 years, dyspnea decreased, and health-related quality of life improved in the NIV group compared with the LTOT group. In an Australian study, 144 patients were randomized to either NIPPV with LTOT (n = 72) or to LTOT alone (n = 72).[36] Although the applied inspiratory pressures in this study were low (mean of 13 cm H_2O), NIPPV did improve sleep quality and sleep-related hypercapnia. In addition, the NIV patients showed good compliance with NIV therapy, with a mean nightly use 4.5 hours. Compared with LTOT alone, NIV showed an improvement in survival, however, at the cost of a worsened quality of life. The previously mentioned meta-analysis also investigated the long-term benefits from the RCTs.[31,32] Despite the previously mentioned positive results, the overall meta-analysis did not find any significant benefits of NIPPV compared with controls.

VENTILATORY SUPPORT DURING SLEEP COMBINED WITH REHABILITATION

Pulmonary rehabilitation has emerged as a recommended standard of care for patients with lung diseases, as it has been shown to improve exercise tolerance, improve quality of life, reduce respiratory symptoms, and reduce the number of hospitalizations.[37] In patients with severe COPD and respiratory failure, NIV can improve gas exchange,[8,11,16–18] lung function,[16,17,38] functional capacity,[18,38] and sleep quality.[3,36] NIV as an adjunct to pulmonary rehabilitation has been used in 2 different settings: (1) NIV during the exercise training, a topic that will not be discussed further here, and (2) NIV during the night while exercise training is performed during the daytime.

The first study investigating the effect of nocturnal NIV used negative pressure ventilation with a pulmowrap ventilator and showed no additional effects of this combination on lung function, inspiratory muscle pressure, exercise tolerance, and clinical improvement. However, the program lasted only for 3 weeks.[39] The first study using nocturnal domiciliary NIPPV in conjunction with a pulmonary rehabilitation program showed promising results despite low ventilator compliance (median use of 2.08 h/d) and the inclusion of only mildly hypercapnic patients (mean $Paco_2$ 45.6 mm Hg).[40] This study showed a significantly improved exercise tolerance and quality of life after 3 months of NIPPV with rehabilitation compared with the rehabilitation alone. The positive effects became especially apparent after 4 weeks, indicating that a certain duration of this combination therapy is necessary to achieve benefits. However, effects on gas exchange were minimal, with no change in $Paco_2$, indicating that no true improvement in ventilation was achieved. Therefore, the authors suggested that other mechanisms should have caused the improvement, and as they found a small increase in maximal inspiratory pressure only in the NIPPV with rehabilitation group, they speculated that relief of respiratory muscle fatigue caused the improvements.

Positive findings were also found in a longer-term study, showing that NIPPV with rehabilitation as compared to rehabilitation alone had a significant beneficial effect on quality of life, daytime arterial blood gases, exercise tolerance, functional activity, and lung function.[38] Although effects on quality of life, blood gases, and daily activity level were already apparent after 3 months of the combined therapy, the positive effects in terms of increased exercise tolerance and lung function continued to increase over time, possibly because the deterioration occurring in the rehabilitation alone group could have been prevented in the NIPPV with rehabilitation group. Importantly, in this study there was proof that NIPPV actually reversed nocturnal hypoventilation measured by nocturnal arterial blood gases, as well as daytime gas. This might be a consequence of better compliance (median use of NIPPV 6.9 h/d) and higher settings (mean IPAP 23 cm H_2O). It is possible that improved gas exchange played an important role in improving quality of life and exercise tolerance, as better blood gases probably give patients a more favorable condition to train.

Thus, to achieve beneficial effects of the addition of nocturnal NIPPV to rehabilitation, a good compliance, higher inspiratory pressures leading to changes in gas exchange, and a certain length of the treatment period seem to be important predictive factors. Although it seems that the longer the treatment period the more benefit, it is obvious that careful implementation of the NIPPV with close initial observation of patients leads to a better starting point and probably earlier and better results. In the study of Köhnlein and colleagues,[41] careful implementation led to improvements in as little as 3 to 5 weeks, although no strict conclusion can be drawn from this study, as it was only observational using a historical control group. In contrast, when NIV is instituted without extra attention to details, it will not lead to physiologic changes or objective benefits.

NIPPV on top of rehabilitation compared with rehabilitation alone has been shown to be able to increase FEV_1[38] and decrease hyperinflation.[41] Possible mechanisms for this lung function improvement are reduced airway obstruction due to improved hypercapnia-induced airway edema, reduced inflammation, and increased small airway recruitment. Lung function improvement has been shown in conjunction with blood gas improvements, but also without obvious changes in gas exchange, indicating that different mechanisms might be important.

To conclude, although evidence is not extensive yet, RCTs have shown that NIPPV on top of rehabilitation is of benefit in severe COPD patients. Important aspects to achieve benefits are careful implementation with sufficient high pressures, assuring that true improvements of gas exchange are achieved by careful monitoring, good compliance, and a sufficiently long period of treatment.

VENTILATORY SUPPORT DURING SLEEP AFTER ACUTE RESPIRATORY FAILURE

It is known that 80% of the patients who receive NIV during acute respiratory failure will be rehospitalized within 12 months after discharge and that 50% of these patients will die in this period.[42] Therefore, the application of chronic NIV might be effective in this situation. In an uncontrolled study, Tuggey and colleagues[43] investigated the benefits of chronic NIV in a group of patients who were admitted frequently because of acute respiratory failure and needed NIV in this situation. They showed that in the year after they started chronic NIV, there was a significant reduction in the number of admissions and total days in hospital. It has to be mentioned, however, that this was in a highly selective group of patients who were compliant with the ventilator and were motivated to use it at home. A randomized pilot trial was carried out by Cheung and colleagues[44] comparing chronic home NIV to placebo NIV (continuous positive airway pressure [CPAP] of 5 cm H_2O). Primary outcome was recurrent severe COPD exacerbation with acute hypercapnic respiratory failure (AHRF) resulting in need for NIV, intubation, or death within the following year. At 1 year, the proportion of patients developing this composite outcome was 38.5% in the NIPPV group versus 60.2% in the placebo CPAP group ($P = .04$). Although the mean IPAP in the NIPPV group was low (15 cm H_2O), the adherence to both types of therapy was high. However, dropout rates were also high, especially in the NIPPV group (35%). At present, there are 2 international RCTs underway investigating the benefits of chronic NIV after acute respiratory failure. The results of these trials have to be awaited to know whether chronic NIV has a place in this specific situation.

IMPORTANT ISSUES IN PROVIDING ADEQUATE VENTILATORY SUPPORT DURING SLEEP

Although the evidence for providing routine chronic NIV to COPD patients is still lacking, much has been learned from the studies that have been published. This section will elaborate on the different aspects that seem important to provide effective chronic ventilatory support.

Selection of Patients

Both Meecham Jones[3] and Clini[34] reported significant benefits of NIV by including patients with a $Paco_2$ of more than 6.6 kPa (49.5 mm Hg) in contrast to other studies. In addition, Meecham Jones and colleagues showed that patients who had an increase in $Paco_2$ during the night before they were on NIPPV experienced the most benefit in terms of decreasing daytime $Paco_2$ after starting NIV. In a recent meta-analysis based on individual data, it was also shown that patients who were more hypercapnic at baseline ($Paco_2$ >55 mm Hg) showed more reduction in their daytime $Paco_2$ compared with patients who were less hypercapnic.[31]

Adequacy of Ventilation

Monitoring seems to be more important to confirm whether ventilation was effective or not than the type of ventilation. While Strumpf and colleagues[28] monitored CO_2 using end tidal CO_2, which is an unreliable measure in patients with COPD, Meecham Jones and colleagues[3] monitored the effectiveness of ventilation by transcutaneous CO_2. The authors' group[18] monitored the effectiveness of ventilation by nocturnal arterial blood gases. In the last-mentioned controlled studies in which the effectiveness of NIPPV during sleep was confirmed reliably with either transcutaneous CO_2 or arterial blood gases, higher mean inspiratory pressures were used, and probably not surprisingly, these studies showed positive effects in most outcomes.[3,18] It is highly likely that appropriate CO_2 monitoring leads to higher pressures needed to achieve effective ventilation; this effect was also shown in a recent retrospective trial using mean inspiratory pressures of 28 cm H_2O.[17] This was also shown in the recent update of a meta-analysis showing that higher levels of IPAP (higher than 18 cm H_2O) lead to a larger reduction in daytime $Paco_2$. Nevertheless, it is not known whether more effective reduction in daytime $Pa CO_2$ leads to clinically important benefits (**Fig. 1**).[31]

Number of Hours on NIV

Because the optimal duration of ventilatory support is not known, different approaches have been used. Two randomized controlled studies treating patients with COPD explored shorter duration of time daytime ventilatory support.[12,16] In 1 study, the patients received bilevel PAP for 2 hours daily for 5 days a week, while in the other study, bilevel PAP was given for 3 hours daily, 5 days a week for 3 consecutive weeks. Despite these short periods of bilevel PAP support, significant benefits in clinical parameters and changes in Pao_2 and $Paco_2$ were found. This finding may be due to the fact that patients adjust to the NIV device during daytime more easily, and mask leakage is less. Other studies found positive outcomes by applying considerably more hours of bilevel PAP. Clini and colleagues[34] showed positive results with a mean number of hours on bilevel PAP of 9 hours, while Meecham Jones and colleagues[3] and the authors' group[38] showed positive outcomes by a median number of hours of bilevel PAP use of 6.9 hours.[3] A recent update of a meta-analysis of chronic NIPPV showed that the largest decrease in $Paco_2$ was found in patients who used the ventilator for more than 5 hours per night (see **Fig. 1**).[31]

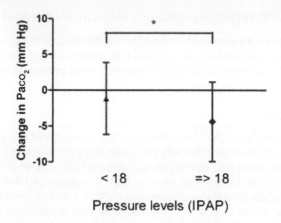

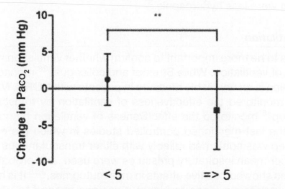

Fig. 1. Change in Paco$_2$ after 3 months of NIPPV (Paco$_2$ baseline - Paco$_2$ after 3 months) for high and low inspiratory positive airway pressure (< 18 and => 18 IPAP) and high and low compliance (< 5 and => 5 ventilation hours per night). Figures display mean change scores and 95% confidence intervals. Significant difference: *: $p<0.05$, **$p<0.01$. (*From* Struik FM, Lacasse Y, Goldstein RS, et al. Nocturnal noninvasive positive pressure ventilation in stable COPD: a systematic review and individual patient data meta-analysis. Respir Med 2014;108: 334; with permission.)

SUMMARY

In conclusion, currently there is no conclusive evidence that NIV should be provided routinely to stable patients with COPD. Nevertheless, patients who are clearly hypercapnic, who receive confirmed effective ventilation by applying higher inspiratory pressures, and have a better compliance might show clinical benefits. The combination of rehabilitation and nocturnal ventilatory support seems to provide more benefits than rehabilitation alone, so this might be a situation in which chronic NIV is effective.

ACKNOWLEDGMENTS

The authors kindly thank Elsevier for using the table and figure as were in Respiratory Medicine in 2014.[33]

REFERENCES

1. Collop N. Sleep and sleep disorders in chronic obstructive pulmonary disease. Respiration 2010;80:78–86.
2. McNicholas WT, Verbraecken J, Marin JM. Sleep disorders in COPD: the forgotten dimension. Eur Respir Rev 2013;22:365–75.
3. Meecham Jones DJ, Paul EA, Jones PW, et al. Nasal pressure support ventilation plus oxygen compared with oxygen therapy alone in hypercapnic COPD. Am J Respir Crit Care Med 1995;152:538–44.
4. Hill NS. Noninvasive ventilation. Does it work, for whom, and how? Am Rev Respir Dis 1993;147:1050–5.
5. Creese R. Bicarbonate ion and striated muscle. J Physiol 1949;110:450–7.
6. Rafferty GF, Lou Harris M, Polkey MI, et al. Effect of hypercapnia on maximal voluntary ventilation and diaphragm fatigue in normal humans. Am J Respir Crit Care Med 1999;160:1567–71.
7. Nizet TA, Heijdra YF, van den Elshout FJ, et al. Respiratory muscle strength and muscle endurance are not affected by acute metabolic acidemia. Clin Physiol Funct Imaging 2009;29:392–9.
8. Windisch W, Dreher M, Storre JH, et al. Nocturnal non-invasive positive pressure ventilation: physiological effects on spontaneous breathing. Respir Physiol Neurobiol 2006;150:251–60.
9. Elliott MW. Noninvasive ventilation in chronic ventilatory failure due to chronic obstructive pulmonary disease. Eur Respir J 2002;20:511–4.
10. Duiverman ML, van Fykern LA, Vennik PW, et al. Reproducibility and responsiveness of a noninvasive EMG technique of the respiratory muscles in COPD patients and in healthy subjects. J Appl Physiol 2004;96:1723–9.
11. Lukácsovits J, Carlucci A, Hill N, et al. Physiological changes during low- and high-intensity noninvasive ventilation. Eur Respir J 2012;39:869–75.
12. Renston JP, DiMarco AF, Supinski GS. Respiratory muscle rest using nasal BiPAP ventilation in patients with stable severe COPD. Chest 1994;105:1053–60.
13. Bégin P, Grassino A. Chronic alveolar hypoventilation helps to maintain the inspiratory muscle effort of COPD patients within sustainable limits. Chest 2000;117: 271S–3S.
14. Schönhofer B, Polkey MI, Suchi S, et al. Effect of home mechanical ventilation on inspiratory muscle strength in COPD. Chest 2006;130:1834–8.
15. Guilleminault C, Cummiskey J. Progressive improvement of apnea index and ventilatory response to CO2 after tracheostomy in obstructive sleep apnea syndrome. Am Rev Respir Dis 1982;126:14–20.
16. Díaz O, Bégin P, Andresen M, et al. Physiological and clinical effects of diurnal noninvasive ventilation in hypercapnic COPD. Eur Respir J 2005;26:1016–23.
17. Windisch W, Kostić S, Dreher M, et al. Outcome of patients with stable COPD receiving controlled noninvasive positive pressure ventilation aimed at a maximal reduction of Pa(CO2). Chest 2005;128:657–62.
18. Duiverman ML, Wempe JB, Bladder G, et al. Nocturnal non-invasive ventilation in addition to rehabilitation in hypercapnic patients with COPD. Thorax 2008;63: 1052–7.
19. Burns GP, Gibson GJ. A novel hypothesis to explain the bronchoconstrictor effect of deep inspiration in asthma. Thorax 2002;57:116–9.
20. De Backer LA, Vos WG, Salgado R, et al. Functional imaging using computer methods to compare the effect of salbutamol and ipratropium bromide in patient-specific airway models of COPD. Int J Chron Obstruct Pulmon Dis 2011;6:637–46.

21. Rossi A. Noninvasive ventilation has not been shown to be ineffective in stable COPD. Am J Respir Crit Care Med 2000;161:688–9.
22. Hill NS. Noninvasive ventilation has been shown to be ineffective in stable COPD. Am J Respir Crit Care Med 2000;161:689–90.
23. Schonhofer B. Non-invasive positive pressure ventilation in patients with stable hypercapnic COPD: light at the end of the tunnel? Thorax 2010;65:765–7.
24. Perrin C, El Far Y, Vandenbos F, et al. Domiciliary nasal intermittent positive pressure ventilation in severe COPD: effects on lung function and quality of life. Eur Respir J 1997;10:2835–9.
25. Sivasothy P, Smith IE, Shneerson JM. Mask intermittent positive pressure ventilation in chronic hypercapnic respiratory failure due to chronic obstructive pulmonary disease. Eur Respir J 1998;1:34–40.
26. Jones SE, Packham S, Hebden M, et al. Domiciliary nocturnal intermittent positive pressure ventilation in patients with respiratory failure due to severe COPD: long-term follow up and effect on survival. Thorax 1998;53:495–8.
27. Dreher M, Storre JH, Schmoor C, et al. High–intensity versus low intensity non invasive ventilation in patients with stable hypercapnic COPD: a randomsied cross-over trial. Thorax 2010;65:303–8.
28. Strumpf DA, Millman RP, Carlisle CC, et al. Nocturnal positive-pressure ventilation via nasal mask in patients with severe chronic obstructive pulmonary disease. Am Rev Respir Dis 1991;144(6):1234–9.
29. Gay PC, Hubmayr RD, Stroetz RW. Efficacy of nocturnal nasal ventilation in stable, severe chronic obstructive pulmonary disease during a 3-month controlled trial. Mayo Clin Proc 1996;71(6):533–42.
30. Lin CC. Comparison between nocturnal nasal positive pressure ventilation combined with oxygen therapy and oxygen monotherapy in patients with severe COPD. Am J Respir Crit Care Med 1996;154(2 Pt 1):353–8.
31. Struik FM, Lacasse Y, Goldstein RS, et al. Nocturnal noninvasive positive pressure ventilation in stable COPD: a systematic review and individual patient data meta-analysis. Respir Med 2014;108:329–37.
32. Struik FM, Lacasse Y, Goldstein R, et al. Nocturnal noninvasive positive pressure ventilation for stable COPD. Cochrane Database Syst Rev 2013;(6):CD002878.
33. Casanova C, Celli BR, Tost L, et al. Long-term controlled trial of nocturnal nasal positive pressure ventilation in patients with severe COPD. Chest 2000;118:1582–90.
34. Clini E, Sturani C, Rossi A, et al. The Italian multicentre study on noninvasive ventilation in chronic obstructive pulmonary disease patients. Eur Respir J 2002;20:529–38.
35. Sin DD, Wong E, Mayers I, et al. Effects of nocturnal noninvasive mechanical ventilation on heart rate variability of patients with advanced COPD. Chest 2007;131:156–63.
36. McEvoy RD, Pierce RJ, Hillman D, et al. Nocturnal non-invasive nasal ventilation in stable hypercapnic COPD: a randomised controlled trial. Thorax 2009;64:561–6.
37. Ries AL, Bauldoff GS, Carlin BW, et al. Pulmonary rehabilitation: joint ACCP/AACVPR evidence-based clinical practice guidelines. Chest 2007;131:4S–42S.
38. Duiverman ML, Wempe JB, Bladder G, et al. Two year home based nocturnal non invasive ventilation added to rehabilitation in COPD patients: a randomized controlled trial. Respir Res 2011;12:112–22.
39. Celli B, Lee H, Criner G, et al. Controlled trial of external negative pressure ventilation in patients with severe chronic airflow obstruction. Am Rev Respir Dis 1989;140:1251–6.

40. Garrod R, Mikelsons C, Paul EA, et al. Randomized controlled trial of domiciliary noninvasive positive pressure ventilation and physical training in severe chronic obstructive pulmonary disease. Am J Respir Crit Care Med 2000;162:1335–41.
41. Köhnlein T, Schönheit-Kenn U, Winterkamp S, et al. Non invasive ventilation in pulmonary rehabilitation in COPD patients. Respir Med 2009;103:1329–36.
42. Chu CM, Chan VL, Lin AW, et al. Readmission rates and life threatening events in COPD survivors treated with non-invasive ventilation for acute hypercapnic respiratory failure. Thorax 2004;59:1020–5.
43. Tuggey JM, Plant PK, Elliott MW. Domiciliary non-invasive ventilation for recurrent acidotic exacerbations of COPD: an economic analysis. Thorax 2003;58(10): 867–71.
44. Cheung AP, Chan VL, Liong JT, et al. A pilot trial of non-invasive ventilation after acute respiratory failure in COPD. Int J Tuberc Lung Dis 2010;14(5):642–9.

Anxiety, Depression, and Cognitive Impairment in Patients with Chronic Respiratory Disease

Vincent S. Fan, MD, MPH[a],*, Paula M. Meek, RN, PhD[b]

KEYWORDS

• Anxiety • Depression • Cognitive impairment • Chronic respiratory disease

KEY POINTS

• Depression, anxiety and cognitive impairment are common among persons with COPD, and psychological symptoms are associated with worse outcomes.
• Psychological symptoms may affect adherence to pulmonary rehabilitation programs, and screening for these symptoms should be considered.
• Pulmonary rehabilitation may improve depression and anxiety symptoms although the effect on cognitive function is not as clear.

INTRODUCTION

Feelings, beliefs, and expectations are important influences on the outcomes from pulmonary rehabilitation. Depression, anxiety, and cognitive impairment are common among patients with chronic obstructive pulmonary disease (COPD) and may both affect the delivery of pulmonary rehabilitation and be modified by pulmonary rehabilitation. Evaluation for these conditions should therefore be considered during the baseline assessment for pulmonary rehabilitation.[1,2]

There has been increasing awareness that depression is a common feature of many chronic illnesses, including respiratory conditions.[3] In lung disease, the psychological comorbidity of anxiety also seems to play an important role, given the relationship between anxiety and dyspnea. In recent years, the links between chronic illness,

This article originally appeared in *Clinics in Chest Medicine*, Volume 35, Issue 2, June 2014.
VA Statement: The views expressed in this article are those of the authors and do not necessarily reflect the position or policy of the Department of Veterans Affairs or the United States Government. *This material is the result of work supported by resources from the VA Puget Sound Health Care System, Seattle, Washington.*
[a] Veterans Affairs Puget Sound Health Care System, Department of Medicine, University of Washington, Seattle, WA, USA; [b] College of Nursing, University of Colorado, CO, USA
* Corresponding author.
E-mail address: Vincent.fan@va.gov

decreases in cognitive function, and these emotional states have begun to be made. The interrelationships among the physiologic aspects of pulmonary rehabilitation and these psychological and cognitive concerns are complex. In addition, it is not clear how and to what degree pulmonary rehabilitation modifies, ameliorates, or eliminates these emotional states or decreases in cognitive function.

A goal of pulmonary rehabilitation is to change patient health behaviors. This change can be facilitated by increasing physical activity in a supervised setting, ideally maintaining this increased physical activity after the formal pulmonary rehabilitation sessions are complete. Changing health behaviors in chronic illness is challenging, and there is increasing evidence that addressing comorbid psychological symptoms such as depression is an important component of health behavior change.[4]

In this article, the prevalence of depression, anxiety, and cognitive impairment in persons with COPD, and the extent to which these conditions limit or modify the effectiveness of pulmonary rehabilitation, are reviewed; in addition, whether pulmonary rehabilitation may ameliorate these psychological and cognitive impairments is discussed.

Depression

Depression is an adjustment disorder that exists on a continuum from feelings of being blue or sad to major depressive illness. Simple mood disturbance such as mild anxiety or depression is typically associated with an identifiable life stressor, which is commonplace in chronic disease. An individual with a simple mood disturbance who begins pulmonary rehabilitation should be able to adequately participate in the program and, with encouragement, have positive outcomes. However, someone with a major depressive disorder needs to be treated aggressively within and beyond the rehabilitation program. Unless this major depression is recognized and addressed, patients probably do not realize their potential gains in pulmonary rehabilitation outcomes.

The defined criteria for the diagnosis of a major depressive disorder are that at least 5 of the symptoms in **Box 1** must be present nearly every day during a 2-week period.

Box 1
Symptoms used to diagnose a major depressive disorder

- Depressed mood most of the day or markedly diminished interest or pleasure in all, or almost all, activities most of the day (must be one of the symptoms)
- Significant weight loss when not dieting or weight gain (eg, 5%) or decrease or increase in appetite
- Insomnia or hypersomnia
- Psychomotor agitation or retardation
- Fatigue or loss of energy
- Feelings of worthlessness or excessive or inappropriate guilt (not merely self-reproach or guilt about being sick)
- Diminished ability to think or concentrate
- Recurrent thoughts of death (not just fear of dying), recurrent suicidal ideation without a specific plan, or a suicide attempt or a specific plan

Data from Diagnostic and statistical manual of mental disorders, fourth edition text revision. Washington, DC: American Psychiatric Association; 2000.

To meet the diagnostic criteria for depression, these symptoms need to have caused clinically significant distress or impairment in social, occupational, or other important areas of functioning. If one of these symptoms existed previously, then it must have changed from the previous occurrence to be considered in the assessment. The symptoms must not be caused by the direct physiologic effects of a substance or a general medical condition or be associated with bereavement unless it has persisted for 2 months.

Some of the symptoms of depression such as poor appetite, sleep disturbance and fatigue are also associated with COPD and, therefore, may present a challenge to providers who are evaluating patients. Also, few studies of the impact of depressive symptoms on COPD outcomes have used strict *Diagnostic and Statistical Manual of Mental Disorders* (DSM) criteria for depression but instead have relied on symptom scales such as the Hospital Anxiety and Depression Scale (HADS)[5] or the Beck Depression Inventory (BDI) scale.[6]

PREVALENCE OF DEPRESSION

Depression and anxiety are the most common psychosocial concerns seen in chronic pulmonary patients enrolled in pulmonary rehabilitation.[7] Estimates of the prevalence of depression range from 10% to close to 80% (depending on the instrument and method used to screen), although the prevalence is most commonly reported as between 25% and 50%.[8–10] The higher percentages likely reflect the presence of symptom burden rather than clinically defined disease. Also, the prevalence of depression may be higher in patients with more severe COPD.[11,12] Some estimates suggest that patients with COPD are 2.5 times more likely to have anxiety and depression than healthy individuals.[11] Cross-sectional studies suggest that women, those with a body mass index less than 21 kg/m^2, and those who experience more significant dyspnea or disability are more likely to have symptoms of depression.[3,13] Patients with COPD without depression also are more than twice as likely to subsequently develop depression compared with those without COPD.[14]

Depressive symptoms in COPD are associated with worse clinical outcomes, including worse health-related quality of life,[9,15] decreased functional performance measured with the 6-minute walk test,[16] increased risk of COPD exacerbations,[17] and a higher risk of death.[18–20] Although it is not known whether treatment of depression may decrease the risk of these adverse outcomes, because there are effective treatments, it seems reasonable to address as an important potentially modifiable comorbid condition in COPD.

Psychological disorders such as depression are also common among patients with other lung diseases undergoing rehabilitation, including interstitial lung disease[21,22] and pulmonary hypertension.[23–25] It is therefore important to understand that depression is common in individuals with chronic lung disease, and most likely, it is an issue for all those enrolled in pulmonary rehabilitation.

Depression Treatment

In general, outside the setting of pulmonary rehabilitation, patients with depression are typically treated with either antidepressant medications or psychotherapy. Although a complete review of antidepressant therapy is beyond the scope of this article, there are few randomized trials specifically assessing the efficacy of antidepressants in COPD. An early study[26] found that nortriptyline improved depressed mood and anxiety. A small randomized trial[27] of a serotonin selective reuptake inhibitor, paroxetine, in 28 patients with COPD found no improvement during the 6-week trial, but improvement in depression and quality of life in a 3-month follow-up open-labeled period. In terms of psychotherapy, cognitive behavioral therapy has been studied in COPD, and the results have been mixed, with 1 randomized trial[28] showing no benefit compared with education alone, and another[29] showing significant improvements in anxiety and depression, which were maintained at 8 months. Although there are limited data of treating depression in COPD specifically,[30] the data on treating depression in older adults with other chronic illness[31] suggest that a comprehensive intervention with antidepressants and psychotherapy is likely to be effective in this population.

DOES DEPRESSION AFFECT PARTICIPATION AND THE LIKELIHOOD OF BENEFITTING FROM PULMONARY REHABILITATION?

Depression may affect patients' ability to engage in self-care behaviors,[32] and in diabetes and heart disease depression, it is associated with worse adherence to medications used to treat the disease.[33,34] In COPD, it is not known whether depression affects adherence to medications, but there is increasing evidence that depression affects whether patients initiate or complete a pulmonary rehabilitation program. For example, an analysis of participants in a large randomized controlled trial of lung volume reduction surgery (National Emphysema Treatment Trial)[35] showed that baseline mild depression and anxiety were both associated with decreased likelihood to complete the 10 required pulmonary rehabilitation sessions: 27% did not complete all of the sessions, and those with mild depressive symptoms (BDI$\geq$5) were less likely to complete the pulmonary rehabilitation program. Depression measured with the HADS was also found to be associated with noncompletion of both a 7-week[36] and an 8-week pulmonary rehabilitation program[37] and with decreased likelihood to be adherent to home pulmonary rehabilitation at 1 year.[38] Although not all studies have found that depression decreases adherence to pulmonary rehabilitation,[39] these results indicate that depressed patients may be less likely to initiate and complete a pulmonary rehabilitation program.

There is also evidence that patients with depression may require more intensive self-management interventions than nondepressed patients. A randomized trial of dyspnea self-management combined with either 4 weeks or 24 weeks of supervised exercise found that those with significant depressive symptoms (Center for Epidemiologic Studies Depression [CES-D] Scale >15) experienced a significant reduction in dyspnea with 24 weeks of exercise, whereas those without depression improved with only 4 weeks.[40]

The finding that depression may adversely affect COPD self-management behaviors by potentially decreasing the participation and completion of pulmonary rehabilitation is consistent with evidence from a recent large randomized controlled trial of patients with depression who also had either diabetes or heart disease.[4] In this trial, concurrent treatment of both depression and chronic medical illness improved both depressive symptoms and the management of the chronic illness. Treatment of depression may therefore have the potential to improve clinical outcomes and also to improve self-management and increase participation in pulmonary rehabilitation programs.

Improvement in Depressive Symptoms as a Result of Pulmonary Rehabilitation

By improving dyspnea, increasing exercise tolerance, and reducing disability, pulmonary rehabilitation may itself contribute to improvement in psychological symptoms such as depression. Pulmonary rehabilitation programs often incorporate education and self-management components to improve patients' ability to manage their dyspnea and stress, which may also contribute to improved psychological symptoms. Several instruments have been used to measure psychological outcomes after a pulmonary rehabilitation program. Desirable instruments are tools that do not rely on physical symptoms (such as fatigue or tiredness), so that the mood and emotional issues can be separated from physical changes that typically result from the disease and the exercise components of pulmonary rehabilitation.

Some of the possible tools include the CES-D,[41] the BDI,[42] the Geriatric Depression Scale (GDS),[43] and the HADS.[5] The CES-D, a 20-item tool using a 0 (rarely) to 3 (most of the time) scoring, also has limited physical items and follows the DSM-III (DSM third edition) criteria.[41] A score less than 16 is considered normal, 16 to 24 shows borderline increase of depressed symptoms and should be considered for referral, and 24 and higher must be immediately referred for evaluation. The BDI has 21 items and has a score with a range from 0 to 63 with a score of 10 or higher corresponding to mild to moderate depressive symptoms. The BDI has been used extensively in the cardiovascular literature, as well as in pulmonary studies.[20] However, a disadvantage of both the BDI and the CES-D instruments is that they were not designed specifically for patients with chronic disease.

The HADS and the GDS are examples of depression symptom scales designed for chronically ill older adults. The GDS is a 15-item tool that is answered with yes or no, so it is quick to administer.[43] A score on the GDS of 5 or greater should trigger further evaluation, whereas a score of 10 or greater requires immediate referral. The HADS has 14 questions (7 depression related and 7 anxiety related), and the depression scale ranges from 0 to 21, with 8 or higher corresponding to mild symptoms, and 11 or higher corresponding to moderate to severe depression.

Several randomized controlled trials of pulmonary rehabilitation have assessed depressive symptoms before and after completion of the intervention program. An early 3-arm trial compared exercise combined with stress management education, stress management education alone, and usual care.[44] This study found that only the group who received the combined exercise and stress management program had a reduction in depression and anxiety. Another small study[45] randomized 24 patients to either an 8-week pulmonary rehabilitation program or control, and found that the intervention group had significant improvement in depressive symptoms measured with the BDI, and improvement in anxiety measured with the Spielberger State-Trait Anxiety Index (STAI). A larger trial of 200 patients with COPD[46] compared pulmonary rehabilitation (including stress management) with usual care and found improvement in both depression and anxiety measured with the HADS at 6 weeks; it also found that depression continued to be improved compared with the intervention group at 1 year. A meta-analysis in 2007 and updated in 2009 that included 5 clinical trials[47,48] also found that comprehensive pulmonary rehabilitation improved depressive and anxiety symptoms among older patients with COPD. Clinical trial data therefore suggest that a comprehensive pulmonary rehabilitation program that includes stress management can improve psychological outcomes in COPD.

A small randomized trial of 30 patients[49] specifically addressed the question of whether 24 sessions of pulmonary rehabilitation combined with 12 sessions of psychotherapy would improve psychological outcomes compared with pulmonary rehabilitation alone and found that the addition of psychotherapy sessions resulted in a greater reduction in depression and anxiety measured with the BDI and Beck Anxiety Inventory. This finding therefore supports the approach of treating psychological symptoms at the same time as the exercise program and incorporating staff with expertise in psychotherapy to the pulmonary rehabilitation team to improve depressive and anxiety symptoms. This approach requires corroboration from further studies.

Several nonrandomized observational studies have been performed using a pre-post study design to address whether patients' depressive symptoms improve with pulmonary rehabilitation. Two observational studies[36,50] found no improvement in HADS depression or HADS anxiety scores after pulmonary rehabilitation. In contrast, several studies have found improvement in depression or anxiety,[37,51,52] and improvement was seen regardless of severity of COPD.[53] These observational data seem to support the general finding that psychological symptoms may improve after pulmonary rehabilitation.

An important consideration when assessing whether pulmonary rehabilitation improves psychological outcomes is the proportion of participants with depression or anxiety on entry into the program. A study of 334 patients with COPD who completed a pulmonary rehabilitation program found an improvement in mean HADS anxiety and depression scores after completion of the rehabilitation program, although these were less than the traditional minimum clinically important difference (MCID) of 1.5.[39] However, when the results were stratified by whether the baseline HADS scores were abnormal (≥ 8), it was found that those with abnormal baseline HADS anxiety or HADS depression scores had a significant improvement in their postpulmonary rehabilitation HADS scores. These findings are supported by another large study of 257 patients who completed a pulmonary rehabilitation program, in which the mean HADS anxiety and depression scores improved significantly, although the anxiety scores did not meet the MCID threshold.[37] However, when the investigators focused on abnormal anxiety or depression scores (HADS ≥ 10 for both scales) at baseline, they found that the proportion of anxious patients decreased from 25% to 9% ($P<.001$), and the proportion of patients with depressive symptoms decreased from 17% to 6% (<0.001) after the intervention.

These 2 studies make the compelling case that the effect of pulmonary rehabilitation on psychological outcomes is likely underestimated, because patients without baseline depression or anxiety who are unlikely to experience an improvement in these areas are included in the analysis. To more rigorously assess whether pulmonary rehabilitation improves depression or anxiety, randomized controlled trials should avoid looking at mean improvement in psychological symptom for all patients regardless of whether they have significant depression or anxiety at baseline. Instead, studies should consider analyzing data by looking at whether the proportion of patients with significant depressive or anxiety symptoms decreases with pulmonary rehabilitation or should restrict the analysis to those who had significant depressive or anxiety symptoms at baseline.

Should Screening for Depression be Performed Before Entry into a Pulmonary Rehabilitation Program?

Given the potential effect of depressive symptoms on completion of pulmonary rehabilitation programs as well as the potential beneficial effect of pulmonary rehabilitation on depressive symptoms, the American Thoracic Society (ATS)/European Respiratory Society statement on the key concepts of pulmonary rehabilitation states that "screening questionnaires for anxiety, depression, and/or cognitive impairment may be undertaken."[2] Little is known in the United States or Europe about whether pulmonary rehabilitation programs consistently screen for and treat depression. A survey of 22 programs in Australia[54] found that most were not using depression-specific or anxiety-specific instruments to screen for psychological comorbidity, and 36% did not offer specific psychological support. Of those programs that did provide support, 41% offered informal support (patients were referred to mental health), and only 5 (23%) provided formal psychological support. A greater awareness in pulmonary rehabilitation programs of the potential benefits of screening for depression is needed to ensure that patients are referred to licensed health professionals for accurate diagnosis and for consideration of antidepressant medications or psychotherapy.

In the United States, the US Preventative Services Taskforce review on screening for depression lists several potential depression screen instruments, which include the BDI, the GDS, and the Primary Care Evaluation of Mental Disorders (PRIME-MD).[55] The PRIME-MD brief screen includes 2 questions that are able to adequately screen those who need further evaluation.[56,57] These 2 questions are:

In the past month, have you felt bothered a lot by:

1. Little interest or pleasure in doing things?

2. Feeling down, depressed or hopeless?

These questions have proved to be sensitive and reasonably predictive of depression that requires further evaluation. An affirmative answer to either or both of these questions should trigger a further evaluation by a mental health professional. Although it is not known whether screening for depression among patients referred to pulmonary rehabilitation changes outcomes, screening with the PRIME-MD or another depression symptom measure used in chronically ill adults such as the GDS or HADS should be considered.

Anxiety

Like depression, anxiety can be considered on a continuum from generalized anxiety to panic disorder. Anxiety can frequently be present along with depression, and some recent reports have suggested that they may be interrelated. Generalized anxiety can be defined as an apprehensive anticipation of danger or a stressful situation. It may be associated with excessive feelings of somatic stress, such as fatigue, restlessness, irritability, rapid speech, sleep disturbances, tachycardia, dyspnea, and sweating. Generalized anxiety would be present if these symptoms and the apprehension are present more days than not over a 6-month period. Because respiratory patients commonly have fatigue, dyspnea, tachycardia, and sleep disturbance, their interpretation in the context of anxiety assessment can be problematic.

An additional difficulty is that there is also a condition called an adjustment disorder with generalized anxiety, which is adjustment to major life events (eg, recent severe exacerbation of a disease requiring hospitalization). The problematic piece is that there may not have been 6 months between the event and when the individual is enrolled in a pulmonary rehabilitation program. In this case, it is important to ascertain whether there were troubling symptoms present for a substantial period before hospitalization.

Panic attacks are further along the continuum, defined as intense episodes of acute anxiety, with dyspnea and cognitive fears. The dyspnea associated with a panic attack must be separated from an acute, severe episode of dyspnea resulting from underlying physical illness, but this may be difficult. A panic disorder is recurrent unexpected episodes (panic attacks) that are coupled with persistent concern about other attacks and worry about implications of such attacks. Panic attacks and panic disorder are serious issues that require further evaluation and treatment outside pulmonary rehabilitation. They can clearly interfere with maximizing benefits from rehabilitation. However, with appropriate support, the rehabilitation environment can be therapeutic to these patients.

Prevalence of Anxiety in COPD

In general, there has been less literature on the role of anxiety in COPD and therefore fewer studies to estimate the prevalence of this condition. The estimated prevalence varies widely, from 6% and 74%, and similar to studies of depression, most studies have used symptom measures and not a clinical diagnosis of anxiety,[58] and the prevalence varies with the severity of COPD and the instrument used to measure anxiety symptoms. Although the results are not consistent, anxiety may increase with worsening disease severity, as measured with a multidimensional index of COPD severity.[59]

What is the Relationship Between Anxiety and Pulmonary Rehabilitation?

Several of the studies that have already been mentioned in this article also assessed the impact of anxiety on adherence to pulmonary rehabilitation. In NETT (National Emphysema Treatment Trial), anxiety was measured with the STAI, which has a range of 20 to 80.[35] Patients with an STAI trait score of more than 36 were less likely to complete pulmonary rehabilitation after adjusting for disease severity. However, in a different study,[38] anxiety measured with the HADS anxiety scale was not associated with adherence to pulmonary rehabilitation in study of long-term follow-up. Anxiety affects patients' ability to exercise, and there is evidence that those with increased anxiety have decreased results on the 6-minute walk test after adjusting for disease severity.[59,60] Although there are fewer studies in this area, the literature suggests that anxiety may lead to worse adherence to pulmonary rehabilitation and limit functional performance measured with the 6-minute walk test.

As described earlier for depression, participants in pulmonary rehabilitation may have an improvement in anxiety symptoms at the end of the intervention period. Many of the studies that have shown improvements in depressive symptoms after pulmonary rehabilitation have also reported a beneficial impact on anxiety symptoms.[44,45,49] Pulmonary rehabilitation therefore seems to improve both depressive and anxiety symptoms for patients with COPD.

Screening for Panic Disorder and Generalized Anxiety

As with depression, it is important to be aware of diagnostic criteria for anxiety, although the diagnosis is generally made by a licensed professional. The ATS statement on key concepts and advances in pulmonary rehabilitation states that "management of anxiety/panic in pulmonary rehabilitation has the potential to reduce such events and improve patient outcomes." To determine whether patients referred to pulmonary rehabilitation have significant anxiety symptoms, adequately screening for anxiety is important. The same study that used the PRIME-MD to screen for depression also successfully used the following 3 questions to adequately screen those who need further evaluation for significant anxiety.[56,57] The first 2 questions are similar to the depression screening questions, but the third question attempts to capture more severe episodes such as panic attacks.

In the past month, have you felt bothered a *lot* by:

1. "Nerves" or feeling anxious or edge?

2. Worrying about a lot of different things?

In the last month:

3. Have you had an anxiety attack (suddenly feeling fear or panic)?

An affirmative answer to any one of these questions should prompt the pulmonary rehabilitation staff to refer the patient for further evaluation by a mental health professional. These questions are also sensitive, with reasonable predictive properties for the detection of generalized anxiety that requires further evaluation. The controlled exercise sessions associated with pulmonary rehabilitation are a perfect venue to help determine if panic attacks are a feature associated with dyspnea episodes and should also be considered part of an assessment of anxiety.

Measures Used to Assess Anxiety as an Outcome in Pulmonary Rehabilitation

Although the 3 PRIME-MD questions are adequate screening questions for rehabilitation programs, there are established anxiety measures that can be used both to screen for anxiety and to assess anxiety outcomes after pulmonary rehabilitation. A recent tool developed for use in primary care holds promise for screening and outcome measurement, the General Anxiety Disorder-7 (GAD-7).[61] The GAD-7 is a 7-item tool that is answered on a 0 to 3 (nearly every day) scale, with an eighth question on how distressing the symptoms are. A score on the GAD-7 of 5 or greater indicates mild anxiety and a score of 10 or greater indicates the need for referral. The Penn State Worry Questionnaire is also a public domain questionnaire that could be used to screen and measure outcomes.[62] The tool originally had 16 items scored on a 1 (not at all typical of me) to 4 (very typical of me) scale, but recent analysis has reduced it to 8 items.[63] The 8-item tool has performed well, but does not have a clear cutoff score, although a mean score of 30 is considered normal for the 16-item version. Other measures that have been used in COPD include the HADS-anxiety scale with 7 questions and a score between 0 and 21 with a cutoff of 8 or more for mild symptoms and 10 or more for moderate to severe symptoms.[5] The STAI has also been used, which has a range of 20 to 80.[64] Symptom measures may also be used successfully as a screening and an outcome variable.

Cognitive function

Cognitive function can be defined as the mental process of knowing, including awareness, perception, reasoning, and judgment. Cognitive function improves as we develop from childhood, then declines as we age. Normal aging has been associated with declines in cognitive function involving memory, language, thinking, and judgment but does not interfere with overall functioning. Mild cognitive impairment is an intermediate stage between the expected cognitive decline of normal aging and dementia. Mild cognitive impairment goes beyond slips of the memory or not being able to find the right word, and many individuals may be aware that their memory or mental function has slipped or it may be noticed by family and friends. In general, normal aging changes and even mild cognitive impairment may not be severe enough to interfere with a person's day-to-day life or their ability to self-manage their illness or affect their usual activities.

However, chronic illness such as COPD can accelerate the normal aging process and lead to important deficits. Clearly, cognitive impairments have implications for pulmonary rehabilitation in terms of education and self-management strategies. Some have suggested that cognitive impairment should be considered a primary component of hypoxemic COPD and not a mere comorbidity of this disease. Hypoxemia can influence cognitive decline but is neither sufficient nor required for an individual with COPD to show decline.

Prevalence of cognitive decline in COPD

Deficits in cognitive function are prevalent in COPD and can be complicated by chronic hypoxemia.[65–68] Cognitive deficiencies worsen along with disease progression,[69] with some reporting abnormalities (such as scores <24 in the Mini-Mental State Examination [MMSE]) in 64% of those with severe COPD.[70] The percentage of patients with abnormalities in the MMSE included verbal recall (26%), construction (39%), attention (31%), language (13%), and orientation (current date or location, 24%). In addition, impairment in test performance that requires a drawing task, such as producing an analog clock with a set time, or other complex goal-directed tasks indicates problems associated with judgment and complexity[71] and has been proposed to be prognostic in hypoxemic patients with COPD.[72]

A recent investigation in nonhypoxemic individuals with COPD that combined multiple modes to assess cognitive function including magnetic resonance imaging and standard neuropsychological tests found reduced white matter integrity, disturbance in the function of gray matter, and lower neuropsychiatric test scores compared with age-related controls.[73] In this investigation, there were deficits in processing speed and executive function as well as episodic and working memory, which corresponds to the deficits seen on the MMSE. Recent findings from the Rotterdam Study[74] have found on high-resolution magnetic resonance imaging greater frequency of cerebral microbleeds in individuals with COPD. This finding supports the proposition that the cognitive function changes seen are at least in part caused by cerebral microbleeds, a novel marker for cerebral small-vessel disease. Although all the cognitive function changes found are important, working memory is particularly relevant to individuals who participate in pulmonary rehabilitation programs; this topic is reviewed in the next section.

Working memory

Working memory in the past was referred to as short-term memory; however, its functions are more complex than first proposed.[75–78] Originally, it was believed that short-term memory collected all sensory information to be stored in a single collection. We know now that there are different systems for different types of information, such as visual and verbal.[79] Working memory consists of a central executive that controls and coordinates the operation of 2 subsystems that process and store information: one for spoken and written material and one for visual or spatial information.[80] Also, the central executive is involved in other cognitive tasks like problem solving and mental arithmetic. Working memory becomes critical in any intervention designed to increase knowledge and change behavior as it applies to real-life tasks. Specifically, working memory is essential to reading and understanding educational materials and navigation of daily activities requiring visual and spatial processing and problem solving central to self-care.

There is some evidence that working memory is linked to the ability to focus attention on a task or information and disregard distractions.[81,82] However, some of the literature that tested working memory training has been drawn into question, and improvements may simply be caused by increasing ability to focus. One study did show improvements in working memory by high-intensity exercise. In this study of both sedentary and active young women,[83] the participants were exercised to the point of exhaustion and working memory was measured during, immediately after, and on recovery. Working memory in these participants decreased during and immediately after the exercise but increased after recovery.

Although specific working memory training has not been performed in individuals with COPD, general cognitive training aimed at stimulating attention, learning, and logical-deductive thinking has been attempted without success.[84] Consequently, it is not clear that extensive cognitive training as opposed to classic strategies that improve the quality of educational materials and improve working memory strategies such as focusing attention is any better. In general, working memory is improved via increased attention to task or information, limitation of distraction, and, potentially, exercise.

Pulmonary rehabilitation as an intervention to improve depression, anxiety, and cognitive impairment

Pulmonary rehabilitation has a real advantage when it comes to treating many psychosocial concerns, because exercise is one of the best interventions for anxiety, depression, and stress relief. Even a short course of pulmonary rehabilitation has shown improvements in depression, verbal memory, and visuospatial functioning.[85]

Besides participating in the exercise portion of the rehabilitation program, there are specific medications and psychotherapy interventions that may improve depression and lower anxiety. The specific medications are not reviewed here, but most of these medications do not take immediate effect and can take as long as several weeks before the individual feels the impact. Unless otherwise indicated by the individual's health care provider, participation in a program should not be restricted. However, anxiety, depression, and cognitive impairments can all affect the individual's ability to focus and learn from any formal educational classes. Care must be given to individualizing the program when the individual has these psychosocial concerns.

It seems that exercise training produces little if any improvement in cognitive function in hypoxic COPD. Therefore, it may be necessary to adapt and tailor the program so that individuals with cognitive impairment can obtain the essential knowledge needed to self-manage their disease. If the individual's cognitive impairments are such that retention of information and judgment are impaired, then a significant other or caregiver needs to be an integral part of the rehabilitative process. Further, the age-old strategy of repetition, repetition, repetition can go a long, long, long way toward helping reinforce information retention.

REFERENCES

1. Nici L, Donner C, Wouters E, et al. American Thoracic Society/European Respiratory Society statement on pulmonary rehabilitation. Am J Respir Crit Care Med 2006;173(12):1390–413.
2. Spruit MA, Singh SJ, Garvey C, et al. An official American Thoracic Society/European Respiratory Society statement: key concepts and advances in pulmonary rehabilitation. Am J Respir Crit Care Med 2013;188(8):e13–64.
3. Schane RE, Walter LC, Dinno A, et al. Prevalence and risk factors for depressive symptoms in persons with chronic obstructive pulmonary disease. J Gen Intern Med 2008;23(11):1757–62.
4. Katon WJ, Lin EH, Von Korff M, et al. Collaborative care for patients with depression and chronic illnesses. N Engl J Med 2010;363(27):2611–20.
5. Zigmond AS, Snaith RP. The hospital anxiety and depression scale. Acta Psychiatr Scand 1983;67(6):361–70.
6. Beck AT, Ward CH, Mendelson M, et al. An inventory for measuring depression. Arch Gen Psychiatry 1961;4:561–71.
7. Maurer J, Rebbapragada V, Borson S, et al. Anxiety and depression in COPD: current understanding, unanswered questions, and research needs. Chest 2008;134(Suppl 4):43S–56S.
8. Ng TP, Niti M, Tan WC, et al. Depressive symptoms and chronic obstructive pulmonary disease: effect on mortality, hospital readmission, symptom burden, functional status, and quality of life. Arch Intern Med 2007;167(1):60–7.
9. Norwood R. Prevalence and impact of depression in chronic obstructive pulmonary disease patients. Curr Opin Pulm Med 2006;12(2):113–7.

10. van Ede L, Yzermans CJ, Brouwer HJ. Prevalence of depression in patients with chronic obstructive pulmonary disease: a systematic review. Thorax 1999;54(8): 688–92.

11. van Manen JG, Bindels PJ, Dekker FW, et al. Risk of depression in patients with chronic obstructive pulmonary disease and its determinants. Thorax 2002;57(5): 412–6.

12. Watz H, Waschki B, Boehme C, et al. Extrapulmonary effects of chronic obstructive pulmonary disease on physical activity: a cross-sectional study. Am J Respir Crit Care Med 2008;177(7):743–51.

13. Chavannes NH, Huibers MJ, Schermer TR, et al. Associations of depressive symptoms with gender, body mass index and dyspnea in primary care COPD patients. Fam Pract 2005;22(6):604–7.

14. Polsky D, Doshi JA, Marcus S, et al. Long-term risk for depressive symptoms after a medical diagnosis. Arch Intern Med 2005;165(11):1260–6.

15. Yohannes AM, Roomi J, Waters K, et al. Quality of life in elderly patients with COPD: measurement and predictive factors. Respir Med 1998;92(10):1231–6.

16. Al-shair K, Dockry R, Mallia-Milanes B, et al. Depression and its relationship with poor exercise capacity, BODE index and muscle wasting in COPD. Respir Med 2009;103(10):1572–9.

17. Xu W, Collet JP, Shapiro S, et al. Independent effect of depression and anxiety on chronic obstructive pulmonary disease exacerbations and hospitalizations. Am J Respir Crit Care Med 2008;178(9):913–20.

18. Almagro P, Calbo E, Ochoa de Echaguen A, et al. Mortality after hospitalization for COPD. Chest 2002;121(5):1441–8.

19. de Voogd JN, Wempe JB, Koeter GH, et al. Depressive symptoms as predictors of mortality in patients with COPD. Chest 2009;135(3):619–25.

20. Fan VS, Ramsey SD, Giardino ND, et al. Sex, depression, and risk of hospitalization and mortality in chronic obstructive pulmonary disease. Arch Intern Med 2007;167(21):2345–53.

21. Akhtar AA, Ali MA, Smith RP. Depression in patients with idiopathic pulmonary fibrosis. Chron Respir Dis 2013;10(3):127–33.

22. Ryerson CJ, Arean PA, Berkeley J, et al. Depression is a common and chronic comorbidity in patients with interstitial lung disease. Respirology 2012;17(3): 525–32.

23. Harzheim D, Klose H, Pinado FP, et al. Anxiety and depression disorders in patients with pulmonary arterial hypertension and chronic thromboembolic pulmonary hypertension. Respir Res 2013;14(1):104.

24. McCollister DH, Beutz M, McLaughlin V, et al. Depressive symptoms in pulmonary arterial hypertension: prevalence and association with functional status. Psychosomatics 2010;51(4):339–339.e8.

25. Batal O, Khatib OF, Bair N, et al. Sleep quality, depression, and quality of life in patients with pulmonary hypertension. Lung 2011;189(2):141–9.

26. Borson S, McDonald GJ, Gayle T, et al. Improvement in mood, physical symptoms, and function with nortriptyline for depression in patients with chronic obstructive pulmonary disease. Psychosomatics 1992;33(2):190–201.

27. Eiser N, Harte R, Spiros K, et al. Effect of treating depression on quality-of-life and exercise tolerance in severe COPD. COPD 2005;2(2):233–41.

28. Kunik ME, Veazey C, Cully JA, et al. COPD education and cognitive behavioral therapy group treatment for clinically significant symptoms of depression and anxiety in COPD patients: a randomized controlled trial. Psychol Med 2008; 38(3):385–96.

29. Hynninen MJ, Bjerke N, Pallesen S, et al. A randomized controlled trial of cognitive behavioral therapy for anxiety and depression in COPD. Respir Med 2010; 104(7):986–94.
30. Alexopoulos GS, Kiosses DN, Sirey JA, et al. Personalised intervention for people with depression and severe COPD. Br J Psychiatry 2013;202(3):235–6.
31. Unutzer J, Katon W, Callahan CM, et al. Collaborative care management of late-life depression in the primary care setting: a randomized controlled trial. JAMA 2002;288(22):2836–45.
32. Katon WJ. Clinical and health services relationships between major depression, depressive symptoms, and general medical illness. Biol Psychiatry 2003;54(3): 216–26.
33. Ciechanowski PS, Katon WJ, Russo JE. Depression and diabetes: impact of depressive symptoms on adherence, function, and costs. Arch Intern Med 2000;160(21):3278–85.
34. Carney RM, Freedland KE, Eisen SA, et al. Major depression and medication adherence in elderly patients with coronary artery disease. Health Psychol 1995;14(1):88–90.
35. Fan VS, Giardino ND, Blough DK, et al. Costs of pulmonary rehabilitation and predictors of adherence in the National Emphysema Treatment Trial. COPD 2008; 5(2):105–16.
36. Lewko A, Bidgood PL, Jewell A, et al. Evaluation of multidimensional COPD-related subjective fatigue following a pulmonary rehabilitation programme. Respir Med 2014;108(1):95–102.
37. Bhandari NJ, Jain T, Marolda C, et al. Comprehensive pulmonary rehabilitation results in clinically meaningful improvements in anxiety and depression in patients with chronic obstructive pulmonary disease. J Cardiopulm Rehabil Prev 2013; 33(2):123–7.
38. Heerema-Poelman A, Stuive I, Wempe JB. Adherence to a maintenance exercise program 1 year after pulmonary rehabilitation: what are the predictors of dropout? J Cardiopulm Rehabil Prev 2013;33(6):419–26.
39. Harrison SL, Greening NJ, Williams JE, et al. Have we underestimated the efficacy of pulmonary rehabilitation in improving mood? Respir Med 2012;106(6): 838–44.
40. Nguyen HQ, Carrieri-Kohlman V. Dyspnea self-management in patients with chronic obstructive pulmonary disease: moderating effects of depressed mood. Psychosomatics 2005;46(5):402–10.
41. Radloff L. The CES-D Scale: a self-report depression scale for research in the general population. Appl Psychol Meas 1977;1:385–401.
42. Beck AT, Steer RA, Garbin M. Psychometric properties of the Beck depression inventory: twenty-five years of evaluation. Clin Psychol Rev 1988;8:77–100.
43. Yesavage JA, Brink TL, Rose TL, et al. Development and validation of a geriatric depression screening scale: a preliminary report. J Psychiatr Res 1982;17(1):37–49.
44. Emery CF, Schein RL, Hauck ER, et al. Psychological and cognitive outcomes of a randomized trial of exercise among patients with chronic obstructive pulmonary disease. Health Psychol 1998;17(3):232–40.
45. Paz-Diaz H, Montes de Oca M, Lopez JM, et al. Pulmonary rehabilitation improves depression, anxiety, dyspnea and health status in patients with COPD. Am J Phys Med Rehabil 2007;86(1):30–6.
46. Griffiths TL, Burr ML, Campbell IA, et al. Results at 1 year of outpatient multidisciplinary pulmonary rehabilitation: a randomised controlled trial. Lancet 2000; 355(9201):362–8.

47. Coventry PA, Hind D. Comprehensive pulmonary rehabilitation for anxiety and depression in adults with chronic obstructive pulmonary disease: systematic review and meta-analysis. J Psychosom Res 2007;63(5):551–65.
48. Coventry PA. Does pulmonary rehabilitation reduce anxiety and depression in chronic obstructive pulmonary disease? Curr Opin Pulm Med 2009;15(2): 143–9.
49. de Godoy DV, de Godoy RF. A randomized controlled trial of the effect of psychotherapy on anxiety and depression in chronic obstructive pulmonary disease. Arch Phys Med Rehabil 2003;84(8):1154–7.
50. Bentsen SB, Wentzel-Larsen T, Henriksen AH, et al. Anxiety and depression following pulmonary rehabilitation. Scand J Caring Sci 2013;27(3):541–50.
51. Pirraglia PA, Casserly B, Velasco R, et al. Association of change in depression and anxiety symptoms with functional outcomes in pulmonary rehabilitation patients. J Psychosom Res 2011;71(1):45–9.
52. von Leupoldt A, Taube K, Lehmann K, et al. The impact of anxiety and depression on outcomes of pulmonary rehabilitation in patients with COPD. Chest 2011; 140(3):730–6.
53. Tselebis A, Bratis D, Pachi A, et al. A pulmonary rehabilitation program reduces levels of anxiety and depression in COPD patients. Multidiscip Respir Med 2013; 8(1):41.
54. Doyle C, Dunt D, Ames D, et al. Managing mood disorders in patients attending pulmonary rehabilitation clinics. Int J Chron Obstruct Pulmon Dis 2013;8:15–20.
55. O'Connor EA, Whitlock EP, Gaynes B, et al. Screening for Depression in Adults and Older Adults in Primary Care: An Updated Systematic Review [Internet]. Rockville (MD): Agency for Healthcare Research and Quality (US); 2009 Dec. Report No.: 10-05143-EF-1. U.S. Preventive Services Task Force Evidence Syntheses, formerly Systematic Evidence Reviews. PMID: 20722174 [PubMed].
56. Kunik ME, Azzam PN, Souchek J, et al. A practical screening tool for anxiety and depression in patients with chronic breathing disorders. Psychosomatics 2007; 48(1):16–21.
57. Spitzer RL, Williams JB, Kroenke K, et al. Utility of a new procedure for diagnosing mental disorders in primary care. The PRIME-MD 1000 study. JAMA 1994;272(22):1749–56.
58. Yohannes AM, Willgoss TG, Baldwin RC, et al. Depression and anxiety in chronic heart failure and chronic obstructive pulmonary disease: prevalence, relevance, clinical implications and management principles. Int J Geriatr Psychiatry 2010; 25(12):1209–21.
59. Eisner MD, Blanc PD, Yelin EH, et al. Influence of anxiety on health outcomes in COPD. Thorax 2010;65(3):229–34.
60. Giardino ND, Curtis JL, Andrei AC, et al. Anxiety is associated with diminished exercise performance and quality of life in severe emphysema: a cross-sectional study. Respir Res 2010;11:29.
61. Spitzer RL, Kroenke K, Williams JB, et al. A brief measure for assessing generalized anxiety disorder: the GAD-7. Arch Intern Med 2006;166(10):1092–7.
62. Meyer TJ, Miller ML, Metzger RL, et al. Development and validation of the Penn State Worry Questionnaire. Behav Res Ther 1990;28(6):487–95.
63. Hopko DR, Stanley MA, Reas DL, et al. Assessing worry in older adults: confirmatory factor analysis of the Penn State Worry Questionnaire and psychometric properties of an abbreviated model. Psychol Assess 2003;15(2):173–83.
64. Spielberger CE, Goruch RL. Manual for the state-trait anxiety inventory. Palo Alto (CA): Consulting Psychologists Press; 1970.

65. Incalzi RA, Gemma A, Marra C, et al. Verbal memory impairment in COPD: its mechanisms and clinical relevance. Chest 1997;112(6):1506–13.
66. Incalzi RA, Gemma A, Marra C, et al. Chronic obstructive pulmonary disease. An original model of cognitive decline. Am Rev Respir Dis 1993;148(2):418–24.
67. Kozora E, Filley CM, Julian LJ, et al. Cognitive functioning in patients with chronic obstructive pulmonary disease and mild hypoxemia compared with patients with mild Alzheimer disease and normal controls. Neuropsychiatry Neuropsychol Behav Neurol 1999;12(3):178–83.
68. Chang SS, Chen S, McAvay GJ, et al. Effect of coexisting chronic obstructive pulmonary disease and cognitive impairment on health outcomes in older adults. J Am Geriatr Soc 2012;60(10):1839–46.
69. Li J, Huang Y, Fei GH. The evaluation of cognitive impairment and relevant factors in patients with chronic obstructive pulmonary disease. Respiration 2013;85(2): 98–105.
70. Ozge C, Ozge A, Unal O. Cognitive and functional deterioration in patients with severe COPD. Behav Neurol 2006;17(2):121–30.
71. Royall DR. Double jeopardy. Chest 2006;130(6):1636–8.
72. Antonelli-Incalzi R, Corsonello A, Pedone C, et al. Drawing impairment predicts mortality in severe COPD. Chest 2006;130(6):1687–94.
73. Dodd JW, Chung AW, van den Broek MD, et al. Brain structure and function in chronic obstructive pulmonary disease: a multimodal cranial magnetic resonance imaging study. Am J Respir Crit Care Med 2012;186(3):240–5.
74. Lahousse L, Vernooij MW, Darweesh SK, et al. Chronic obstructive pulmonary disease and cerebral microbleeds. The Rotterdam Study. Am J Respir Crit Care Med 2013;188(7):783–8.
75. Baddeley AD. Working memory. Oxford (United Kingdom), New York: Clarendon Press, Oxford University Press; 1986.
76. Hitch GJ, Baddeley AD. Verbal reasoning and working memory. Q J Exp Psychol 1976;28:603–21.
77. Dales RE, Cakmak S, Leech J, et al. The association between personal care products and lung function. Ann Epidemiol 2013;23(2):49–53.
78. Vogiatzis I, Zakynthinos S. The physiological basis of rehabilitation in chronic heart and lung disease. J Appl Physiol (1985) 2013;115(1):16–21.
79. Baddeley AD, Hitch GJ, Allen RJ. Working memory and binding in sentence recall. J Mem Lang 2009;61(3):438–56.
80. Polkey MI, Spruit MA, Wouters E, et al. Reply: minimal or maximal clinically important difference: using death to define MCID. Am J Respir Crit Care Med 2013; 187(12):1392.
81. Zanto TP, Gazzaley A. Neural suppression of irrelevant information underlies optimal working memory performance. J Neurosci 2009;29(10):3059–66.
82. Berry AS, Zanto TP, Rutman AM, et al. Practice-related improvement in working memory is modulated by changes in processing external interference. J Neurophysiol 2009;102(3):1779–89.
83. Bue-Estes CL, Willer B, Burton H, et al. Short-term exercise to exhaustion and its effects on cognitive function in young women. Percept Mot Skills 2008;107(3):933–45.
84. Incalzi RA, Corsonello A, Trojano L, et al. Cognitive training is ineffective in hypoxemic COPD: a six-month randomized controlled trial. Rejuvenation Res 2008; 11(1):239–50.
85. Kozora E, Tran ZV, Make B. Neurobehavioral improvement after brief rehabilitation in patients with chronic obstructive pulmonary disease. J Cardiopulm Rehabil 2002;22(6):426–30.

Comorbidities and Systemic Effects of Chronic Obstructive Pulmonary Disease

Gourab Choudhury, MBBS, MRCP(UK)*,
Roberto Rabinovich, MBBS, MD, PhD,
William MacNee, MBChB, MD, FRCP(G), FRCP(E)

KEYWORDS

- Chronic obstructive pulmonary disease • Comorbidities • Systemic effects
- Inflammation • Management strategy

KEY POINTS

- Definitive types of systemic effects and co-morbidities have been seen in COPD patients.
- There are possible contributory mechanisms to these effects.
- There are clinical implications of these co-morbidities in the cohort.
- Novel therapies reduce the burden of observed effects.

INTRODUCTION

Chronic obstructive pulmonary disease (COPD) is a major cause of morbidity and mortality worldwide. It has been projected to move from the sixth to the third most common cause of death worldwide by 2020, while rising from fourth to third in terms of morbidity within the same time frame.[1]

The prevalence of COPD in the general population is estimated to be around 1% of the adult population, but rises sharply among those 40 years and older. The prevalence continues to climb appreciably higher with age.[2]

COPD is known primarily to affect the lung structure and function, resulting in emphysematous destruction of lung tissue and large and small airway disease that occur in varying proportion and severity within individuals.[3]

Besides the lung abnormalities, COPD is now recognized to be a condition that has an impact on other organs, the so-called systemic effects and comorbidities of

---

This article originally appeared in *Clinics in Chest Medicine*, Volume 35, Issue 1, March 2014.
ELEGI and COLT Laboratories, Queen's Medical Research Institute, 47 Little France Crescent, EH16 4TJ Edinburgh, UK
* Corresponding author.
E-mail address: gchoudhu@staffmail.ed.ac.uk

COPD.[4–6] Conventionally, comorbidity has been defined as a disease coexisting with the primary disease of interest. In COPD, however, the definition becomes more perplexing, as certain coexisting illnesses may be a consequence of the patients' underlying COPD when it could termed as more of a systemic effect.

It is as yet unclear whether these associations are a consequence of shared risk factors such as cigarette smoking or poor physical activity, or whether COPD is a true causal factor. Nevertheless, these extrapulmonary features of COPD add to the challenge and burden of assessing and managing the disease.

This article reviews the types, possible mechanisms, and clinical implications of these systemic effects and comorbidities on COPD patients.

CLASSIFICATION

Table 1 lists the systemic effects and comorbidities associated with COPD. Table 2 summarizes the results of a PubMed search investigating the prevalence of COPD and comorbidities in various studies performed in the past.

CARDIOVASCULAR DISEASE

COPD is now well known to be a risk factor for the development of atherosclerosis and consequent cardiovascular complications.[7,8]

Prevalence

Cardiovascular disease is undoubtedly the most significant nonrespiratory contributor to both morbidity and mortality in COPD.

In a large cohort of patients with COPD admitted to a Veterans Administration Hospital or clinic, the prevalence of coronary artery disease was 33.6%, appreciably higher than the 27.1% prevalence seen in a matched cohort without COPD.[9] In the Lung Health Study,[10] which assessed deaths and hospitalizations over a 5-year period in a cohort of COPD patients, mortality in 5887 patients aged 35 to 46 years with COPD with mild to moderate airways obstruction was 2.5%, of whom 25% died of cardiovascular complications. Moreover, in these patients with relatively mild COPD, cardiovascular disease accounted for 42% of the first hospitalization and 44% of the second hospitalization over a follow-up period of 5 years. By comparison, only 14% of the hospitalizations in this cohort were from respiratory causes.

Divo and colleagues[11] looked at 1664 patients with COPD over 4 years to evaluate COPD comorbidities and mortality risk. Using a multivariate analysis, they generated a COPD comorbidity index (COPD-specific comorbidity test) based on the comorbidities that increase mortality risk. The prevalence of coronary artery disease in this study was unsurprisingly highest at 30.2%, with congestive heart failure (HF) and

Table 1	
Observed systemic effects and comorbidities in the COPD population	
Systemic Effects of COPD[4–6]	Comorbidities in COPD[4–6]
Muscle dysfunction	Cardiovascular disease
Cachexia	Lung cancer
Anemia	Osteoporosis
Muscle dysfunction	Diabetes
Autonomic dysfunction	Psychological issues: anxiety/depression
Systemic inflammation	Obstructive sleep apnea

Table 2
Data from various studies (PubMed search) looking at the prevalence of COPD and comorbidities

First Author	Journal	Type of Study	Patient Size (n)	Cardiac (%)	Hypertension (%)	Diabetes (%)	Psychiatric (%)	Cancer (%)	Osteoporosis (%)
van Manen et al	J Clin Epidemiol	Observational	1145	13	23	5	9	6	—
Almagro et al	Chest	Retrospective matched cohort	2699	22	—	—	10	4	—
Sidney et al	Chest	Retrospective matched cohort	45,966	18	18	2	—	—	—
Schnell et al	BMC Pulm Med	Cross-Sectional	995	12.7	—	—	20.6	16.5	16.9
Feary et al	Thorax	Cross-Sectional	29,870	28	—	12.2	—	—	—

— signifies no data available.

dysrhythmias making up another 15.7% and 13% of the cases, respectively, and correlated strongly with the association for increased risk of death ($P<.05$).

Holguin and colleagues[12] assessed the prevalence of COPD deaths in United States between 1979 and 2001, and found approximately 47 million hospital discharges (8.5% of all hospitalizations in adults) with a primary or secondary diagnosis of COPD (21% and 79%, respectively). The reported hospital mortality in this cohort was related to heart disease in 43%, taking the major share for the cause of death, compared with 37% related to respiratory failure and another 25% related to pneumonia.

Forced expiratory volume in 1 second (FEV_1) is also known to be an independent predictor of cardiovascular complications in COPD patients. In the Lung Health Study, for every 10% decrease in FEV_1, cardiovascular mortality increased by approximately 28% and nonfatal coronary events increased by approximately 20% in mild to moderate COPD.[10] Even a moderate reduction of expiratory flow volumes multiplies the risk of cardiovascular morbidity and sudden cardiac deaths by 2 to 3 times, independent of other risk factors.[13-16]

COPD patients also have shown evidence of atherosclerotic plaque burden as assessed by increased carotid intimal medial thickening (CIMT),[17] and are associated with increased cardiovascular and all-cause mortality.[18]

Pathogenesis

The pathogenesis of atherosclerosis in COPD is multifactorial.[19] **Box 1** summarizes the potential mechanisms that have been linked directly or indirectly to the cardiovascular complications seen in this cohort. **Fig. 1** summarizes the presumed mechanisms for cardiovascular disease in COPD patients.

Inflammation

Inflammation is considered to be a potential pathogenic mechanism in atherosclerosis. Recent studies, however, indicate that sustained systemic inflammation occurs only in a proportion of patients with COPD, and its relationship to the development of cardiovascular disease has as yet not been fully established.[20] Patients with COPD and coexistent cardiovascular disease nevertheless tend to have higher systemic levels of biomarkers, such as interleukin (IL)-6 and fibrinogen, than those without this comorbidity.[21] In addition, systemic inflammation increases exacerbations of COPD when there is an increased risk of cardiovascular events.[22,23]

The specific cellular mechanisms by which systemic inflammation plays a role in the pathogenesis of cardiovascular disease are complex. However, studies have revealed the importance of inflammation in atherosclerotic plaque initiation, development, and rupture (see **Fig. 1**).[24,25]

[18]F-Fluorodeoxyglucose positron emission tomography imaging has also shown direct evidence of inflammation in the vascular wall of the aorta, presumably

---

Box 1
Potential pathogenic mechanisms of cardiovascular disease in COPD

- Systemic and lung inflammation
- Hypoxia: both alveolar and tissue hypoxia
- Hypercapnic acidosis
- Endothelial dysfunction/vessel wall abnormalities
- Polycythemia

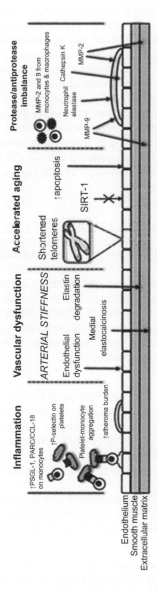

Fig. 1. The putative mechanisms for the pathogenesis of cardiovascular disease in COPD. MMP, matrix metalloproteinase; PARC/CCL-18, pulmonary and activation-regulated chemokine CC chemokine ligand 18; PSGL, P-selectin glycoprotein ligand 1; SIRT, sirtuin 1. (*From* Maclay JD, MacNee W. Cardiovascular disease in COPD: mechanisms. Chest 2013;143(3):798–807. http://dx.doi.org/10.1373/chest.12-0938; with permission.)

associated with atherosclerotic plaques, in patients with COPD when compared with smoking control subjects.[26]

Systemic inflammation is discussed in more details later in this article.

Hypoxia

Patients with COPD are subjected to hypoxia: either sustained hypoxia in patients with severe disease, or intermittent hypoxia during exercise or exacerbations. There are several effects of hypoxia that can influence atherogenesis, including systemic inflammation and oxidative stress, upregulation of cell-adhesion molecules, and hemodynamic stress.[27–29] Animal studies have shown hypoxia to be a contributor to atherosclerosis in the presence of dyslipidemia, as increased lipid peroxidation, a marker of oxidative stress, and reduced levels of the antioxidant superoxide dismutase are found in the myocardial tissue of rats exposed to hypoxic environments.[30,31]

Hypoxia also induces hemodynamic stress, increasing the heart rate and cardiac index,[32] and affects the renal circulation, reducing renal blood flow and activating the renin-angiotensin system, resulting in increased peripheral vasoconstriction and oxidative stress.[33] Respiratory failure in patients with COPD is also associated with activation of the sympathetic nervous system,[34] which is associated with an increased risk for cardiovascular disease.[35]

Effect of cigarette smoking

Chronic cigarette smoking is an independent risk factor for the development of cardiovascular complications in COPD patients.[36] Possible mechanisms include increased systemic oxidative stress, altered nitric oxide (NO) bioavailability, endothelial dysfunction, and influence on the levels of other major risk factors, such as blood pressure.[37–39]

However, studies have also shown that independent of current smoking, plasma levels of fibrinogen and other markers of coagulation are significantly higher in patients with stable COPD than in healthy subjects.[40,41] This amplified procoagulant activity in COPD may principally be a consequence of inflammation, initiating the coagulation cascade by promoting tissue factor gene expression in endothelial cells, hence contributing to increased thrombotic events.[42]

Polycythemia

Secondary polycythemia is a known complication of COPD, and occurs mainly as a result of chronic hypoxemia. A prospective study by Cote and colleagues,[43] however, had shown that only 6% of their 683 COPD patients developed secondary polycythemia, perhaps because the development of polycythemia in COPD has been less common in recent times, and is thought to be due to more effective management of hypoxia in COPD such as the use of long-term oxygen therapy (LTOT) in patients who meet the criteria.

However, when present in COPD polycythemia can contribute to the development of pulmonary hypertension and pulmonary endothelial dysfunction with reduced cerebral and coronary blood flow, thus adding to the pathogenic cascade.[44]

Hypercapnic acidosis

Respiratory acidosis resulting from hypercapnia is a well-known occurrence in patients with COPD, particularly in the advanced phase. A recent study by Minet and colleagues[45] has shown that respiratory acidosis could be one of the potent mechanisms behind endothelial dysfunction, adding to the burden of cardiovascular complications.

Abnormalities in vascular endothelial function/vessel wall

Some,[46,47] but not all studies[48] have demonstrated abnormal endothelial function in COPD patients in comparison with smokers who have not developed COPD.

Arterial stiffness can be assessed using carotid-femoral pulse-wave velocity (PWV), a measure that is predictive of cardiovascular events in healthy individuals and in patients with ischemic heart disease.[49] Arterial stiffness is increased in COPD patients in comparison with healthy smokers[50,51] and is associated with the FEV_1 percent predicted emphysema and systemic inflammation,[52] and may result from increased elastolysis in the vessel wall.[53]

Common Cardiovascular Complications

HF is common in COPD patients, and COPD is common in HF patients. In a survey of COPD patients in primary care, 20% had previously unrecognized HF,[54] which is associated with a worse prognosis in COPD patients.[55]

A study of 186 consecutive patients with left ventricular systolic dysfunction in an HF clinic found that 39% had COPD diagnosed by spirometry, and those patients with HF and severe COPD had a worse prognosis than the HF patients with mild to moderate COPD or normal lung function.[56] Higher mortality was again reported among patients with COPD when compared with individuals without lung disease in a study of 4132 patients hospitalized with cardiac failure in Norway.[57]

In another prospective prognostic study performed as part of the EchoCardiography and Heart Outcome Study (ECHOS), 532 patients admitted with a clinical diagnosis of HF were studied.[58] The prevalence of COPD in these patients was found to be 35% and was associated with a worse prognosis.

COPD is indeed a predictor of mortality in HF.[30] Studies have shown 5-year survival in HF patients with COPD to be as low as 31%, compared with 71% in its absence.[57] HF in COPD patients has often been postulated to be secondary to increased intrathoracic pressure–induced impaired low-pressure ventricular filling, as is expected with hyperinflated lungs in this population.[59] However, Barr and colleagues[60] have shown that computed tomography (CT)-quantified emphysema scores negatively correlated with ventricular filling even in a group without COPD and minor emphysema, in whom hyperinflation is unlikely to play a role. The investigators hypothesized that endothelial dysfunction associated with emphysema could contribute to impaired left ventricular filling and the consequent failure cascade.

Patients with COPD also have increased risk for cardiac arrhythmias.[61] Following surgery for non–small cell lung carcinoma, patients with spirometric evidence of COPD had an increased risk for supraventricular tachycardia, and were found to be refractory to first-line treatment.[62] Atrial fibrillation (AF) is also more common in COPD following coronary artery bypass grafting.[63] In a study conducted in Finland on 738 patients with COPD, AF was found to be an independent predictor of increased mortality and poor health-related quality of life (HRQoL) in comparison with the general population.[64]

Coronary artery disease is also common and is undertreated in patients with COPD.[65] In a group of healthy Japanese men, CIMT (a surrogate measure strongly associated with atherosclerotic plaque burden) was significantly increased in individuals who smoked and had airflow limitation compared with matched smokers and nonsmokers.[17] This finding suggests that smokers with a spirometric-based diagnosis of COPD may have evidence of subclinical atherosclerosis independent of cigarette smoking.

The presence of COPD in patients with myocardial infarction (MI) is also associated with a poorer prognosis. In a study of 14,703 patients with acute MI, all-cause mortality was 30% in patients with COPD versus 19% in those without COPD.[66] Campo and colleagues[14] assessed 11,118 consecutive patients with ST-elevation MI (STEMI) stratified according to the presence or absence of COPD. At the 3-year follow-up,

COPD was found to be an independent predictor of mortality (hazard ratio [HR] 1.4, 95% confidence interval [CI] 1.2–1.6). Hospital readmissions from recurrent MI (10% vs 6.9%, $P<.01$) and HF (10% vs 6.9%, $P<.01$) were significantly more frequent in patients with COPD when compared with those without. Also hospital readmission for COPD was found to be a strong independent risk factor for recurrence of MI (HR 2.1, 95% CI 1.4–3.3) and HF (HR 5.8, 95% CI 4.6–7.5).

In a study of exacerbations of COPD from the United Kingdom Health Improvement Database, the incidence rate of MI was 1.1 per 100 patient-years, with a 2.27-fold increased risk of MI 1 to 5 days after exacerbation.[67]

In another prospective study, 242 COPD patients admitted to hospital with an exacerbation were studied to observe the prevalence of MI following hospitalization.[22] Twenty-four patients (10%) were found to have elevated troponin, among whom 20 (8.3%; 95% CI 5.1%–12.5%) had chest pain and/or serial electrocardiographic changes, in keeping with MI. Overall, 1 in 12 patients met the criteria for MI.

Interventions to Reduce Cardiovascular Complications

Smoking cessation
A recent meta-analysis assessing the impact of smoking has shown a decline of acute coronary syndrome risk in 30 of 35 estimates with a 10% (95% CI 6–14, $P<.001$) pooled relative risk reduction, supporting the fact that smoking is an independent risk factor toward development of cardiovascular complications.[68] Smoking cessation therefore unsurprisingly remains one of the primary cornerstones of cardiovascular risk management.

Effective management of COPD
It is well known that for every 10% decrease in FEV_1, cardiovascular mortality increases by about 28%, and nonfatal coronary events increase by about 20% in mild to moderate COPD.[16] Therefore, early detection and effective management of the disease is of importance in reducing the associated complications of this condition.

The use of current medications to treat COPD, however, has not been shown to be definitive toward reduction of cardiovascular events. Whereas observational studies have suggested that inhaled corticosteroids (ICS) may potentially confer benefit on cardiovascular events or mortality,[69] randomized controlled trials (RCTs) have failed to show any significant effect of ICS therapy on MI or cardiovascular death. The use of long-acting inhaled β-agonists does not appear to produce an increased risk of cardiovascular deaths.[70] The long-acting antimuscarinic, tiotropium, appears to confer an increased risk of cardiovascular death when used in a higher dose in the Respimat inhaler but not in the Handihaler formulation,[71] which may even be associated with a decrease in cardiovascular mortality.[72]

Cardiovascular drugs
Medications currently associated with cardiovascular risk reduction, such as β-blockers (BB), angiotensin-converting enzyme (ACE) inhibitors, statins, and angiotensin II receptor blockers (ARBs), have been shown in retrospective pharmacoepidemiologic studies to have an impact on the clinical outcome of COPD patients by reducing the cardiovascular events and mortality.[73–75] These observational studies, however, suffer from immortal time bias, and prospective studies are required to definitively assess the benefits of these drugs in this population.

BB are known to improve survival of patients within a large spectrum of cardiovascular diseases, including ischemic heart disease and HF.[76–80] In a large observational study involving 2230 COPD patients, the association of BB usage with all-cause mortality and risk of exacerbation was studied.[81] Use of BB was found to be associated with a reduction in mortality as well as the risk of exacerbations in a broad spectrum of patients with COPD with concurrent cardiovascular disease. Importantly in a subgroup analyses, including patients with COPD but without overt cardiovascular disease, but with hypertension as the main remaining indication for the prescription of BB, similar outcomes were noted. This result further indicates the potential protective benefit of BB in COPD even in those with no known history of heart disease.

However, BB have been underprescribed in patients with COPD cardiovascular disease,[82] largely because of the potential to worsen airflow limitation and consequent theoretical respiratory side effects (namely bronchospasm).

A recent meta-analysis of studies in COPD patients has shown that cardioselective BB, given as a single dose or for longer duration, produced no change in FEV_1 or respiratory symptoms when compared with placebo, and did not affect the FEV_1-guided treatment response to β2-agonists.[83]

Another recent study also explored the association between BB therapy and outcomes in patients hospitalized with acute exacerbations of COPD with underlying ischemic heart disease, HF, or hypertension. The study accounted for the problem of immortal time bias, and found no improvement or worse mortality in COPD patients using BB.[84] Judicious use of BB may therefore be warranted in patients with severe COPD and respiratory failure on LTOT in whom the use of BB was associated, in one study, with increased mortality.[85]

Similarly, statins, ACE inhibitors, and ARBs are also widely used for the treatment and prevention of cardiovascular disease, and their potential role in other disease states has become increasingly recognized. Mortensen and colleagues[86] studied the association of prior outpatient use of statins and ACE inhibitors on mortality for subjects of 65 years or older who were hospitalized with acute COPD exacerbations. A total of 11,212 subjects with a mean age of 74.0 years were studied in this group, of whom 32.0% were using ACE inhibitors or ARBs, the use of which was associated with significant reduction in 90-day mortality (odds ratio [OR] 0.55, 95% CI 0.46–0.66). A similar pharmacoepidemiologic study done by Mancini and colleagues[75] suggested that statins in combination with either ACE inhibitors or ARBs improved cardiovascular and pulmonary outcomes not only in the high-risk but also in the low-risk COPD populations.

SKELETAL MUSCLE EFFECTS

A striking systemic consequence of COPD is the reduction in peripheral muscle mass, resulting in muscle wasting and dysfunction. Muscle dysfunction, with or without evidence of atrophy, can be defined physiologically as the failure to achieve the basic muscle functions of strength and resistance, the latter being inversely related to an increase in the fatigability of the muscle.

Reduced quadriceps strength in COPD is associated with reduced exercise capacity,[87,88] compromised health status,[89] increased need for health care resources,[90] and mortality independent of airflow obstruction.[91] Skeletal muscle weakness, particularly quadriceps weakness, has also recently been shown to be a feature of early disease,[92] and its development is likely to be multifactorial with inflammation and oxidative stress[93] being the predominant factors, coupled with physical inactivity.[94,95] Several other factors such as protein synthesis/degradation imbalance and hypoxia have also been postulated to explain the initiation and the progression of muscle wasting in COPD patients.[88,96]

Prevalence

Eighteen percent to 36% of COPD patients present with net loss of muscle mass, which is responsible for weight loss in 17% to 35% of such patients.[97] However, muscle wasting is also present in 6% to 21% of patients of normal weight.[98] The reductions in mass and cross-sectional area of limb muscles of COPD patients have been linked to the impaired muscle strength seen in these patients. When limb-muscle strength is normalized per unit of mass or cross-sectional area, no differences can be observed between control subjects and COPD patients, suggesting that atrophy is indeed an important causative factor in the reduced limb-muscle strength and endurance in COPD.[97] Hence, it could be argued that muscle wasting is a better predictor of HRQoL and survival than is body weight.[99]

Unintentional loss of muscle mass, unsurprisingly, has a significant impact on the quality of life, and can be associated with premature death.[100]

Fig. 2 illustrates the various pathophysiologic changes that are observed in skeletal muscles of COPD patients and the possible mechanisms implicated.

Pathophysiologic Changes Associated with Muscle Dysfunction/Wasting

Fiber redistribution results in an increase in the number of type IIx muscle fibers,[101,102] which, in turn, is associated with significant muscle atrophy.[102]

Alterations in muscle bioenergetics in skeletal limb muscle of COPD patients correlate with exercise tolerance. For example, the early lactate release that occurs during exercise, the increased phosphate/phosphocreatine relationship during submaximal exercise, and the reduced activity of oxidative enzymes in these patients all indicate a change in muscle bioenergetics.[103]

Altered capillary structuration has also been found in the skeletal muscle of COPD patients. Electron and optic microscopy studies show reduced capillary density and the number of contacts between capillaries and fibers in skeletal muscles of COPD patients.[104]

Factors Contributing to Muscle Dysfunction

Several factors, such as protein synthesis/degradation imbalance, hypoxia, inactivity, inflammation, and oxidative stress, have been proposed to explain the initiation and the progression of muscle wasting in COPD.[96,97] Mitochondrial dysfunction, apoptosis, and oxidative stress have all also been implicated to the wasting and dysfunction observed in COPD.

Mitochondrial dysfunction is manifested as reduced citrate synthase activity that correlates with time to fatigue of the muscle,[105] while reduced mitochondrial oxidative phosphorylation and coupling have been associated with reduced muscle mass and endurance.[106]

Other factors that contribute to this muscle dysfunction include the following.

- Abnormal protein metabolism. A substantial proportion of COPD patients is characterized by low fat-free mass with altered muscle and plasma amino acid levels, suggesting abnormal protein metabolism.[107] The signaling pathways that govern muscle hypertrophy and/or atrophy have yet to be fully defined. However, several key factors have been identified. **Fig. 3** summarizes the salient pathways governing skeletal muscle metabolism. Marked activation of the ubiquitin-proteasome pathway is found in muscle of patients with COPD, and is thought to be one of the key factors in muscle atrophy and dysfunction as seen in COPD patients.[108,109]

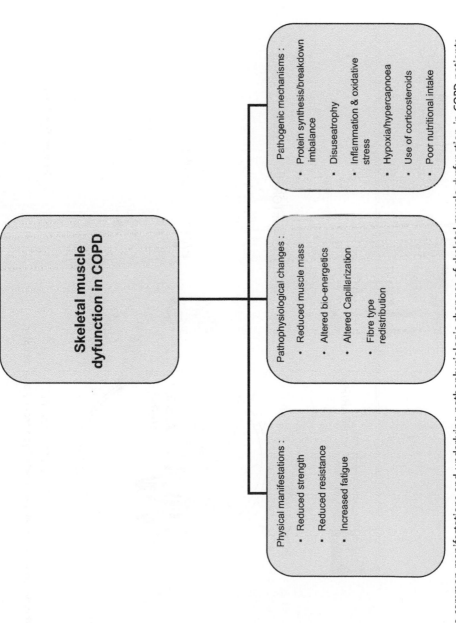

Fig. 2. The common manifestations and underlying pathophysiologic changes of skeletal muscle dysfunction in COPD patients.

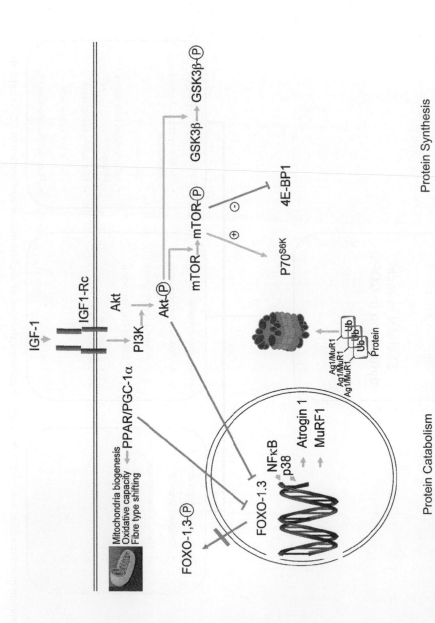

Fig. 3. Pathways governing skeletal muscle hypertrophy and atrophy.

- Poor nutritional intake and unmatched calorie expenditure are further factors contributing to muscle wasting in COPD patients. Chronic usage of oral corticosteroids is also a well-known contributor to myopathy in this group.[110] Previous studies have shown that the histology of steroid-induced myopathy in patients with COPD is of global myopathy affecting both type IIa and IIb fibers, and type I fibers to a lesser extent.[111] However, administration of corticosteroids for relatively short periods of time, for example during an exacerbation, has not been shown to cause any significant deleterious effect on the skeletal muscle of COPD patients.[112]
- Hypoxia is implicated in mitochondrial biogenesis, oxidative stress, inflammation, and autophagy. It results in enhanced cytokine production by macrophages, contributing to the activation of the tumor necrosis factor (TNF) system. Significant inverse correlations between partial pressure of arterial oxygen and circulating TNF-α and soluble TNF-receptor levels have been reported in patients with COPD,[113] limiting the production of energy and possibly affecting the protein synthesis also.[114]
- Hypercapnic acidosis can inhibit the oxidative enzymes, further contributing to protein degradation and the process of muscle wasting.[115]
- Inflammation, as in cardiovascular complications, is another mechanism contributing to skeletal muscle dysfunction in COPD patients. Relatively fewer data are currently available on the concentration of cytokines in muscle of COPD patients, the most studied being TNF-α. High levels of TNF-α protein in serum have been associated with quadriceps weakness,[116] and COPD patients with low fat-free mass (FFM) are reported to show high mRNA levels of TNF-α in the quadriceps, together with lower body mass index (BMI).[117] Of interest, high levels of C-reactive protein (CRP) have been found to be inversely related to the distance covered in a 6-minute walking test in COPD patients, suggesting a role for chronic inflammation in these patients.[118]

Interventions to Improve Skeletal Muscle Dysfunction

- Exercise training is the single most important therapeutic intervention to treat muscle dysfunction/wasting in patients with COPD.[119] Improving exercise tolerance by enhancing muscle strength, with consequent improved endurance and reduced fatigue, have all proved to be very effective.[119] Exercise training improves body weight by improving FFM, enhancing oxygen delivery to the muscle mitochondria and fiber-type redistribution.[119,120]
- Oxygen therapy and consequent correction of hypoxia in suitable candidates have also been shown to improve the mitochondrial oxidative capacity in COPD patients.[120,121]
- Smoking cessation is likely to be an important aspect in improving muscle dysfunction. Chronic smoking has been associated with diverse mitochondrial respiratory chain (MRC) dysfunction in lymphocytes. In a study of MRC function in peripheral lymphocytes of 10 healthy chronic smokers before and after cessation of smoking,[122] smokers showed a significant decrease in complex IV MRC activity and respiration compared with control lymphocytes, which returned to normal values after cessation of tobacco smoking.
- Other novel therapies such as the antioxidant N-acetylcysteine[123] and peroxisome proliferator-activated receptors (such as polyunsaturated fatty acids)[120,124] are potential interventions that may improve muscle insufficiency in COPD patients, and are currently in the process of being tried and tested.

OSTEOPOROSIS

Osteoporosis is a systemic skeletal disorder characterized by low bone mineral density (BMD) and microarchitectural changes, leading to impaired bone strength and increased risk of fracture.[4]

Low BMI, advanced age, female sex, chronic use of oral corticosteroids, and endocrinologic disorders such as hyperthyroidism and primary hyperparathyroidism have all been implicated as risk factors in the development of osteoporosis in the general population.[125] Predictably, osteoporosis is a well-recognized comorbidity of COPD patients and is an important area of consideration for therapeutic interventions.[126]

The most commonly used tool to measure BMD is dual-energy x-ray absorptiometry (DEXA), which is used to define osteoporosis and provides a useful estimate of fracture risk.[127] The T score is one of the principal parameters used to measure BMD, and is calculated by subtracting the mean BMD of a young-adult reference population from the patient's BMD and dividing it by the standard deviation of the reference population. According to the World Health Organization (WHO), a T score greater than −1 is accepted as normal, T scores between −1 and −2.5 are classified as osteopenia, and T scores of less than −2.5 are defined as osteoporosis.[127]

Prevalence of Osteoporosis in COPD

The prevalence of osteoporosis in COPD varies between 4% and 59%, depending on the diagnostic methods used and the severity of the COPD population.[128]

A recent systematic review calculated an overall mean prevalence of osteoporosis of 35% from 14 articles by measuring BMD in a COPD population. The individuals in these studies had a mean age of 63 and a mean FEV_1 percent predicted of 47%.[128]

More than half of the patients with COPD recruited for the large TORCH (Toward a Revolution in COPD Health) trial (6000 patients) had osteoporosis or osteopenia as determined by DEXA scan.[129]

In another cross-sectional study, the prevalence of osteoporosis was 75% in patients with Global Initiative for Chronic Obstructive Lung Disease (GOLD) stage IV disease, and strongly correlated with reduced FFM.[130,131] Another important finding in this study was that the prevalence rate was high even for males, with an even higher incidence in postmenopausal women.

Another large cohort of 1634 COPD subjects was studied longitudinally with 259 smoker and 186 nonsmoker controls[132] in a study evaluating CT bone attenuation of the thoracic and lumber vertebrae, the extent of emphysema and coronary artery calcification on CT scans, and clinical parameters and outcomes. Bone attenuation was lower in the COPD patients than in control subjects, and correlated positively with FEV_1 ($P = .014$), FEV_1/forced vital capacity ratio ($P<.001$), FFM index ($P<.001$), and CRP ($P<.001$), and negatively with the extent of emphysema ($P<.001$). Lower CT bone attenuation was also found to be associated with higher exacerbation ($P = .022$) and hospitalization rates ($P = .002$).

In a Norwegian cross-sectional study of 1004 consecutively admitted COPD patients attending a 4-week rehabilitation program, the prevalence of vertebral deformities was found to be significantly higher in COPD patients than in the control group ($P<.0001$).[133] An increase in severity of airflow limitation from GOLD stage II to stage III was associated with an almost 2-fold increase in the average number of vertebral deformities. Of note, significant differences between COPD patients and controls were also found for pack-years ($P<.0001$), and use of calcium/vitamin D ($P<.0001$) and oral corticosteroids ($P<.0001$).

Potential Contributors to Osteoporosis in COPD

Corticosteroids

Oral glucocorticosteroids (OGCS) have both direct adverse effects on bone and indirect effects attributable to muscle weakening and atrophy.[134] OGCS are known to cause a decrease in vascular endothelial growth factor, skeletal angiogenesis, bone hydration, and strength.[135] These effects are both dose-dependent and duration-dependent. Fewer adverse effects are seen in episodic usage of OGCS in comparison with continuous use, but lower continuous doses have fewer detrimental effects on bone than frequent high-dose therapy,[136] because systemic usage of corticosteroids can cause rapid bone loss within the first few months of treatment, followed by a slower 2% to 5% loss per year with chronic use.[137] However, ICS have not been shown to aggravate the bone mineral loss in COPD patients.[138]

Inflammation

Studies suggest that COPD and associated systemic inflammation is a risk factor for osteoporosis independent of other potentiators such as age and oral corticosteroid therapy.[50,139] In a Chinese study, the presence of systemic inflammation was associated with a greater likelihood of low BMD, and multivariate logistic regression analysis showed that TNF-α and IL-6 were independent predictors of low BMD.[139] Both these factors are known to stimulate osteoclasts and increase bone resorption through receptor activator of nuclear factor (NF)-κB ligand (RANKL)-mediated bone resorption in vitro.[50,140] In addition, many other cytokines have been found to interact with the osteoprotegerin/RANKL system, supporting the concept that inflammatory mediators possibly contribute to the regulation of bone remodeling in COPD patients.[141]

Calcification paradox

Mounting data support a calcification paradox, whereby reduced BMD is associated with increased vascular calcification. Furthermore, BMD is more prevalent in older persons with lower BMI.[142] Therefore, although BMI and coronary artery calcification (CAC) exhibit a positive relationship in younger persons, it is predicted that in older persons and/or those at risk for osteoporosis, an inverse relationship between BMI and CAC may apply. Kovacic and colleagues[142] studied 9993 subjects who underwent percutaneous coronary intervention. Index lesion calcification (ILC) was analyzed with respect to BMI. In multivariable modeling, BMI was an independent inverse predictor of moderate to severe ILC (OR 0.967, 95% CI 0.953–0.980; $P<.0001$).

Therapeutic Interventions

Prevention and treatment of osteoporosis involves both pharmacologic and nonpharmacologic interventions.

Nonpharmacologic measures

Nonpharmacologic interventions include simple measures such as smoking cessation, and alcohol consumption in moderation along with good nutrition. As discussed earlier, exercise training, particularly weight-bearing and strengthening exercise performed at least 3 times per week, may be effective for maintaining skeletal health, given the association of reduced physical activity with bone loss and fracture in elderly COPD patients.[136,143,144]

Pharmacologic measures

COPD patients, with or without diagnosed osteoporosis, should be encouraged to take calcium (1000 mg/d) and vitamin D (800 IU/d) supplements routinely, as these have been shown to reduce the risk of fracture in this cohort.[126,136]

Definitive therapy is recommended in documented fragility hip or vertebral (clinical or morphometric) fracture; or T score lower than −2.5; or with less marked bone loss (T score between −1 and −2.5) and 1 major criterion (use of systemic corticosteroids [3 months/year], major fragility fracture [spine-hip] and so forth).[128,139] An oral bisphosphonate, such as alendronate and risedronate, is currently considered as the first line of treatment of osteoporosis together with vitamin D and calcium supplementation.[145,146] Bisphosphonates act by inhibiting bone resorption, and have also been shown to prevent osteoblast and osteocyte apoptosis.[145]

Anabolic drugs such as the human parathyroid hormone (PTH) analogue teriparatide (PTH_{1-34}) are also being increasingly used to treat osteoporosis in COPD patients, particularly in postmenopausal women and men with advanced osteoporosis. These agents act by stimulating bone formation through effects on osteoblasts and osteocytes, and therefore have great relevance predominantly in OGCS-induced osteoporosis.[134,147]

Efforts should be made to detect and treat low BMD in COPD patients to minimize fracture risk. Bone densitometry is widely available and should be used to screen patients at risk of low BMD, particularly those with low BMI, as current rates of detection and treatment of osteoporosis are low. Lehouck and colleagues[126] have suggested a more aggressive approach to the diagnosis and management of low BMD in COPD, and this should be widely implemented to minimize the risk of osteoporotic complications.[148] In this context the term FRAX has been described.[126] FRAX is a computer-based algorithm (http://www.shef.ac.uk/FRAX) that offers models for assessment of fracture likelihood in both men and women from the evidence provided from clinical risk factors such as age, sex, BMI, prior fragility fracture, smoking status, ethanol abuse, and prior use of corticosteroids. With FRAX, the 10-year fracture probability can be derived using these clinical risk factors, alone or in conjunction with femoral neck BMD, to enhance fracture-risk prediction and to differentiate the patients who will benefit most from definitive treatment.[149] It is hoped that FRAX will become an increasingly used tool in the future, but for the moment the identification of patients who need antiresorptive treatment remains based on clinical history, BMD, and prevalent fracture status.

NUTRITIONAL EFFECTS IN COPD

Nutritional abnormalities are also a common problem in COPD patients. There are 3 types of nutritional abnormality that occur in this population: semistarvation (low BMI with normal or above-normal FFM index), muscle atrophy (normal or above-normal BMI with low FFM index), and cachexia (low BMI with low FFM index).[150]

Prevalence and Implications

Weight loss has been reported in about 50% of patients with severe COPD and, although less common, it is still observed in about 10% to 15% of mild to moderate COPD.[5]

Several studies have shown an association between malnutrition and impaired pulmonary status in patients with COPD.[151] Poor nutritional status and consequent weight loss in these patients is known to be associated increased gas trapping, lower diffusing capacity, and lower exercise tolerance compared with their normal nourished counterparts.[152] Impairment of skeletal muscle function along with reduction in diaphragmatic mass, with a decrease in strength and endurance of the respiratory muscle that could occur in a malnourished state, have all been implicated in causing these adverse effects on pulmonary function.

Loss of skeletal muscle bulk is the main contributor to weight loss in COPD, with loss of fat mass contributing to a lesser extent.[153] It is important to recognize that if nutritional assessment includes only body weight and unintentional weight loss, some patients with normal BMI would go undetected despite being depleted of FFM.[154,155] In a cross-sectional study[154] involving 300 COPD patients requiring LTOT, 17% of patients had a low BMI, whereas the prevalence of FFM depletion was 2 times higher (around 38%).

This finding is of therapeutic importance, as improving the nutrition in COPD patients can lead to improvement in anthropometric measures and muscle strength, thus resulting in improved and better quality of life and survival rates in these patients. Post hoc analysis of COPD patients who gain weight has suggested a decrease in mortality.[156] At least one study has reported improved immune function as a result of nutritional support.[157]

Factors Contributing to Nutritional Depletion

The cause of nutritional abnormalities in COPD patients seems to be multifactorial, as with other systemic effects.[5,158] **Box 2** lists the important contributory mechanisms.

Therapeutic Interventions

Dietary intervention following a proper nutritional assessment remains one of the primary cornerstones in the management of this condition.

A meta-analysis of 13 RCTs on the effects of nutritional support in stable COPD patients[151] showed significant improvements in favor of nutritional support for body weight ($P<.001$; in 11 studies) and grip strength ($P<.050$; in 4 studies) associated with greater increases in mean total protein and energy intakes following the intervention.

Similar results have been produced by Ferreira and colleagues,[152] who assessed 17 RCTs from the Cochrane Airways Review Group Trials Register. The meta-analysis showed that nutritional supplementation produced significant weight gain in patients with COPD, especially in those who were malnourished. In the 11 RCTs that studied 325 undernourished patients, there was a mean difference of 1.65 kg (95% CI 0.14–3.16) in favor of supplementation. Nourished patients, however, may not respond to supplemental feeding to the same degree as their undernourished counterparts (1 RCT with 71 participants: standardized mean difference [SMD] of 0.27, 95% CI −0.20–0.73).

Ferreira and colleagues[152] found a significant change from baseline in FFM index (overall SMD 0.57, 95% CI 0.04–1.09), which became even more significant in undernourished patients (3 RCTs, 125 participants: SMD 1.08, 95% CI 0.70–1.47). This study also emphasized the significant improvement in respiratory muscle strength and HRQoL that occurs in undernourished patients following a nutritional intervention.

Box 2
Factors governing the nutritional depletion in COPD

- Poor nutritional intake particularly during exacerbations
- Increased metabolic rate associated with breathing problems resulting from abnormal respiratory dynamics
- Drugs such as β2-agonists increasing metabolic rate
- Chronic systemic inflammation

This nutritional intervention can be in the form of oral supplementation, enteral nutrition, or, in some extreme cases, parenteral nutrition.[158] A diet rich in protein and fat content is desirable, as an increase in fat calories with a decrease in carbohydrate calories helps to limit the amount of carbon dioxide production while still maintaining an adequate intake of protein for lean muscle mass.[158,159]

In addition, the diet of these patients should include a good supply of vitamins, minerals, and antioxidants. In this context, ω-3 fatty acid has been shown to be of some value in combating the anti-inflammatory properties of TNF-α.[158,160] Therefore, this could potentially be of novel therapeutic benefit in achieving good nutritional status in these patients.

OBESITY AND OBSTRUCTIVE SLEEP APNEA IN COPD

The prevalence of obesity, defined as BMI greater than 30 kg/m^2, has multiplied during the last decades, and varies from 10% to 20% in most European countries to 32% in the United States.[161] It plays a major role in the development of the metabolic syndrome, and has been identified as an important risk factor for chronic diseases such as type 2 diabetes mellitus and cardiovascular disease. A link between obesity and COPD is also being increasingly recognized.[162] The risk of developing obesity is increased in patients with COPD as a result of physical inactivity in daily life in these patients in comparison with healthy age-matched controls.[163] In addition, patients with COPD who receive repeated courses of systemic OGCS are at increased risk of truncal obesity as a result of steroid-mediated redistribution of stored energy and the stimulatory effect on intake.[164]

As discussed previously, low BMI is associated with increased all-cause and COPD-related mortality, unrelated to disease severity.[154] By contrast, the relative risk for mortality seems somewhat decreased in overweight and obese patients with COPD, particularly in GOLD stage 3 to 4, imparting a sort of protective effect, the so-called obesity paradox, as mortality is increased in those with disease of GOLD stage 1 to 2 with obesity traits.[156,165]

Chronic low-grade inflammation is also a hallmark of obesity, insulin resistance, and type 2 diabetes.[166,167] Besides the presence of chronic airflow obstruction, low-grade systemic inflammation could therefore be one of the common mechanisms that may be responsible for the observed mortality and morbidity in obese COPD patients.

In this context, mention should also be made of obstructive sleep apnea (OSA). OSA syndrome (ie, OSA and excessive daytime sleepiness) affects at least 4% to 5% of middle-aged persons.[168] Well-recognized risk factors include excess body weight, nasal congestion, alcohol, smoking, and menopause in women.[169]

Epidemiologic studies have shown that 20% of patients with OSA also have COPD, whereas 10% of patients with COPD have OSA independent of disease severity.[170–172] Such bidirectional interplay between OSA and COPD has been given the term overlap syndrome.[172] Possible shared mechanistic links include increased parasympathetic tone, hypoxemia-related reflex bronchoconstriction/vasoconstriction, irritation of upper airway neural receptors, altered nocturnal neurohormonal secretion, proinflammatory mediators, within-breath and interbreath interactions between upper and lower airways, and lung volume–airway dependence.[172]

Management of OSA and COPD

It is currently unclear whether long-term positive airway pressure therapy for COPD patients without OSA affects outcomes. In one such study, 122 COPD patients hospitalized with respiratory failure were randomized to LTOT versus noninvasive nocturnal ventilation (positive airway pressure) plus oxygen therapy. There was an improvement in HRQoL and reduction in length of stay in the intensive care unit in the noninvasive ventilation group, but no difference in mortality or subsequent hospitalizations was found.[173]

Thus the overlap syndrome represents a condition with important phenotypic characterization, and clarifies the frequent association, symptomatic load, and mortality consequences noted. However, the use of positive airway pressure in overlap syndrome needs further assessment.

ANEMIA IN COPD

As discussed earlier, in severe COPD, polycythemia with a raised hematocrit is known to be a common phenomenon. However, just as for other chronic conditions, COPD could also be associated with anemia.

The WHO defines anemia as a disease associated with low hemoglobin (males <13.0 g/dL and females <12 g/dL).[174]

Prevalence

Key findings of studies of anemia in COPD are summarized in **Table 3**.

A study by Rutten and colleagues[177] in the Netherlands involved 321 patients with COPD admitted for pulmonary rehabilitation, and found anemia in 20% of the patients and polycythemia in another 8%. There was no difference in disease-related outcomes or other comorbidities in the patients with and without anemia. However, after adjustment for confounders, anemia was found to be an independent determinant for higher CRP levels and lower BMD.

Low blood count can also be defined by hematocrit (<39% in men and <36% in women). In a French study involving severe COPD patients who required LTOT, a reduced hematocrit level was associated with increased mortality, whereas a raised hematocrit level was protective, independent of other markers of mortality.[176]

Pathogenesis

The anemia of chronic illness is typically a normocytic anemia and is most commonly observed in patients with infectious disease, and inflammatory or neoplastic diseases.

COPD fulfills the criteria of a chronic, inflammatory, multisystem disease that would be expected to result in anemia. John and colleagues[175] studied 101 COPD patients and determined the prevalence of anemia and its relationship to body mass and weight loss, inflammatory parameters, and erythropoietin levels. Anemia was diagnosed in 13 patients (12.8%). These patients showed elevated erythropoietin levels and had increased systemic inflammation markers (raised CRP) in comparison with the nonanemic patients. This finding raises the possibility that erythropoietin resistance, as is possible in the COPD cohort, is potentially mediated by chronic inflammation.

Management

As for any other anemia of chronic disease, treatment of the underlying disease is the therapeutic approach of choice for anemia in COPD.[178]

The level of hemoglobin is strongly and independently associated with increased functional dyspnea and poorer exercise tolerance, and is therefore an important contributor to poor quality of life.[43] Schönhofer and colleagues[179] demonstrated that correction of anemia with blood transfusions (among 20 patients with severe COPD) significantly reduced disease-related elevations in minute ventilation and

Table 3
PubMed search: anemia/anemia AND COPD OR chronic obstructive pulmonary disease in title/abstract

Authors,Ref. Year	Journal	Study Type	Prevalence (%)	Outcome	Comment
John et al,[175] 2005	Chest	Prospective (N = 101)	13/101 = 13	No outcome data EPO resistance?	Outpatients
John et al, 2006	Int J Cardiol	Retrospective hospital records (N = 312)	23	No outcome data	COPD hospitalized
Cote et al,[43] 2007	Eur Respir J	Prospective cohort (N = 677)	116/677 = 17	Independent predictor dyspnea	COPD outpatients
Chambellan et al,[176] 2005	Chest	Retrospective database (N = 2524)	M: 12.6, F: 8.2	Hb as outcome predictor	LTOT
Krishnan et al, 2006	BMC Pulm Med	Post hoc analysis from general population (N = 495)	7.5	Anemia associated with worse HRQoL	No outcome
Schonhofer et al, 1998	Crit Care Med	Prospective 20 anemic adults (10 COPD)	—	Correction of Hb improves breathing pattern and efficacy	No outcome
Kollert et al, 2011	IJCP	Retrospective hospital record database (N = 326)	14.7	Determinants of anemia: pH, $Pa{O_2}$	No outcome
Boutou et al, 2011	Respiration	Prospective, 283 stable COPD	10	Association with dyspnea and exercise capacity	Good patient selection
Rasmussen et al, 2010	Clin Epidemiol	Retrospective hospital records (N = 222)	42/222 = 18	Increased mortality at 90 d	Mechanically ventilated
Markoulaki et al, 2011	Eur J Intern Med	Prospective observational 93 acute exacerbated COPD	NA	Hb decreased, EPO increased	No outcome
Similkowski et al, 2006	Eur Respir J	NA	10–15	Mechanisms of anemia Therapeutic implications	Review
Barnes & Celli,[6] 2009	Eur Respir J	NA	15–30	Impaired functional capacity Mortality predictor	Review

Abbreviations: EPO, erythropoietin; Hb, hemoglobin; HRQoL, health-related quality of life; LTOT, long-term oxygen therapy; NA, no data available; $Pa{O_2}$, partial pressure of oxygen in arterial blood.

work of breathing, suggesting that anemia correction may be beneficial in alleviating dyspnea and improving exercise capacity. Therefore, blood transfusion in selected cases may be necessary, as erythropoietin is unlikely to work in this cohort because of end-organ resistance. Iron supplements, likewise, are unlikely to be useful and possibly could have a deleterious effect by adding to the burden of systemic oxidative stress.[6]

Autonomic Dysfunction

The autonomic nervous system (ANS) controls physiologic processes such as regulation of the airway smooth muscle tone, fluid transport through the airway epithelium, capillary permeability, bronchial circulation, and release of mediators from inflammatory cells.[180] Autonomic dysfunction (AD) is a known phenomenon in COPD patients,[181] and may be an important factor in the pathogenesis of the disease because of the multiple parameters that are under control of the ANS such as the arterial and cardiac baroreceptors,[182] the bronchopulmonary C fibers, and pulmonary stretch receptors, which are capable of triggering ventilation, bronchomotor, and cardiovascular effects.[183,184]

Recurrent hypoxemia, hypercapnea, increased intrathoracic pressure swings resulting from airway obstruction, increased respiratory effort, and systemic inflammation along with the use of β-sympathomimetics have all been implicated as trigger factors for AD as observed in COPD.[181]

Prevalence and Clinical Implications

Tug and colleagues[185] assessed the prevalence of AD according to disease severity in 35 stable COPD patients. Sympathetic system (SS) was evaluated with sympathetic skin response (SSR), and QT- and QTc-interval (milliseconds) analyses. The parasympathetic system was evaluated with the variations in heart-rate interval. AD was detected in 20 patients (57%), parasympathetic dysfunction (PD) in 14 (40%), mixed-type dysfunction in 5 (14%), and sympathetic dysfunction (SD) in only 1 patient (3%). For the 12 patients with mild COPD, there were cases of isolated SD in 1 patient (8.5%), isolated PD in 5 (42%), and AD in 6 (50%). For the 23 moderate to severe COPD patients, mixed AD was detected in 5 patients (22%), isolated PD in 9 (39%), and AD in 14 (61%).

This imbalance in the autonomic nervous activity can contribute to airway narrowing via an effect on the airway smooth muscle, bronchial vessels, and mucous glands in the bronchial wall, and therefore could add to disease progression and severity.

Correction of hypoxia and control of the systemic inflammation seem reasonable target strategies that may help to improve health status in COPD patients.

LUNG CANCER AND COPD

With a shared common environmental risk factor in exposure to cigarette smoke, it is understandable why lung cancer is one of the most frequent comorbidities and one of the commonest causes of death in COPD patients.

Prevalence

Previous studies have shown that COPD is an independent risk factor for the development of lung cancer and that having moderate to severe COPD can increase the risk of developing lung cancer up to almost 5-fold.[186,187]

Thirty-eight percent of deaths in individuals with mild to moderate airflow limitation in the Lung Health Study died of lung cancer.[10] In addition to these 57 deaths, another 35 participants were diagnosed with the disease but survived to the end of follow-up.

An inverse correlation between the degree of airflow obstruction and the risk for lung cancer was demonstrated in an analysis of 22-year follow-up data of 5402 participants from the first National Health and Nutrition Examination Survey (NHANES I), including a total of 113 cases of lung cancer.[188] Tockman and colleagues[189] and Skillrud and colleagues[190] have previously demonstrated that the incidence of lung cancer increased in individuals with COPD as their FEV_1 declined, a relationship that with-stood correction for lifetime cigarette smoke dosage.

Fig. 4 summarizes the inverse relationship observed between lung cancer and lung function values as seen in COPD patients.[188] Unsurprisingly, lung cancer along with cardiovascular diseases comprises two-thirds of all deaths in COPD patients.[191]

Recent studies also indicate that emphysema and airflow limitation are risk factors for lung cancer, independent of exposure to cigarette smoke.[192] Cross-sectional studies have shown that after allowing for cigarette-smoke exposure, reduced FEV_1 (as seen in COPD) is the single most important risk factor for lung cancer, and that these 2 diseases are linked by more than smoking exposure alone.[188,193]

An Italian study has also shown that airflow limitation is primarily a risk factor for squamous cell lung cancer (95% CI 1.63–18.5; $P = .006$), whereas symptoms of chronic bronchitis without COPD is a risk factor (risk greater than 4-fold) for adenocarcinoma of the lung. In a subset analysis, the association of concurrent bronchitic symptoms and COPD imparted a 3-fold increased risk for squamous cell carcinoma of the lung, further consolidating the link between these 2 conditions.[194]

Pathogenesis and Clinical Implications of Lung Cancer in COPD

The pathogenic mechanism linking these conditions remains unclear, although like other comorbidities in COPD it seems to be multifactorial.

Inflammation and oxidative stress seem to play important roles. The process of epithelial-to-mesenchymal transition (EMT), in which cells undergo a switch from an epithelial phenotype to a mesenchymal phenotype, is an important phenomenon that occurs in both patients with lung cancer and COPD patients.[195,196]

Studies have also shown that inflammation directly promotes EMT by inducing the expression of E-cadherin transcriptional repressors, which could explain the

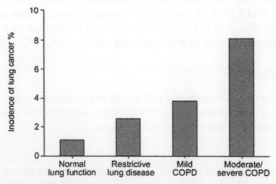

Fig. 4. Inverse relationship between degree of lung function obstruction and incidence of lung cancer. (*Reproduced* with permission of the European Respiratory Society. Sin DD, Anthonisen NR, Soriano JB, et al. Mortality in COPD: role of comorbidities. Eur Respir J 2006;28(6);1250; http://dx.doi.org/10.1183/09031936.00133805.)

connecting link between these 2 conditions.[187,196] An exaggerated inflammatory response, leading to aberrant airway epithelial and matrix remodeling characterized by excessive growth factor release and elevated matrix metalloproteinases (MMP), has also been postulated as a possible mechanism connecting the 2 conditions.[197,198]

NF-κB activation has also been suggested as a link between inflammation and lung cancer.[199] Synergistic effects of latent infection and cigarette smoking cause chronic airway inflammation through enhanced expression of cytokines and adhesion molecules, possibly through NF-κB–mediated activation.[200,201] Some of the cytokines can also inhibit apoptosis, interfering with cellular repair and promoting angiogenesis.[202]

Retrospective studies have also suggested that reducing pulmonary inflammation with ICS or systemic inflammation with statin therapy may reduce the risk of lung cancer in COPD patients, adding further support for a role for inflammation as a common link in both of these conditions.[203,204]

Studies have also suggested specific candidate gene loci as potential genetic links connecting lung cancer and COPD.[205,206] The genes identified in these studies suggest that this common genetic susceptibility may be mediated through receptors expressed on the bronchial epithelium that implicate common molecular pathways underlying both COPD and lung cancer.

The transcription factor, nuclear factor erythroid 2-related factor 2 (Nrf2), which regulates multiple antioxidant and detoxifying genes, has been shown to be downregulated in COPD lungs[207] and may contribute to the increased susceptibility of COPD patients to lung cancer, because Nrf2 plays an important role in defense against carcinogens in tobacco smoke by regulating the expression of several detoxifying enzymes.[208] Epidermal growth factor receptor (EGFR), which promotes epithelial proliferation, also has increased expression in the lungs of COPD patients, which could promote carcinogenesis.[209]

As the increased risk of lung cancer in COPD may be a reflection of increased inflammation and oxidative stress in the lungs, anti-inflammatory therapies or antioxidants should hypothetically diminish the risk of lung cancer.

PSYCHOLOGICAL EFFECTS IN COPD

Anxiety and depression are common in patients with COPD, and have an impact on the psychosocial aspects of the management of this disease. Prognostic studies involving patients with COPD have mostly focused on physiologic variables, with less attention given to the psychological aspects of the disease.

Prevalence

The prevalence of generalized anxiety disorder in COPD patients ranges between 10% and 33%, and that of panic attacks or panic disorder between 8% and 67%.[210] Disease severity in COPD has not clearly been associated with the magnitude of anxiety/depression.[211,212]

Estimates of the prevalence of depression and depressive symptoms vary in COPD patients, ranging from 6% to 60%.[213–215] Hanania and colleagues[216] studied the prevalence and determinants of depression in COPD patient in the ECLIPSE study. The study cohort consisted of 2118 subjects with COPD, 335 smokers without COPD (smokers), and 243 nonsmokers without COPD (nonsmokers). A total of 26%, 12%, and 7% of COPD, smokers, and nonsmokers, respectively, suffered from depression. Using a multivariate logistic regression model, increased fatigue, higher score for St George's Respiratory Questionnaire for COPD patients, younger age, female sex, history of cardiovascular disease, and current smoking status were all significantly associated with depression in this cohort.

Clinical Implications

Depression in COPD might result from a vicious cycle of sedentary lifestyle, smoking habits, and poor nutritional and health status. There is increasing evidence that inflammation itself could be a mediator of depression in COPD patients.[217] Depressive symptoms were found to be strong predictors of mortality (OR 1.9, 3.6, and 2.7, respectively), independent of other markers of disease severity and risk factors, in COPD patients in 3 studies,[218–220] whereas one other study found no association between mortality and depression after adjustment for disease severity.[221]

Therefore, the effect of depression on function in COPD patients and the early recognition and treatment of symptoms remain inherent important aspects in the management of this cohort.

DIABETES AND METABOLIC SYNDROME IN COPD
Prevalence and Pathogenesis

Studies have shown prevalence rates for diabetes of between 1% and 16% in patients with COPD.[222,223] Large population studies have also shown that there is an increased prevalence of diabetes among COPD patients (risk ratio [RR] 1.5–1.8), even in patients with mild disease.[6,224]

Poulain and colleagues[225] looked at a cohort of 28 male patients with COPD, and divided patients according to their body habitus. The study showed that presence of obesity, particularly abdominal obesity, was associated with metabolic and inflammatory abnormalities that are typically associated with the development of cardiovascular diseases and diabetes, such as increased levels of insulin, TNF-α, and IL-6, and may mediate insulin resistance by blocking signaling through the insulin receptor. This finding further cements the common inflammatory pathway theory in the pathogenesis of the systemic effects of COPD.

Rana and colleagues[224] also performed a prospective cohort study in which they looked at the relationship of COPD and asthma with the development of type 2 diabetes. During 8 years of follow-up, a total of 2959 new cases of type 2 diabetes were documented. The risk was significantly higher for patients with COPD than for those without (multivariate RR 1.8, 95% CI 1.1–2.8), but this was not the case among the asthmatics. This finding would further corroborate the fact that COPD is potentially a risk factor for the development of diabetes.

Management and Clinical Implications

Hyperglycemia, especially during acute exacerbations of COPD, is associated with poorer outcomes of acute noninvasive ventilation,[226] longer inpatient stay, and higher rates of in-hospital mortality.[148,227] Therefore, it is important to identify underlying hyperglycemic status in COPD patients to reduce the burden of morbidity and mortality as well as unnecessary utilization of health care resources.

The metabolic syndrome is a complex disorder and an emerging clinical challenge, recognized clinically by the findings of abdominal obesity, elevated triglycerides, atherogenic dyslipidemia, elevated blood pressure, and high blood glucose and/or insulin resistance.[228] It is also associated with a prothrombotic state and a proinflammatory state. Patients with COPD often have 1 or more components of the metabolic syndrome,[228] which are, at least in part, independent of treatment with steroids and/or physical inactivity.[229]

Clini and colleagues[230] also postulated that the metabolic syndrome was more likely to be present in COPD patients, as augmented levels of circulatory proinflammatory proteins from both the lung and adipose tissue (adipokines) overlap in these patients. This coexistence perhaps rests on several factors including the presence of physical inactivity, systemic inflammation partly related to smoking habit, sedentary lifestyle, airway inflammation, adipose tissue, and inflammatory marker activation, among others.

Apart from the risks per se from high glucose level already described, COPD patients with hyperglycemia are likely to have more than one species of bacteria grown from sputum, suggesting impaired immunity.[148] Although some nondiabetic COPD patients have hyperglycemia induced by systemic corticosteroids during exacerbations, this is more likely in the context of diabetes, therefore oral hypoglycemic medications or insulin may be a necessity.

Preventive measures include lifestyle advice including dietary guidance, and regular screening of those at higher risk, given the higher prevalence and adverse clinical impact of diabetes on COPD patients. This approach would potentially enable earlier diagnosis and prevention of complications.

There should also be more focus on global interventions intended at altering factors such as physical deconditioning and obesity, as such an approach may help slow the metabolic complications seen in COPD patients, particularly those with features of the metabolic syndrome.

SYSTEMIC INFLAMMATION IN COPD

As described earlier, systemic inflammation is a well-established occurrence in COPD patients. Numerous studies have provided evidence of systemic inflammation in COPD patients, as shown by the presence of inflammatory mediators such as acute-phase proteins, as well as markers of oxidative stress and immune responses that are increased in the peripheral blood in COPD patients in comparison with smokers who have not developed the disease.[231–233]

However, the presence of systemic inflammation is poorly defined in COPD patients; most studies have been cross-sectional and indicate that not all COPD patients have a systemic inflammatory response. Systemic inflammation, as already discussed, is a known risk factor for developing many of the conditions described conventionally as comorbidities of COPD.[222,231,234,235] Smoking, a major cause of airway inflammation in COPD, is known to be associated with systemic inflammation, and is a potential link between the pulmonary and systemic inflammation in COPD and its comorbidities.[232,236–240] Smoking and reduced FEV_1 also have been found to have an additive effect on systemic inflammatory markers.[241]

While increasing evidence suggests that the systemic inflammatory pathway provides the common link between COPD and its comorbidities,[234,236,239,242] the mechanisms by which the systemic inflammation arises are unclear. There is much debate around whether the systemic inflammation in COPD arises from a spill-over of inflammatory mediators from lung inflammation,[6,231,243] or whether the systemic inflammation in COPD represents a systemic component of the disease that develops in parallel with, or before, pulmonary inflammation.[231,243] The absence of a relationship between inflammatory biomarkers in the sputum and blood of COPD patients has provided some evidence against the spill-over theory.[231,237,244] Smoking, lung hyperinflation, tissue hypoxia, skeletal muscle, bone marrow stimulation, immunologic disorders, and infections are all cited as possible sources of systemic inflammation as seen in COPD.[231,242,245]

Several studies and meta-analyses have shown that in patients with stable COPD there are often elevated levels of systemic inflammatory markers, such as increased circulating leukocytes, CRP, IL-6, IL-8, fibrinogen, and TNF-α.[233,234,245–247] **Table 4** summarizes the various inflammatory mediators as described in COPD.

However, the prevalence of systemic inflammation in COPD has not been well studied, and many of the earlier published data are derived from short-term, cross-sectional studies with small sample sizes.[256] These studies show a wide intersubject validation in systemic biomarkers. Moreover, there is no agreed consensus on the type, number, and value of inflammatory biomarkers needed to define systemic inflammation. These cross-sectional studies are unable to fully establish the relationship between biomarkers and key health outcomes, owing to the chronic nature of COPD and its comorbidities. Data from the Evaluation of COPD Longitudinally to Identify Predictive Surrogate Endpoints (ECLIPSE) study[257] in more than 2000 COPD patients, control smokers, and nonsmokers assessed longitudinally over 3 years was used to evaluate systemic inflammatory biomarkers. Many systemic inflammatory biomarkers were found to be reproducible over time, with fibrinogen being the most repeatable.[258] As shown in other studies, differences in several biomarkers can be

Table 4
Mediators of systemic inflammation in COPD

	Mediators	Actions
Cytokines	Interleukin (IL)-6	Cardiovascular and skeletal muscle dysfunction[6,21]
	Tumor necrosis factor (TNF)-α	Metabolic and skeletal muscle dysfunction (SMD)[113,114,139]
	IL-1β	Cachexia in COPD[6]
	CXCL8 (IL-8) and other CXC chemokines	Neutrophil and monocyte recruitment and also contributes to SMD[6]
	Adipokines such as leptins	Possible role in cachexia in COPD[6]
Acute-phase proteins	C-reactive protein	Raised in infective exacerbations potentiates cardiovascular effects and SMD[4,118]
	Fibrinogen	Cardiovascular complications[40,41]
	Surfactant protein D	Derived from lung tissue; is a good marker of lung inflammation[248]
	Serum amyloid A (SA-A)	Released by circulating proinflammatory cytokines, SA-A levels are raised during acute exacerbations of COPD and its concentrations are correlated with the severity of exacerbation[6,249]
Circulating cells	Neutrophils	Inverse correlation between neutrophil numbers in the circulation and FEV$_1$,[250] increased turnover in smokers,[6] enhanced production of reactive oxygen species[251]
	Monocytes	Increase macrophage accumulation in the lungs with defective phagocytic property,[6] increase matrix metalloproteinase-9 production compared with nonsmokers[252]
	Lymphocytes	Increased apoptosis of peripheral T lymphocytes from COPD patients, with increased expression of Fas, TNF-α, and transforming growth factor β,[6,253] increase in apoptosis of CD8$^+$ T cells in COPD[254]
	Natural killer (NK) cells	Reduction of cytotoxic and phagocytic function of circulating NK cells has been reported in COPD[6,255]

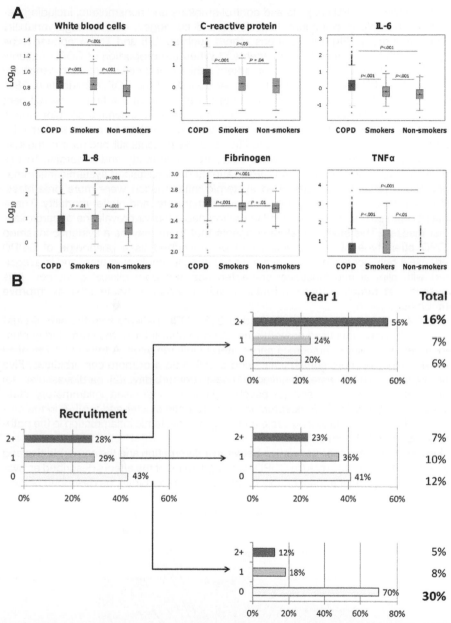

Fig. 5. (*A*) Box plot (log scale) of the different biomarkers determined at baseline in COPD patients, smokers with normal lung function (S), and nonsmokers (NS). IL, interleukin; TNF, tumor necrosis factor. (*B*) Proportion of patients with no, 1, or 2 (or more) biomarkers (white blood cell count, C-reactive protein, interleukin-6, and fibrinogen) in the upper quartile of the COPD distribution, at baseline (*left bars*) and after 1 year of follow-up (*right bars*). (*From* Agusti A, Edwards LD, Rennard SI, et al. Persistent systemic inflammation is associated with poor clinical outcomes in COPD: a novel phenotype. PLoS One 2012;7(5):e37483.)

shown between COPD subjects and control smokers and nonsmokers, including peripheral white blood cell count, IL-6, CRP, and fibrinogen, despite large variability within each group (**Fig. 5**A), whereas others such as IL-8 and TNF-α appear to be higher in smokers than in COPD patients.[20] When the proportion of COPD patients with 0, 1, or 2 (or more) of these biomarkers (white blood cell count, high-sensitivity CRP, IL-6, and fibrinogen) were in the upper quartile of the COPD distribution, 28% of patients had 2 or more of these biomarkers elevated at the time of recruitment and 56% of these subjects still had 2 or more systemic inflammatory biomarkers elevated at 1 year (see **Fig. 5**B), whereas 43% of patients had no raised systemic inflammatory biomarkers at baseline and 70% of these patients still had none of the systemic biomarkers elevated at 1 year. Thus, from this study and according to this definition, approximately 16% of COPD patients have sustained systemic inflammation. Those patients with sustained systemic inflammation were more breathless, with poorer exercise capacity, higher exacerbation rate, and higher mortality. Those patients with sustained systemic inflammation had a higher prevalence of cardiovascular disease. This study therefore suggests that there may be a systemic inflamed COPD phenotype of COPD, which can be described as a phenotype of COPD because it only occurs in a percentage of patients, is stable over time, and is associated with clinical and functional characteristics and poor clinical outcomes. It is possible that targeting these individuals with appropriate treatment may improve outcomes.

Vanfleteren and colleagues[259] looked at 213 COPD patients with the aim of clustering 13 clinically identified comorbidities, and to characterize the comorbidity clusters in terms of clinical outcomes and systemic inflammation. A total of 97.7% of all patients had 1 or more comorbidities and 53.5% had 4 or more comorbidities. Five comorbidity clusters were identified: (1) less comorbidity, (2) cardiovascular, (3) cachectic, (4) metabolic, and (5) psychological. An increased inflammatory state was observed only for TNF receptors in the metabolic cluster and for IL-6 in the cardiovascular cluster, suggesting a role for low-grade systemic inflammation in the pathogenesis of COPD comorbidities.

Fig. 6 summarizes the interrelation between inflammation and the comorbidities and systemic effects as observed in COPD, although some of the effects described as systemic could also be interchangeably described as comorbidity, as described earlier.

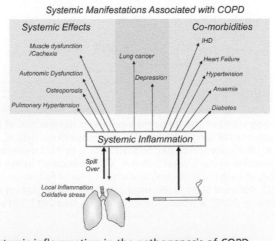

Fig. 6. Role of systemic inflammation in the pathogenesis of COPD.

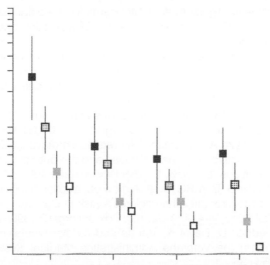

Fig. 7. The impact of comorbidities on all-cause mortality in COPD patients. Prediction of all-cause mortality within 5 years of COPD patients by modified GOLD category and the presence of no (▦), 1 (□), 2 (▨), or 3 (■) comorbid diseases (diabetes, hypertension, or cardiovascular disease). The reference group (normal) was subjects with normal lung function for each comorbid disease. Models were adjusted for age, sex, race, smoking status, education level, and body mass index. Subjects were from the Atherosclerosis Risk in Communities Study during 1986 to 1989 and the Cardiovascular Health Study during 1989 to 1990. GOLD 3/4: forced expiratory volume in 1 second (FEV_1)/forced vital capacity (FVC) <0.70 and FEV_1 <50% predicted; GOLD 2: FEV_1/FVC <0.70 and FEV_1 ≥50 to <80% predicted; GOLD 1: FEV_1/FVC <0.70 and FEV_1 ≥80% predicted; restricted (R): FEV_1/FVC ≥0.70 and FVC <80% predicted; GOLD 0: presence of respiratory symptoms in the absence of any lung function abnormality and no lung disease. (*Reproduced* with permission of the European Respiratory Society. Mannino DM, Thorn D, Swensen A, et al. Prevalence and outcomes of diabetes, hypertension and cardiovascular disease in COPD. Eur Respir J 2008;32(4):967; http://dx.doi.org/10.1183/09031936.00012408.)

SUMMARY

The extrapulmonary effects of COPD are truly multifarious, and have an adverse effect on function and outcomes in COPD.

Fig. 7 summarizes the impact of comorbidities on all-cause mortality in COPD patients.

The clinical management of this condition should therefore be directed toward identifying and treating these extrapulmonary effects, which may lead to improved outcomes for this condition. Novel therapies particularly targeted toward the inflammation associated with COPD should be developed.

REFERENCES

1. Murray CJ, Lopez AD. Alternative projections of mortality and disability by cause 1990-2020: Global Burden of Disease Study. Lancet 1997;349:1498–504.
2. Chapman KR, Mannino DM, Soriano JB, et al. Epidemiology and costs of chronic obstructive pulmonary disease. Eur Respir J 2006;27:188–207. http://dx.doi.org/10.1183/09031936.06.00024505.

3. Celli BR, MacNee W, Agusti A, et al. Standards for the diagnosis and treatment of patients with COPD: a summary of the ATS/ERS position paper. Eur Respir J 2004;23(6):932–46.

4. MacNee W. Systemic inflammatory biomarkers and co-morbidities of chronic obstructive pulmonary disease. Ann Med 2012;45:291–300.

5. Agusti AG. Systemic effects of chronic obstructive pulmonary disease. Proc Am Thorac Soc 2005;2(4):367–70 [discussion: 371–2].

6. Barnes PJ, Celli BR. Systemic manifestations and comorbidities of COPD. Eur Respir J 2009;33:1165–85. http://dx.doi.org/10.1183/09031936.00128008.

7. Ghoorah K, De Soyza A, Kunadian V. Increased cardiovascular risk in patients with chronic obstructive pulmonary disease and the potential mechanisms linking the two conditions: a review. Cardiol Rev 2013;21:196–202.

8. Agarwal SK, Heiss G, Barr RG, et al. Airflow obstruction, lung function, and risk of incident heart failure: the Atherosclerosis Risk in Communities (ARIC) study. Eur J Heart Fail 2012;14(4):414–22. http://dx.doi.org/10.1093/eurjhf/hfs016.

9. Mapel DW, Dedrick D, Davis K. Trends and cardiovascular co-morbidities of COPD patients in the Veterans Administration Medical System, 1991-1999. COPD 2005;2(1):35–41.

10. Anthonisen NR, Connett JE, Enright PL, et al, Lung Health Study Research Group. Hospitalizations and mortality in the Lung Health Study. Am J Respir Crit Care Med 2002;166(3):333–9.

11. Divo M, Cote C, de Torres JP, et al. Comorbidities and risk of mortality in patients with chronic obstructive pulmonary disease. Am J Respir Crit Care Med 2012; 186(2):155–61. http://dx.doi.org/10.1164/rccm.201201-0034OC.

12. Holguin F, Folch E, Redd SC, et al. Comorbidity and mortality in COPD-related hospitalizations in the United States, 1979 to 2001. Chest 2005;128:2005–11.

13. Bang KM, Gergen PJ, Kramer R, et al. The effect of pulmonary impairment on all-cause mortality in a national cohort. Chest 1993;103(2):536–40.

14. Campo G, Guastaroba P, Marzocchi A, et al. Impact of chronic obstructive pulmonary disease on long-term outcome after ST-segment elevation myocardial infarction receiving primary percutaneous coronary intervention. Chest 2013. http://dx.doi.org/10.1378/chest.12-2313.

15. Hole DJ, Watt GC, Davey-Smith G, et al. Impaired lung function and mortality risk in men and women: finding from the Renfrew and Paisley prospective population study. BMJ 1996;313:711–5 [discussion: 715–6].

16. Sin DD, Man SF. Why are patients with chronic obstructive pulmonary disease at increased risk of cardiovascular diseases? The potential role of systemic inflammation in chronic obstructive pulmonary disease. Circulation 2003;107(11): 1514–9.

17. Iwamoto H, Yokoyama A, Kitahara Y, et al. Airflow limitation in smokers is associated with subclinical atherosclerosis. Am J Respir Crit Care Med 2009;179(1): 35–40.

18. van Gestel YR, Flu WJ, van Kuijk JP, et al. Association of COPD with carotid wall intima-media thickness in vascular surgery patients. Respir Med 2010;104(5): 712–6.

19. Ross R. The pathogenesis of atherosclerosis: a perspective for the 1990s. Nature 1993;362(6423):801–9.

20. Agusti A, Edwards LD, Rennard SI, et al, Evaluation of COPD Longitudinally to Identify Predictive Surrogate End-points (ECLIPSE) Investigators. Persistent systemic inflammation is associated with poor clinical outcomes in COPD: a novel phenotype. PLoS One 2012;7(5):e37483.

21. Celli BR, Locantore N, Yates J, et al, ECLIPSE Investigators. Inflammatory bio-markers improve clinical prediction of mortality in chronic obstructive pulmonary disease. Am J Respir Crit Care Med 2012;185(10):1065–72.
22. McAllister DA, Maclay JD, Mills NL, et al. Diagnosis of myocardial infarction following hospitalisation for exacerbation of COPD. Eur Respir J 2012;39: 1097–103. http://dx.doi.org/10.1183/09031936.00124811.
23. Hurst JR, Donaldson GC, Perera WR, et al. Use of plasma biomarkers at exac-erbation of chronic obstructive pulmonary disease. Am J Respir Crit Care Med 2006;174(8):867–74.
24. Maclay JD, MacNee W. Cardiovascular disease in COPD: mechanisms. Chest 2013;143(3):798–807. http://dx.doi.org/10.1378/chest.12-0938.
25. Libby P, Theroux P. Pathophysiology of coronary artery disease. Circulation 2005;111(25):3481–8.
26. Coulson JM, Rudd JH, Duckers JM, et al. Excessive aortic inflammation in chronic obstructive pulmonary disease: an 18 F-FDG PET pilot study. J Nucl Med 2010;51(9):1357–60.
27. Lattimore J, Wilcox I, Nakhla S, et al. Repetitive hypoxia increases lipid loading in human macrophages—a potentially atherogenic effect. Atherosclerosis 2005; 179(2):255–9.
28. Ichikawa H, Flores S, Kvietys PR, et al. Molecular mechanisms of anoxia/reoxygenation-induced neutrophil adherence to cultured endothelial cells. Circ Res 1997;81(6):922–31.
29. Hartmann G, Tschöp M, Fischer R, et al. High altitude increases circulating interleukin-6, interleukin-1 receptor antagonist and C-reactive protein. Cytokine 2000;12(3):246–52.
30. Savransky V, Nanayakkara A, Li J, et al. Chronic intermittent hypoxia induces atherosclerosis. Am J Respir Crit Care Med 2007;175(12):1290–7.
31. Chen L, Einbinder E, Zhang Q, et al. Oxidative stress and left ventricular func-tion with chronic intermittent hypoxia in rats. Am J Respir Crit Care Med 2005; 172(7):915–20.
32. Thomson AJ, Drummond GB, Waring WS, et al. Effects of short-term isocapnic hyperoxia and hypoxia on cardiovascular function. J Appl Physiol 2006;101: 809–16.
33. Skwarski KM, Morrison D, Barratt A, et al. Effects of hypoxia on renal hormonal balance in normal subjects and in patients with COPD. Respir Med 1998;92(12): 1331–6.
34. Heindl S, Lehnert M, Criée CP, et al. Marked sympathetic activation in patients with chronic respiratory failure. Am J Respir Crit Care Med 2001;164: 597–601.
35. Curtis BM, O'Keefe JH Jr. Autonomic tone as a cardiovascular risk factor: the dangers of chronic fight or flight. Mayo Clin Proc 2002;77:45–54.
36. Cordero A, Bertomeu-Martínez V, Mazón P, et al. Clinical features and hospital complications of patients with acute coronary syndromes according to smoking habits. Med Clin (Barc) 2012;138(10):422–8. http://dx.doi.org/10.1016/j.medcli. 2011.01.016.
37. Bernhard D, Wang XL. Smoking, oxidative stress and cardiovascular dis-eases—do anti-oxidative therapies fail? Curr Med Chem 2007;14:1703–12.
38. Brook RD, Rajagopalan S. Particulate matter, air pollution, and blood pressure. J Am Soc Hypertens 2009;3:332–50.
39. Talukder MA, Johnson WM, Varadharaj S, et al. Chronic cigarette smoking causes hypertension, increased oxidative stress, impaired NO bioavailability,

endothelial dysfunction, and cardiac remodeling in mice. Am J Physiol Heart Circ Physiol 2011;300(1):H388–96.

40. Alessandri C, Basili S, Violi F, et al. Chronic Obstructive Bronchitis and Haemostasis Group. Hypercoagulability state in patients with chronic obstructive pulmonary disease. Thromb Haemost 1994;72(3):343–6.

41. Ashitani JI, Mukae H, Arimura Y, et al. Elevated plasma procoagulant and fibrinolytic markers in patients with chronic obstructive pulmonary disease. Intern Med 2002;41(3):181–5.

42. Libby P. Inflammation in atherosclerosis. Nature 2002;420(6917):868–74.

43. Cote C, Zilberberg MD, Mody SH, et al. Haemoglobin level and its clinical impact in a cohort of patients with COPD. Eur Respir J 2007;29:923–9.

44. Weber FP. The prognostic significance of secondary polycythaemia in cardio-pulmonary cases. Proc R Soc Med 1913;6:83–98.

45. Minet C, Vivodtzev I, Tamisier R, et al. Reduced six-minute walking distance, high fat-free-mass index and hypercapnia are associated with endothelial dysfunction in COPD. Respir Physiol Neurobiol 2012;183(2):128–34. http://dx.doi.org/10.1016/j.resp.2012.06.017.

46. Barr RG, Mesia-Vela S, Austin JH, et al. Impaired flow mediated dilation is associated with low pulmonary function and emphysema in ex-smokers: the Emphysema and Cancer Action Project (EMCAP) Study. Am J Respir Crit Care Med 2007;176:1200–7.

47. Eickhoff P, Valipour A, Kiss D, et al. Determinants of systemic vascular function in patients with stable chronic obstructive pulmonary disease. Am J Respir Crit Care Med 2008;178:1211–8.

48. Maclay JD, McAllister DA, Mills NL, et al. Vascular dysfunction in chronic obstructive pulmonary disease. Am J Respir Crit Care Med 2009;180:513–20.

49. Vlachopoulos C, Aznaouridis K, Stefanadis C. Prediction of cardiovascular events and all-cause mortality with arterial stiffness: a systematic review and meta-analysis. J Am Coll Cardiol 2010;55:1318–27.

50. Sabit R, Bolton CE, Edwards PH, et al. Arterial stiffness and osteoporosis in chronic obstructive pulmonary disease. Am J Respir Crit Care Med 2007;175(12):1259–65.

51. Mills NL, Miller JJ, Anand A, et al. Increased arterial stiffness in patients with chronic obstructive pulmonary disease: a mechanism for increased cardiovascular risk. Thorax 2008;63(4):306–11.

52. McAllister DA, Maclay JD, Mills NL, et al. Arterial stiffness is independently associated with emphysema severity in patients with chronic obstructive pulmonary disease. Am J Respir Crit Care Med 2007;176:1208–14.

53. Maclay JD, McAllister DA, Rabinovich R, et al. Systemic elastin degradation in chronic obstructive pulmonary disease. Thorax 2012;67:606–12.

54. Rutten FH, Cramer MJ, Grobbee DE, et al. Unrecognized heart failure in elderly patients with stable chronic obstructive pulmonary disease. Eur Heart J 2005;26(18):1887–94.

55. Boudestein LC, Rutten FH, Cramer MJ, et al. The impact of concurrent heart failure on prognosis in patients with chronic obstructive pulmonary disease. Eur J Heart Fail 2009;11(12):1182–8. http://dx.doi.org/10.1093/eurjhf/hfp148.

56. Mascarenhas J, Lourenco P, Lopes R, et al. Chronic obstructive pulmonary disease in heart failure. Prevalence, therapeutic and prognostic implications. Am Heart J 2008;155:521–5.

57. De Blois J, Simard S, Atar D, et al. COPD predicts mortality in heart failure: the Norwegian Heart Failure Registry. J Card Fail 2010;16:225–9.

58. Iversen KK, Kjaergaard J, Akkan D, et al. The prognostic importance of lung function in patients admitted with heart failure. Eur J Heart Fail 2010;12(7): 685–91. http://dx.doi.org/10.1093/eurjhf/hfq050.
59. Watz H, Waschki B, Meyer T, et al. Decreasing cardiac chamber sizes and associated heart dysfunction in COPD, role of hyperinflation. Chest 2010;138(1): 32–8.
60. Barr RG, Bluemke DA, Ahmed FS, et al. Percent emphysema, airflow obstruction, and impaired left ventricular filling. N Engl J Med 2010;362(3):217–27.
61. Shih H, Webb C, Conway W, et al. Frequency and significance of cardiac arrhythmias in chronic obstructive lung disease. Chest 1988;94:44–8.
62. Sekine Y, Kesler KA, Behnia M, et al. COPD may increase the incidence of refractory supraventricular arrhythmias following pulmonary resection for non-small cell lung cancer. Chest 2001;120:1783–90.
63. Mathew JP, Fontes ML, Tudor IC, et al. A multicenter risk index for atrial fibrillation after cardiac surgery. JAMA 2004;291:1720–9.
64. Ryynänen OP, Soini EJ, Lindqvist A, et al. Bayesian predictors of very poor health related quality of life and mortality in patients with COPD. BMC Med Inform Decis Mak 2013;13:34. http://dx.doi.org/10.1186/1472-6947-13-34.
65. Reed RM, Eberlein M, Girgis RE, et al. Coronary artery disease is under-diagnosed and under-treated in advanced lung disease. Am J Med 2012; 125(12):1228.e13–22. http://dx.doi.org/10.1016/j.amjmed.2012.05.018.
66. Hawkins NM, Huang Z, Pieper KS, et al. Chronic obstructive pulmonary disease is an independent predictor of death but not atherosclerotic events in patients with myocardial infarction: analysis of the Valsartan in Acute Myocardial Infarction Trial (VALIANT). Eur J Heart Fail 2009;11(3):292–8. http://dx.doi.org/10. 1093/eurjhf/hfp001.
67. Donaldson GC, Hurst JR, Smith CJ, et al. Increased risk of myocardial infarction and stroke following exacerbation of COPD. Chest 2010;137(5):1091–7.
68. Mackay DF, Irfan MO, Haw S, et al. Meta-analysis of the effect of comprehensive smoke-free legislation on acute coronary events. Heart 2010;96:1525–30.
69. Sin DD, Man SF, Marciniuk DD, et al. The effects of fluticasone with or without salmeterol on systemic biomarkers of inflammation in chronic obstructive pulmonary disease. Am J Respir Crit Care Med 2008;177(11):1207–14. http://dx.doi. org/10.1164/rccm.200709-1356OC.
70. Calverley PM, Anderson JA, Celli B, et al. Cardiovascular events in patients with COPD: TORCH study results. Thorax 2010;65(8):719–25. http://dx.doi.org/10. 1136/thx.2010.136077.
71. Verhamme KM, Afonso A, Romio S, et al. Use of tiotropium Respimat(R) SMI vs. tiotropium Handihaler(R) and mortality in patients with COPD. Eur Respir J 2013; 42:606–15.
72. Celli B, Decramer M, Leimer I, et al. Cardiovascular safety of tiotropium in patients with COPD. Chest 2010;137(1):20–30. http://dx.doi.org/10.1378/chest. 09-0011.
73. Dransfield MT, Rowe SM, Johnson JE, et al. Use of beta blockers and the risk of death in hospitalised patients with acute exacerbations of COPD. Thorax 2008; 63(4):301–5.
74. Dobler CC, Wong KK, Marks GB. Associations between statins and COPD: a systematic review. BMC Pulm Med 2009;9:32. http://dx.doi.org/10.1186/1471-2466-9-32.
75. Mancini GB, Etminan M, Zhang B, et al. Reduction of morbidity and mortality by statins, angiotensin-converting enzyme inhibitors, and angiotensin receptor

blockers in patients with chronic obstructive pulmonary disease. J Am Coll Cardiol 2006;47:2554–60.

76. Gottlieb SS, McCarter RJ, Vogel RA. Effect of beta-blockade on mortality among high-risk and low-risk patients after myocardial infarction. N Engl J Med 1998; 339(8):489–97.

77. Hunt SA, Abraham WT, Chin MH, et al. 2009 focused update incorporated into the ACC/AHA 2005 Guidelines for the Diagnosis and Management of Heart Failure in Adults: a report of the American College of Cardiology Foundation/ American Heart Association Task Force on Practice Guidelines developed in collaboration with the International Society for Heart and Lung Transplantation. Circulation 2009;119:e391–479.

78. Poole-Wilson PA, Swedberg K, Cleland JG, et al. Comparison of carvedilol and metoprolol on clinical outcomes in patients with chronic heart failure in the Carvedilol Or Metoprolol European Trial (COMET): randomised controlled trial. Lancet 2003;362:7–13.

79. Heart Failure Society of America, Lindenfeld J, Albert NM, Boehmer JP, et al. HFSA 2010 comprehensive heart failure practice guideline. J Card Fail 2010; 16:e1–194.

80. Andreas S, Anker SD, Scanlon PD, et al. Neurohumoral activation as a link to systemic manifestations of chronic lung disease. Chest 2005;128(5):3618–24.

81. Rutten FH, Zuithoff NP, Hak E, et al. Beta-blockers may reduce mortality and risk of exacerbations in patients with chronic obstructive pulmonary disease. Arch Intern Med 2010;170(10):880–7. http://dx.doi.org/10.1001/archinternmed. 2010.112.

82. Hawkins NM, Jhund PS, Simpson CR, et al. Primary care burden and treatment of patients with heart failure and chronic obstructive pulmonary disease in Scotland. Eur J Heart Fail 2010;12(1):17–24. http://dx.doi.org/10.1093/eurjhf/ hfp160.

83. Salpeter S, Ormiston T, Salpeter E. Cardioselective beta-blockers for chronic obstructive pulmonary disease. Cochrane Database Syst Rev 2005;(4): CD003566.

84. Stefan MS, Rothberg MB, Priya A, et al. Association between β-blocker therapy and outcomes in patients hospitalised with acute exacerbations of chronic obstructive lung disease with underlying ischaemic heart disease, heart failure or hypertension. Thorax 2012;67(11):977–84. http://dx.doi.org/10.1136/ thoraxjnl-2012-201945.

85. Ekström MP, Hermansson AB, Ström KE. Effects of cardiovascular drugs on mortality in severe chronic obstructive pulmonary disease. Am J Respir Crit Care Med 2013;187(7):715–20. http://dx.doi.org/10.1164/rccm.201208- 1565OC.

86. Mortensen EM, Copeland LA, Pugh MJ, et al. Impact of statins and ACE inhibitors on mortality after COPD exacerbations. Respir Res 2009;10:45. http://dx. doi.org/10.1186/1465-9921-10-45.

87. Agusti AG, Noguera A, Sauleda J, et al. Systemic effects of chronic obstructive pulmonary disease. Eur Respir J 2003;21:347–60.

88. Gosselink R, Troosters T, Decramer M. Peripheral muscle weakness contributes to exercise limitation in COPD. Am J Respir Crit Care Med 1996;153:976–80.

89. Shrikrishna D, Hopkinson NS. Chronic obstructive pulmonary disease: consequences beyond the lung. Clin Med 2012;12:71–4.

90. Decramer M, Gosselink R, Troosters T, et al. Muscle weakness is related to utilization of health care resources in COPD patients. Eur Respir J 1997;10:417–23.

91. Swallow EB, Reyes D, Hopkinson NS, et al. Quadriceps strength predicts mortality in patients with moderate to severe chronic obstructive pulmonary disease. Thorax 2007;62:115–20.
92. Seymour JM, Spruit MA, Hopkinson NS, et al. The prevalence of quadriceps weakness in COPD and the relationship with disease severity. Eur Respir J 2010;36:81–8.
93. Shrikrishna D, Hopkinson NS. Skeletal muscle dysfunction in chronic obstructive pulmonary disease. Respir Med 2009;5:7–13 COPD Update.
94. Hopkinson NS, Polkey MI. Does physical inactivity cause chronic obstructive pulmonary disease? Clin Sci 2010;118:565–72.
95. Shrikrishna D, Patel M, Tanner RJ, et al. Quadriceps wasting and physical inactivity in patients with COPD. Eur Respir J 2012. http://dx.doi.org/10.1183/09031936.00170111.
96. Wust RC, Degens H. Factors contributing to muscle wasting and dysfunction in COPD patients. Int J Chron Obstruct Pulmon Dis 2007;2:289–300.
97. Schols AM, Soeters PB, Dingemans AM, et al. Prevalence and characteristics of nutritional depletion in patients with stable COPD eligible for pulmonary rehabilitation. Am Rev Respir Dis 1993;147:1151–6.
98. Bernard S, LeBlanc P, Whittom F, et al. Peripheral muscle weakness in patients with chronic obstructive pulmonary disease. Am J Respir Crit Care Med 1998; 158:629–34.
99. Mostert R, Goris A, Weling-Scheepers C, et al. Tissue depletion and health related quality of life in patients with chronic obstructive pulmonary disease. Respir Med 2000;94:859–67.
100. Marquis K, Debigare R, Lacasse Y, et al. Midthigh muscle cross-sectional area is a better predictor of mortality than body mass index in patients with chronic obstructive pulmonary disease. Am J Respir Crit Care Med 2002;166: 809–13.
101. Whittom F, Jobin J, Simard PM, et al. Histochemical and morphological characteristics of the vastus lateralis muscle in patients with chronic obstructive pulmonary disease. Med Sci Sports Exerc 1998;30:1467–74.
102. Gosker HR, Engelen MP, van Mameren H, et al. Muscle fiber type IIX atrophy is involved in the loss of fat-free mass in chronic obstructive pulmonary disease. Am J Clin Nutr 2002;76:113–9.
103. Sala E, Roca J, Marrades RM, et al. Effects of endurance training on skeletal muscle bioenergetics in chronic obstructive pulmonary disease. Am J Respir Crit Care Med 1999;159:1726–34.
104. Jobin J, Maltais F, Doyon JF, et al. Chronic obstructive pulmonary disease: capillarity and fiber characteristics of skeletal muscle. J Cardiopulm Rehabil 1998;18: 432–7.
105. Allaire J, Maltais F, Doyon JF, et al. Peripheral muscle endurance and the oxidative profile of the quadriceps in patients with COPD. Thorax 2004;59: 673–8.
106. Rabinovich RA, Bastos R, Ardite E, et al. Mitochondrial dysfunction in COPD patients with low body mass index. Eur Respir J 2007;29:643–50.
107. Engelen MP, Deutz NE, Wouters EF, et al. Enhanced levels of whole-body protein turnover in patients with chronic obstructive pulmonary disease. Am J Respir Crit Care Med 2000;162:1488–92.
108. Plant PJ, Brooks D, Faughnan M, et al. Cellular markers of muscle atrophy in chronic obstructive pulmonary disease (COPD). Am J Respir Cell Mol Biol 2010;42:461–71.

109. Rabinovich RA, Vilaro J. Structural and functional changes of peripheral muscles in chronic obstructive pulmonary disease patients. Curr Opin Pulm Med 2010;16:123–33.
110. Dekhuijzen PN, Decramer M. Steroid-induced myopathy and its significance to respiratory disease: a known disease rediscovered. Eur Respir J 1992;5: 997–1003.
111. Decramer M, de Bock V, Dom R. Functional and histologic picture of steroid-induced myopathy in chronic obstructive pulmonary disease. Am J Respir Crit Care Med 1996;153:1958–64.
112. Hopkinson NS, Man WD, Dayer MJ, et al. Acute effect of oral steroids on muscle function in chronic obstructive pulmonary disease. Eur Respir J 2004;24(1): 137–42.
113. Takabatake N, Nakamura H, Abe S, et al. The relationship between chronic hypoxemia and activation of the tumor necrosis factor-α system in patients with chronic obstructive pulmonary disease. Am J Respir Crit Care Med 2000;161: 1179–84.
114. Preedy VR, Smith DM, Sugden PH. The effects of 6 hours of hypoxia on protein synthesis in rat tissues in vivo and in vitro. Biochem J 1985;228:179–85.
115. Vohwinkel CU, Lecuona E, Sun H, et al. Elevated CO_2 levels cause mitochondrial dysfunction and impair cell proliferation. J Biol Chem 2011;286:37067–76.
116. Yende S, Waterer GW, Tolley EA, et al. Inflammatory markers are associated with ventilatory limitation and muscle dysfunction in obstructive lung disease in well functioning elderly subjects. Thorax 2006;61:10–6.
117. Remels AH, Gosker HR, Schrauwen P, et al. TNF-α impairs regulation of muscle oxidative phenotype: implications for cachexia? FASEB J 2010;24:5052–62.
118. Pinto-Plata VM, Müllerova H, Toso JF, et al. C-Reactive protein in patients with COPD, control smokers and non-smokers. Thorax 2006;61:23–8.
119. Ries AL, Bauldoff GS, Carlin BW, et al. Pulmonary rehabilitation: joint ACCP/AACVPR evidence-based clinical practice guidelines. Chest 2007;131:4S–42S.
120. Meyer A, Zoll J, Charles AL, et al. Skeletal muscle mitochondrial dysfunction during chronic obstructive pulmonary disease: central actor and therapeutic target. Exp Physiol 2013;98:1063–78.
121. MacIntyre NR. Oxygen therapy and exercise response in lung disease. Respir Care 2000;45:194–200.
122. Cardellach F, Alonso JR, López S, et al. Effect of smoking cessation on mitochondrial respiratory chain function. J Toxicol Clin Toxicol 2003;41(3):223–8.
123. Koechlin C, Couillard A, Simar D, et al. Does oxidative stress alter quadriceps endurance in chronic obstructive pulmonary disease? Am J Respir Crit Care Med 2004;169:1022–7.
124. Broekhuizen R, Wouters EF, Creutzberg EC, et al. Polyunsaturated fatty acids improve exercise capacity in chronic obstructive pulmonary disease. Thorax 2005;60:376–82.
125. Ettinger MP. Aging bone and osteoporosis: strategies for preventing fractures in the elderly. Arch Intern Med 2003;163(18):2237–46.
126. Lehouck A, Boonen S, Decramer M, et al. COPD, bone metabolism, and osteoporosis. Chest 2011;139(3):648–57. http://dx.doi.org/10.1378/chest.10-1427.
127. Kanis JA. WHO Study Group Assessment of fracture risk and its application to screening for postmenopausal osteoporosis: synopsis of a WHO report. Osteoporos Int 1994;46:368–81.
128. Graat-Verboom L, Wouters EF, Smeenk FW, et al. Current status of research on osteoporosis in COPD: a systematic review. Eur Respir J 2009;341:209–18.

129. Calverley PM, Anderson JA, Celli B, et al. Salmeterol and fluticasone propionate and survival in chronic obstructive pulmonary disease. N Engl J Med 2007;356: 775–89.
130. Vrieze A, de Greef MH, Wijkstra PJ, et al. Low bone mineral density in COPD patients related to worse lung function, low weight and decreased fat-free mass. Osteoporos Int 2007;18:1197–202.
131. Jorgensen NR, Schwarz P, Holme I, et al. The prevalence of osteoporosis in patients with chronic obstructive pulmonary disease: across sectional study. Respir Med 2007;101:177–85.
132. Romme EA, Murchison JT, Edwards LD, et al. CT measured bone attenuation in patients with chronic obstructive pulmonary disease: relation to clinical features and outcomes. J Bone Miner Res 2013. http://dx.doi.org/10.1002/jbmr.1873.
133. Kjensli A, Falch JA, Ryg M, et al. High prevalence of vertebral deformities in COPD patients: relationship to disease severity. Eur Respir J 2009;33: 1018–24.
134. Mazokopakis EE, Starakis IK. Recommendations for diagnosis and management of osteoporosis in COPD men. ISRN Rheumatol 2011;2011:901416.
135. Weinstein RS, Wan C, Liu Q, et al. Endogenous glucocorticoids decrease skeletal angiogenesis, vascularity, hydration, and strength in aged mice. Aging Cell 2010;9:147–61.
136. Langhammer A, Forsmo S, Syversen U. Long-term therapy in COPD: any evidence of adverse effect on bone? Int J Chron Obstruct Pulmon Dis 2009;4: 365–80.
137. Manolagas SC, Weinstein RS. New developments in the pathogenesis and treatment of steroid-induced osteoporosis. J Bone Miner Res 1999;14(7):1061–6.
138. Mathioudakis AG, Amanetopoulou SG, Gialmanidis IP, et al. Impact of long-term treatment with low-dose inhaled corticosteroids on the bone mineral density of chronic obstructive pulmonary disease patients: aggravating or beneficial? Respirology 2013;18(1):147–53. http://dx.doi.org/10.1111/j.1440-1843.2012. 02265.
139. Liang B, Feng Y. The association of low bone mineral density with systemic inflammation in clinically stable COPD. Endocrine 2012;42(1):190–5. http://dx. doi.org/10.1007/s12020-011-9583-x.
140. Hardy R, Cooper MS. Bone loss in inflammatory disorders. J Endocrinol 2009; 201(3):309–20.
141. Ritchlin CT, Haas-Smith SA, Li P, et al. Mechanisms of TNF-alpha- and RANKL-mediated osteoclastogenesis and bone resorption in psoriatic arthritis. J Clin Invest 2003;111(6):821–31.
142. Kovacic JC, Lee P, Baber U, et al. Inverse relationship between body mass index and coronary artery calcification in patients with clinically significant coronary lesions. Atherosclerosis 2012;221(1):176–82. http://dx.doi.org/10.1016/j. atherosclerosis.2011.11.020.
143. Ebeling PR. Osteoporosis in men. N Engl J Med 2008;358(14):1474–82.
144. Gennari L, Bilezikian JP. Osteoporosis in men. Endocrinol Metab Clin North Am 2007;36(2):399–419.
145. Plotkin LI, Aguirre JI, Kousteni S, et al. Bisphosphonates and estrogens inhibit osteocyte apoptosis via distinct molecular mechanisms downstream of extracellular signal-regulated kinase activation. J Biol Chem 2005;280(8):7317–25.
146. Ringe JD, Faber H, Farahmand P, et al. Efficacy of risedronate in men with primary and secondary osteoporosis: results of a 1-year study. Rheumatol Int 2006;26(5):427–31.

147. Misiorowski W. Parathyroid hormone and its analogues—molecular mechanisms of action and efficacy in osteoporosis therapy. Endokrynol Pol 2011;62(1):73–8.

148. Patel AR, Hurst JR. Extrapulmonary comorbidities in chronic obstructive pulmonary disease: state of the art [review]. Expert Rev Respir Med 2011;5(5):647–62. http://dx.doi.org/10.1586/ers.11.62.

149. Kanis JA, McCloskey EV, Johansson H, et al, National Osteoporosis Guideline Group. Case finding for the management of osteoporosis with FRAX—assessment and intervention thresholds for the UK. Osteoporos Int 2008;19(10):1395–408.

150. Schols AM, Broekhuizen R, Weling-Scheepers CA, et al. Body composition and mortality in chronic obstructive pulmonary disease. Am J Clin Nutr 2005;82(1): 53–9.

151. Collins PF, Elia M, Stratton RJ. Nutritional support and functional capacity in chronic obstructive pulmonary disease: a systematic review and meta-analysis. Respirology 2013. http://dx.doi.org/10.1111/resp.12070.

152. Ferreira IM, Brooks D, White J, et al. Nutritional supplementation for stable chronic obstructive pulmonary disease. Cochrane Database Syst Rev 2012;(12):CD000998. http://dx.doi.org/10.1002/14651858.CD000998.pub3.

153. Schols AM, Gosker HR. The pathophysiology of cachexia in chronic obstructive pulmonary disease. Curr Opin Support Palliat Care 2009;3(4):282–7. http://dx. doi.org/10.1097/SPC.0b013e328331e91c.

154. Cano NJ, Roth H, Court-Ortuné I, et al. Nutritional depletion in patients on long-term oxygen therapy and/or home mechanical ventilation. Eur Respir J 2002;20: 30–7.

155. Vermeeren MA, Creutzberg EC, Schols AM, et al, COSMIC Study Group. Prevalence of nutritional depletion in a large out-patient population of patients with COPD. Respir Med 2006;100:1349–55.

156. Landbo C, Prescott E, Lange P, et al. Prognostic value of nutritional status in chronic obstructive pulmonary disease. Am J Respir Crit Care Med 1999;160: 1856–61.

157. Fuenzalida CE, Petty TL, Jones ML. The immune response to short nutritional intervention in advanced COPD. Am Rev Respir Dis 1990;142(1):49–56.

158. DeBellis HF, Fetterman JW Jr. Enteral nutrition in the chronic obstructive pulmonary disease (COPD) patient. J Pharm Pract 2012;25(6):583–5. http://dx.doi. org/10.1177/0897190012460827.

159. Malone A. Enteral formula selection: a review of selected product categories. Pract Gastroenterol 2005;28:56–8.

160. de Batlle J, Sauleda J, Balcells E, et al. Association between Ω3 and Ω6 fatty acid intakes and serum inflammatory markers in COPD. J Nutr Biochem 2011; 23(7):817–21.

161. World Health Organization. Overweight and obesity: a new nutrition emergency? Monitoring the rapidly emerging public health problem of overweight and obesity: the WHO global database on body mass index. SCN News 2004;5–12.

162. Poulain M, Doucet M, Major GC, et al. The effect of obesity on chronic respiratory diseases: pathophysiology and therapeutic strategies. CMAJ 2006;174: 1293–9.

163. Pitta F, Troosters T, Spruit MA, et al. Characteristics of physical activities in daily life in chronic obstructive pulmonary disease. Am J Respir Crit Care Med 2005; 171:972–7.

164. Dallman MF, la Fleur SE, Pecoraro NC, et al. Minireview: glucocorticoids—food intake, abdominal obesity, and wealthy nations in 2004. Endocrinology 2004; 145:2633–8.

165. Franssen FM, O'Donnell DE, Goossens GH, et al. Obesity and the lung: 5. Obesity and COPD. Thorax 2008;63:1110–7. http://dx.doi.org/10.1136/thx. 2007.086827.
166. Bastard JP, Maachi M, Lagathu C, et al. Recent advances in the relationship between obesity, inflammation, and insulin resistance. Eur Cytokine Netw 2006;17: 4–12.
167. Yudkin JS. Adipose tissue, insulin action and vascular disease: inflammatory signals. Int J Obes Relat Metab Disord 2003;27(Suppl 3):S25–8.
168. Young T, Palta M, Dempsey J, et al. The occurrence of sleep disordered breathing among middle-aged adults. N. Engl. J Med 1993;328:1230–5.
169. Young T, Peppard PE, Gottlieb DJ. Epidemiology of obstructive sleep apnea: a population health perspective. Am J Respir Crit Care Med 2002;165:1217–39.
170. McNicholas WT. Chronic obstructive pulmonary disease and obstructive sleep apnea: overlaps in pathophysiology, systemic inflammation, and cardiovascular disease. Am J Respir Crit Care Med 2009;180:692–700.
171. Fletcher EC. Chronic lung disease in the sleep apnea syndrome. Lung 1990; 168(Suppl):751–61.
172. Ioachimescu OC, Teodorescu M. Integrating the overlap of obstructive lung disease and obstructive sleep apnoea: OLDOSA syndrome. Respirology 2013; 18(3):421–31. http://dx.doi.org/10.1111/resp.12062.
173. Clini E, Sturani C, Rossi A, et al. The Italian multicentre study on noninvasive ventilation in chronic obstructive pulmonary disease patients. Eur Respir J 2002;20:529–38.
174. Butterworth CE, Fielding JF, Finch CA, et al. Nutritional anaemias. Report of a WHO scientific group. World Health Organ Tech Rep Ser 1968;405:5–37.
175. John M, Hoernig S, Doehner W, et al. Anemia and inflammation in COPD. Chest 2005;127(3):825–9.
176. Chambellan A, Chailleux E, Similowski T, et al. Prognostic value of the hematocrit in patients with severe COPD receiving long-term oxygen therapy. Chest 2005;128:1201–8.
177. Rutten EP, Franssen FM, Spruit MA, et al. Anemia is associated with bone mineral density in chronic obstructive pulmonary disease. COPD 2013;10: 286–92.
178. Weiss G. Pathogenesis and treatment of anaemia of chronic disease. Blood Rev 2002;16:87–96.
179. Schönhofer B, Wenzel M, Geibel M, et al. Blood transfusion and lung function in chronically anemic patients with severe chronic obstructive pulmonary disease. Crit Care Med 1998;26:1824–8.
180. Barnes PJ. Neural control of human airways in health and disease. Am Rev Respir Dis 1986;134:1289–314.
181. van Gestel AJ, Steier J. Autonomic dysfunction in patients with chronic obstructive pulmonary disease (COPD). J Thorac Dis 2010;2(4):215–22.
182. Buda AJ, Pinsky MR, Ingles NB, et al. Effect of intrathoracic pressure on left ventricular performance. N Engl J Med 1979;301:453–9.
183. Undem BJ, Kollarik M. The role of vagal afferent nerves in chronic obstructive pulmonary disease. Proc Am Thorac Soc 2005;2:355–60.
184. Dempsey JA, Sheel AW, St Croix CM. Respiratory influences on sympathetic vasomotor outflow in humans. Respir Physiol Neurobiol 2002;130:3–20.
185. Tug T, Terzi SM, Yoldas TK. Relationship between the frequency of autonomic dysfunction and the severity of chronic obstructive pulmonary disease. Acta Neurol Scand 2005;112(3):183–8.

186. Purdue MP, Gold L, Jarvholm B, et al. Impaired lung function and lung cancer incidence in a cohort of Swedish construction workers. Thorax 2007;62(1):51–6.
187. Punturieri A, Szabo E, Croxton TL. Lung cancer and chronic obstructive pulmonary disease: needs and opportunities for integrated research. J Natl Cancer Inst 2009;101(8):554–9.
188. Mannino DM, Aguayo SM, Petty TL, et al. Low lung function and incident lung cancer in the United States: data from the First National Health and Nutrition Examination Survey follow-up. Arch Intern Med 2003;163:1475–80.
189. Tockman MS, Anthonisen NR, Wright EC, et al. Airways obstruction and the risk for lung cancer. Ann Intern Med 1987;106(4):512–8.
190. Skillrud DM, Offord KP, Miller RD. Higher risk of lung cancer in chronic obstructive pulmonary disease. A prospective, matched, controlled study. Ann Intern Med 1986;105(4):503–7.
191. Anthonisen NR, Skeans MA, Wise RA, et al. The effects of a smoking cessation intervention on 14.5-year mortality: a randomized clinical trial. Ann Intern Med 2005;142:233–9.
192. Wilson DO, Weissfeld JL, Balkan A, et al. Association of radiographic emphysema and airflow obstruction with lung cancer. Am J Respir Crit Care Med 2008;178:738–44.
193. Young RP, Hopkins RJ, Christmas T, et al. COPD prevalence is increased in lung cancer independence of age, gender and smoking history. Eur Respir J 2009; 34:380–6.
194. Papi A, Casoni G, Caramori G, et al. COPD increases the risk of squamous histological subtype in smokers who develop non-small cell lung carcinoma. Thorax 2004;59(8):679–81.
195. Jacobson BA, Alter MD, Kratzke MG, et al. Repression of cap-dependent translation attenuates the transformed phenotype in non-small cell lung cancer both in vitro and in vivo. Cancer Res 2006;66(8):4256–62.
196. Krysan K, Lee JM, Dohadwala M, et al. Inflammation, epithelial to mesenchymal transition, and epidermal growth factor receptor tyrosine kinase inhibitor resistance. J Thorac Oncol 2008;3(2):107–10.
197. Brody JS, Spira A. Chronic obstructive pulmonary disease, inflammation and lung cancer. Proc Am Thorac Soc 2006;3:535–8.
198. Yao HW, Rahman I. Current concepts on the role of inflammation in COPD and lung cancer. Curr Opin Pharmacol 2009;9:375–83.
199. Lin WW, Karin M. A cytokine-mediated link between innate immunity, inflammation, and cancer. J Clin Invest 2007;117:1175–83.
200. Wright JG, Christman JW. The role of nuclear factor kappa B in the pathogenesis of pulmonary diseases: implications for therapy. Am J Respir Med 2003;2:211–9.
201. Teramoto S, Kume H. The role of nuclear factor-kappa B activation in airway inflammation following adenovirus infection and COPD. Chest 2001;119:1294–5.
202. O'Byrne KJ, Dalgleish AG. Chronic immune activation and inflammation as the cause of malignancy. Br J Cancer 2001;85:473–83.
203. Parimon T, Chien JW, Bryson CL, et al. Inhaled corticosteroids and risk of lung cancer among patients with chronic obstructive pulmonary disease. Am J Respir Crit Care Med 2007;175:712–9.
204. van Gestel YR, Hoeks SE, Sin DD, et al. COPD and cancer mortality: the influence of statins. Thorax 2009;64:963–7.
205. Young RP, Hopkins RJ. How the genetics of lung cancer may overlap with COPD. Respirology 2011;16(7):1047–55. http://dx.doi.org/10.1111/j.1440-1843.2011.02019.x.

206. Schwartz AG, Ruckdeschel JC. Familial lung cancer: genetic susceptibility and relationship to chronic obstructive pulmonary disease. Am J Respir Crit Care Med 2006;173:16–22.
207. Malhotra D, Thimmulappa R, Navas-Acien A, et al. Decline in Nrf2 regulated antioxidants in COPD lungs due to loss of its positive regulator DJ-1. Am J Respir Crit Care Med 2008;178:592–604.
208. Cho HY, Reddy SP, Kleeberger SR. Nrf2 defends the lung from oxidative stress. Antioxid Redox Signal 2006;8:76–87.
209. Krieken JH, Hiemstra PS. Expression of epidermal growth factors and their receptors in the bronchial epithelium of subjects with chronic obstructive pulmonary disease. Am J Clin Pathol 2006;125:184–92.
210. Hill K, Geist R, Goldstein RS, et al. Anxiety and depression in end-stage COPD. Eur Respir J 2008;31(3):667–77. http://dx.doi.org/10.1183/09031936.00125707.
211. Engstrom CP, Persson LO, Larsson S, et al. Functional status and well being in chronic obstructive pulmonary disease with regard to clinical parameters and smoking: a descriptive and comparative study. Thorax 1996;51:825–30.
212. Dowson C, Laing R, Barraclough R, et al. The use of the Hospital Anxiety and Depression Scale (HADS) in patients with chronic obstructive pulmonary disease: a pilot study. N Z Med J 2001;114:447–9.
213. van Manen JG, Bindels PJ, Dekker FW, et al. Risk of depression in patients with chronic obstructive pulmonary disease and its determinants. Thorax 2002;57: 412–6.
214. van Ede L, Yzermans CJ, Brouwer HJ. Prevalence of depression in patients with chronic obstructive pulmonary disease: a systematic review. Thorax 1999;54: 688–92.
215. Kunik ME, Roundy K, Veazey C, et al. Surprisingly high prevalence of anxiety and depression in chronic breathing disorders. Chest 2005;127:1205–11.
216. Hanania NA, Müllerova H, Locantore NW, et al. Evaluation of COPD Longitudinally to Identify Predictive Surrogate Endpoints (ECLIPSE) study investigators. Determinants of depression in the ECLIPSE chronic obstructive pulmonary disease cohort. Am J Respir Crit Care Med 2011;183(5):604–11. http://dx.doi.org/10.1164/rccm.201003-0472OC.
217. Anisman H, Merali Z, Hayley S. Neurotransmitter, peptide and cytokine processes in relation to depressive disorder: comorbidity between depression and neurodegenerative disorders. Prog Neurobiol 2008;85(1):1–74.
218. Almagro P, Calbo E, Ochoa-de-Echaguen A, et al. Mortality after hospitalization for COPD. Chest 2002;121:1441–8.
219. Ng TP, Niti M, Tan WC, et al. Depressive symptoms and chronic obstructive pulmonary disease: effect on mortality, hospital readmission, symptom burden, functional status, and quality of life. Arch Intern Med 2007;167:60–7.
220. Fan VS, Ramsey SD, Giardino ND, et al. Sex, depression, and risk of hospitalization and mortality in chronic obstructive pulmonary disease. Arch Intern Med 2007;167:2345–53.
221. de Voogd JN, Wempe JB, Koëter GH, et al. Depressive symptoms as predictors of mortality in patients with COPD. Chest 2009;135:619–25. http://dx.doi.org/10.1378/chest.08-0078 Prepublished online November 24, 2008.
222. Mannino DM, Thorn D, Swensen A, et al. Prevalence and outcomes of diabetes, hypertension and cardiovascular disease in COPD. Eur Respir J 2008;32(4): 962–9.
223. Rabinovich RA, MacNee W. Chronic obstructive pulmonary disease and its comorbidities. Br J Hosp Med (Lond) 2011;72(3):137–45.

224. Rana JS, Mittleman MA, Sheikh J, et al. Chronic obstructive pulmonary disease, asthma, and risk of type 2 diabetes in women. Diabetes Care 2004;27:2478–84.
225. Poulain M, Doucet M, Drapeau V, et al. Metabolic and inflammatory profile in obese patients with chronic obstructive pulmonary disease. Chron Respir Dis 2008;5(1):35–41.
226. Chakrabarti B, Angus RM, Agarwal S, et al. Hyperglycaemia as a predictor of outcome during non-invasive ventilation in decompensated COPD. Thorax 2009;64(10):857–62.
227. Baker EH, Janaway CH, Philips BJ, et al. Hyperglycaemia is associated with poor outcomes in patients admitted to hospital with acute exacerbations of chronic obstructive pulmonary disease. Thorax 2006;61(4):284–9.
228. Marquis K, Maltais F, Duguay V, et al. The metabolic syndrome in patients with chronic obstructive pulmonary disease. J Cardiopulm Rehabil 2005;25:226–32.
229. Fabbri LM, Luppi F, Beghe B, et al. Complex chronic comorbidities of COPD. Eur Respir J 2008;31:204–12. http://dx.doi.org/10.1183/09031936.00114307.
230. Clini E, Crisafulli E, Radaeli A, et al. COPD and the metabolic syndrome: an intriguing association. Intern Emerg Med 2013;8(4):283–9.
231. Agusti A. Systemic effects of chronic obstructive pulmonary disease: what we know and what we don't know (but should). Proc Am Thorac Soc 2007;4:522–5.
232. van Eeden SF, Sin DD. Chronic obstructive pulmonary disease: a chronic systemic inflammatory disease. Respiration 2008;75:224–38.
233. Garcia-Rio F, Miravitlles M, Soriano JB, et al. Systemic inflammation in chronic obstructive pulmonary disease: a population-based study. Respir Res 2010; 11:63.
234. Sin DD, Anthonisen NR, Soriano JB, et al. Mortality in COPD: role of comorbidities. Eur Respir J 2006;28(6):1245–57.
235. Gan WQ, Man SF, Sin DD. Association between chronic obstructive pulmonary disease and systemic inflammation: a systematic review and a meta-analysis. Thorax 2004;59:574–80.
236. Fabbri LM, Rabe KF. From COPD to chronic systemic inflammatory syndrome? Lancet 2007;370:797–9.
237. Gea J, Barreiro E, Orozco-Levi M. Systemic inflammation in COPD. Clin Pulm Med 2009;16:233–42.
238. Luppi F, Franco F, Beghe B, et al. Treatment of chronic obstructive pulmonary disease and its comorbidities. Proc Am Thorac Soc 2008;5:848–56.
239. Rennard SI. Inflammation in COPD: a link to systemic comorbidities. Eur Respir Rev 2007;16:91–7.
240. Yanbaeva DG, Dentener MA, Creutzberg EC, et al. Systemic effects of smoking. Chest 2007;131:1557–66.
241. Gan WQ, Man SF, Sin DD. The interactions between cigarette smoking and reduced lung function on systemic inflammation. Chest 2005;127:558–64.
242. Maclay JD, McAllister DA, Macnee W. Cardiovascular risk in chronic obstructive pulmonary disease. Respirology 2007;12:634–41.
243. Sevenoaks MJ, Stockley RA. Chronic obstructive pulmonary disease, inflammation and co-morbidity—a common inflammatory phenotype? Respir Res 2006;7: 70.
244. Donaldson GC, Seemungal TA, Patel IS, et al. Airway and systemic inflammation and decline in lung function in patients with COPD. Chest 2005;128:1995–2004.
245. Eagan TM, Ueland T, Wagner PD, et al. Systemic inflammatory markers in COPD: results from the Bergen COPD Cohort Study. Eur Respir J 2010;35: 540–8.

246. Walter RE, Wilk JB, Larson MG, et al. Systemic inflammation and COPD: the Framingham Heart Study. Chest 2008;133:19–25.
247. Pinto-Plata V, Toso J, Lee K, et al. Use of proteomic patterns of serum biomarkers in patients with chronic obstructive pulmonary disease: correlation with clinical parameters. Proc Am Thorac Soc 2006;3:465–6.
248. Sin DD, Leung R, Gan WQ, et al. Circulating surfactant protein D as a potential lung-specific biomarker of health outcomes in COPD: a pilot study. BMC Pulm Med 2007;7:13.
249. Bozinovski S, Hutchinson A, Thompson M, et al. Serum amyloid A is a biomarker of acute exacerbations of chronic obstructive pulmonary disease. Am J Respir Crit Care Med 2008;177:269–78.
250. Sparrow D, Glynn RJ, Cohen M, et al. The relationship of the peripheral leukocyte count and cigarette smoking to pulmonary function among adult men. Chest 1984;86:383–6.
251. Burnett D, Chamba A, Hill SL, et al. Neutrophils from subjects with chronic obstructive lung disease show enhanced chemotaxis and extracellular proteolysis. Lancet 1987;2:1043–6.
252. Aldonyte R, Jansson L, Piitulainen E, et al. Circulating monocytes from healthy individuals and COPD patients. Respir Res 2003;4:11.
253. Hodge SJ, Hodge GL, Reynolds PN, et al. Increased production of TGF-beta and apoptosis of T lymphocytes isolated from peripheral blood in COPD. Am J Physiol Lung Cell Mol Physiol 2003;285:L492–9.
254. Domagala-Kulawik J, Hoser G, Dabrowska M, et al. Increased proportion of Fas positive CD8+ cells in peripheral blood of patients with COPD. Respir Med 2007;101:1338–43.
255. Fairclough L, Urbanowicz RA, Corne J, et al. Killer cells in chronic obstructive pulmonary disease. Clin Sci (Lond) 2008;114:533–41.
256. Sin DD, Vestbo J. Biomarkers in chronic obstructive pulmonary disease. Proc Am Thorac Soc 2009;6:543–5.
257. Agusti A, Calverley P, Celli B, et al. Characterisation of COPD heterogeneity in the ECLIPSE cohort. Respir Res 2010;11:122–36.
258. Dickens JA, Miller B, Edwards L, et al. For the Evaluation of COPD Longitudinally to Identify Surrogate Endpoints (ECLIPSE) study investigators. Respir Res 2011; 12:146.
259. Vanfleteren LE, Spruit MA, Groenen M, et al. Clusters of comorbidities based on validated objective measurements and systemic inflammation in patients with chronic obstructive pulmonary disease. Am J Respir Crit Care Med 2013; 187(7):728–35. http://dx.doi.org/10.1164/rccm.201209-1665OC.

Patients with Chronic Pulmonary Disease

Caron M. Hong, MD, MSc[a],*, Samuel M. Galvagno Jr, DO, PhD[b]

KEYWORDS

- Postoperative pulmonary complications • Preoperative preparation
- Chronic obstructive pulmonary disease • Anesthesia • Preoperative assessment
- Anesthesia and coexisting pulmonary disease • Asthma • Restrictive lung disease

KEY POINTS

- Preoperative evaluations are essential for individuals with chronic pulmonary disease to minimize postoperative pulmonary complications and perioperative morbidity and mortality.
- A detailed history and physical examination, including an assessment of functional status, is the most important means of predicting and preparing for postoperative pulmonary complications.
- Smoking is a risk factor for cancer, cardiovascular disease, and chronic respiratory disorders and a cessation goal should be 8 weeks before surgery.
- Chronic pulmonary disease, including chronic obstructive pulmonary disease, asthma, restrictive lung disease, obstructive sleep apnea, and obesity, has an associated risk of postoperative pulmonary complications and necessitates specific preoperative assessments to aid in risk reduction and appropriate surgical and anesthetic management.

PREOPERATIVE PATIENT ASSESSMENT

A meticulous preoperative evaluation of the patient with pulmonary disease is indicated because both regional and general anesthesia have the potential to precipitate numerous untoward physiologic effects.[1] These effects are caused by positive pressure ventilation, patient positioning, and the drugs used to induce and maintain general anesthesia.[2] Up to 90% of patients develop some degree of atelectasis during anesthesia.[3] Compression atelectasis results from patient positioning and loss of functional residual capacity (FRC). Hence, obesity and larger proportions of poorly

This article originally appeared in *Medical Clinics*, Volume 97, Issue 6, November 2013.
Disclosures: None.
[a] Department of Anesthesiology, University of Maryland School of Medicine, 22 South Greene Street, S11C0, Baltimore, MD 21201, USA; [b] Department of Anesthesiology, Shock Trauma Center, University of Maryland School of Medicine, 22 South Greene Street, T1R83, Baltimore, MD 21201, USA
* Corresponding author.
E-mail address: chong@anes.umm.edu

aerated lung areas predispose patients to ventilation-perfusion mismatching. Reabsorption atelectasis results when lower tidal volumes are used with a high Fio_2. Oxygen rapidly diffuses across the alveolar membrane, causing a pressure difference that leads to airway collapse.[2] FRC decreases significantly during general anesthesia; a decline of up to 50% of baseline may result because of a loss of inspiratory muscle tone and cephalad displacement of the diaphragm,[4,5] leading to increased shunting, dead space, and hypoxemia.[6] General anesthesia induces numerous other deleterious biologic effects on the respiratory system, including decreased alveolar macrophage activity, inhibition of mucociliary clearance, and decreased surfactant production.[5] All of these effects have the potential to cause precipitous changes in arterial oxygen concentration and postoperative pulmonary complications in patients with preexisting pulmonary disease.

Postoperative pulmonary complications (PPC) occur in approximately 10–30% of all patients who require general anesthesia.[5] PPC increase morbidity and mortality and are more costly than venous thromboembolic, cardiovascular, or infectious complications following surgery.[7] Fortunately, with a careful history and physical examination, many PPCs can be anticipated and potentially prevented.[6]

One of the most important preoperative assessments is a detailed description of the patient's quality of life.[7,8] An adequate activity level, as assessed by a validated questionnaire or simple questions about mobility, ability to climb 2 flights of stairs without dyspnea, and other markers of fitness has been independently associated with improved short-term mortality after major abdominal surgery.[9] Functional status is also assessed as a part of the Postoperative Pneumonia Risk Index.[6,10] This instrument incorporates type of surgery, age, functional status, and blood urea nitrogen level (BUN) to assess the risk of developing postoperative pneumonia (Table 1).

Any patient with dyspnea or cough must be evaluated carefully with a focused history and physical examination. A history of cardiac failure, American Society of Anesthesiologists (ASA) class ≥ 2 (Table 2), advanced age, chronic obstructive pulmonary disease (COPD), or a history of functional dependence have been shown to be significant risk factors for PPC.[6]

The risk for serious PPC, such as acute respiratory distress syndrome, is low (0.2%), but higher in patients with renal failure, COPD, emergency surgery, or in patients who have received numerous anesthetics.[11]

The "cough test" is performed by having the patient take a deep breath and cough once. A positive finding is defined as repeated coughing after the first cough.[6,12] This test has been shown to be a predictor of PPC.[12] Abnormal physical examination findings, such as adventitious lung sounds, have been shown to be highly associated with PPC (OR = 5.8); no individual spirometric variable has been as highly correlated with PPC.[13,14]

PREOPERATIVE TESTING

A general suggested approach to assessing the complaint of dyspnea is outlined in Fig. 1. Although the list of indications for pulmonary function tests (PFTs) is lengthy,[15] PFTs have a limited role in predicting PPC. In general, PFTs are recommended before surgery in patients undergoing lung resection or to classify the degree of lung impairment (ie, COPD) when there is uncertainty about the extent of disease.[5,13] PFTs may also be considered to determine the baseline lung function in patients with myasthenia gravis. PFTs alone do not reliably predict risk better than clinical evaluation alone, and the use of spirometry is fraught with limitations.[13,14,16] Although a postoperative forced expiratory volume in 1 second (FEV_1) greater than 40% has been shown to

Table 1	
The postoperative pneumonia risk index	
Type of surgery	
Abdominal aortic aneurysm repair	15
Thoracic	14
Upper abdominal	10
Neck	8
Neurosurgery	8
Vascular	3
Age	
>80 y old	17
79–79 y old	13
60–60 y old	9
50–59 y old	4
Functional status	
Totally dependent	10
Partially dependent	6
Weight loss >10% in past 6 mo	7
History of COPD	5
General anesthesia	4
Impaired sensorium	4
History of stroke	4
BUN (mg/dL)	
<8	4
22–30	2
>30	3
Other factors	
Blood transfusion >4 U	3
Emergency surgery	3
Steroid use for chronic condition	3
Current smoker within 1 y	3
Alcohol intake >2 drinks/d	2

Scoring: 0–15 points, 0.24%; 16–25 points, 1.18%; 26–40 points, 4.6%; 41–55 points, 10.8%; >55 points, 15.9%.

Data from Canet J, Mazo V. Postoperative pulmonary complications. Minerva Anestesiol 2010;76:138–43; and Arouzullah A, Khuri S, Henderson W, et al. Development and validation of a multifactorial risk index for predicting postoperative pneumonia after major noncardiac surgery. Ann Intern Med 2001;135:847–57.

be associated with fewer PPC, the best assessment is a detailed description of the patient's quality of life.[8,17] In many cases, the FEV_1 alone may be inadequate. If PFTs are obtained, the FEV_1/Q (perfusion) ratio, combined with the FEV_1/Ht (height in centimeters), may be superior for determining functional status in young and old patients with severe lung disease.[16,18]

Laboratory testing is rarely helpful when evaluating patients with respiratory disease. Baseline arterial blood gas determinations have not been shown to help with risk stratification, but if available for a patient with advanced lung disease, may serve

Table 2	
The ASA physical status classification system	
ASA Physical Status 1	A normal healthy patient
ASA Physical Status 2	A patient with mild systemic disease (eg, mild intermittent asthma)
ASA Physical Status 3	A patient with severe systemic disease (eg, advanced COPD, congestive heart failure)
ASA Physical Status 4	A patient with severe systemic disease that is a constant threat to life (eg, active respiratory failure, stage IV COPD)
ASA Physical Status 5	A moribund patient who is not expected to survive without the operation (eg, a severe asthmatic requiring an exploratory laparotomy for necrotic bowel)
ASA Physical Status 6	A declared brain-dead patient whose organs are being removed for donor purposes

Data from American Society of Anesthesiologists. 2011 relative value guide package. Chicago: American Society of Anesthesiologists; 2011.

to establish baseline values for later comparison because therapy is adjusted in the intensive care unit.[5] Elevated levels of BUN (>30 mg/dL) and decreased levels of serum albumin (<3 g/dL) have been shown to predict PPC.[13,19]

Radiographic tests, such as chest computed tomography (CT) or chest radiography, are only useful when attempting to diagnose acute causes of dyspnea. Echocardiography should be considered for patients with heart failure as a cause (see **Fig. 1**).

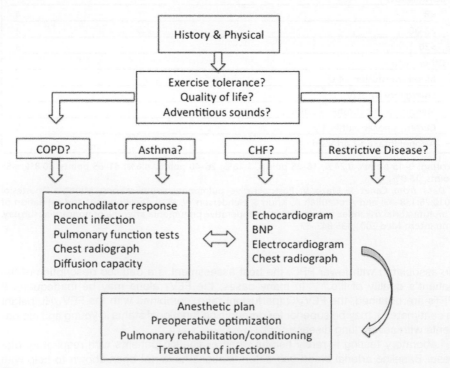

Fig. 1. Suggested general approach to the complaint of dyspnea.

SMOKING CESSATION

Smoking is a well-defined risk factor for PPC and a major independent risk factor for cancer, cardiovascular disease, and chronic respiratory disorders.[20–22] Smoking and comorbidities directly related to tobacco use have been shown to increase airway reactivity, decrease mucociliary clearance, and impede wound healing.[6] Although the cessation of smoking 48 hours before surgery decreases carboxyhemoglobin levels and cyanide levels, sputum production increases and symptoms of cough may worsen acutely.[22] In a recent systematic review that included 25 studies, the risk of PPC was similar in smokers who quit less than 2 or 2–4 weeks before surgery.[23] Ideally, to avoid PPCs, smokers should quit 8 weeks before surgery.[5,21] Smoking cessation has been shown to improve immune function and wound healing in addition to the salutary effects on pulmonary function and avoidance of PPC.[21]

CHRONIC OBSTRUCTIVE PULMONARY DISEASE

COPD is a leading cause of morbidity and mortality worldwide and is responsible for greater than 100,000 deaths per year in the United States.[24,25] COPD is defined by a pulmonary component that is characterized by "persistent airflow limitation" that is not fully reversible and "usually progressive and associated with an enhanced chronic inflammatory response."[24] The pathophysiological effects of COPD are summarized in **Fig. 2**.

Smoking is well-established as the leading risk factor for COPD, but other causes, such as occupational exposures, air pollution, lung development abnormalities, and genetic factors, may be responsible. A postbronchodilator FEV_1/forced vital capacity (FVC) ratio less than 0.70 confirms the presence of airflow limitation and is recommended for the diagnosis and assessment of the severity of COPD.[24] Both the FEV_1 and the FEV_1/FVC ratio are used to classify the stages of COPD according to the Global Initiative for Chronic Obstructive Lung Disease (GOLD-COPD), as listed in **Table 3**.[24] It is unlikely that PFTs will unmask high-stage patients with severe

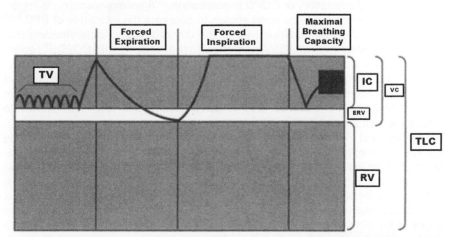

Fig. 2. Representative spirogram for a patient with COPD. ERV, expiratory reserve volume; IC, inspiratory capacity; RV, residual volume; TLC, total lung capacity; TV, tidal volume; VC, vital capacity. In advanced COPD, the inspiratory capacity and expiratory reserve volume are decreased, whereas the residual volume is greatly increased. (*From* Galvagno S. Emergency pathophysiology. Jackson (WY): Teton NewMedia; 2004; with permission.)

Table 3 GOLD-COPD staging, based on severity of postbronchodilator airflow limitation		
Stage 1	Mild	$FEV_1 \geq 80\%$ predicted
Stage 2	Moderate	$50\% \leq FEV_1 < 80\%$ predicted
Stage 3	Severe	$30\% \leq FEV_1 < 50\%$ predicted
Stage 4	Very severe	$FEV_1 < 30\%$ predicted

Data from Vestbo J, Hurd SS, Agusti AG, et al. Global strategy for the diagnosis, management, and prevention of chronic obstructive pulmonary disease: GOLD executive summary. Am J Respir Crit Care Med 2013;187:347–65.

disability, and the level of physical tolerance (ie, stair climbing) has been shown to correlate well with PFT data.[14,26] Furthermore, PFTs do not reliably predict PPC in patients with COPD (see **Table 3**).[13,14]

In stages 1 to 2, the principles of management are centered around prevention, vaccination, pulmonary rehabilitation, and long-acting bronchodilators. In stage 3, inhaled glucocorticoids are added. In stage 4, patients require supplemental oxygen and are often severely physically debilitated.

In addition to a thorough history and physical examination, additional ancillary tests may be considered for high-stage COPD patients. Chest radiographs and chest CT studies are indicated only to rule out infection or other coexisting disease, such as carcinoma. An electrocardiograph (ECG) should be obtained in most COPD patients because signs of right heart strain (ie, right ventricular hypertrophy) may prompt the need for additional testing. Coexisting coronary artery disease is common in COPD patients,[26] and in stage 2 COPD or greater, an ECG or pharmacologic stress test is recommended if the patient reports poor exercise tolerance. Routine laboratory testing is not very helpful, although malnutrition is common in COPD patients, as potentially indicated by a low serum albumin level.

The major preoperative goal of management for patients with COPD involves the prevention of PPC, such as pneumonia, bronchospasm, respiratory failure with prolonged mechanical ventilation, or COPD exacerbation.[26] Smoking cessation is imperative for COPD patients and has been shown to decrease the incidence of PPC.[5,26] Bronchodilators should be continued up to the day of surgery, understanding that bronchodilators rarely improve FEV_1 more than 10% in patients with COPD.[26] Nevertheless, these agents should be continued before, during, and after surgery.[26] Prophylactic use of antibiotics is not recommended, but infections should be treated promptly when identified. Preoperative pulmonary conditioning may be helpful in some high-stage COPD patients, and in some studies this has been shown to decrease the incidence of PPC.

Recognition and treatment of a COPD exacerbation is a primary concern, because progression to surgery during an acute exacerbation will invariably increase the incidence of PPC as well as other systemic complications.[27] An exacerbation is defined as an acute event characterized by worsening of the patient's respiratory status, worse than usual daily variation.[24] One of the most common precipitating factors is a viral or bacterial upper respiratory tract infection. A thorough history will reveal changes in baseline dyspnea, worsening cough, or changes in sputum production beyond normal day-to-day variation.[24] COPD exacerbations are treated with short-acting inhaled β-agonists with or without anticholinergics (ie, ipratropium). Systemic corticosteroids and antibiotics have been shown to improve FEV_1, shorten recovery time, and reduce the length of hospital stay.[24] Similar effects with low-dose compared with high-dose steroids have been observed in at least one study, and preoperative use of corticosteroids has not been shown to increase the risk of wound healing or postoperative pneumonia.[26–28] Ideally, postponement of surgery during a COPD exacerbation is strongly advisable.

ASTHMA

Asthma is one of the most common diseases, affecting more than 300 million people worldwide,[29] in every sector of the population, without prejudice. It is attributed to 1 in 250 deaths, most preventable.[29] Therefore, asthma has been the topic of global public health intervention movements in the past few decades to implement practice guidelines to improve management and prevent morbidity and mortality.

Asthma occurs from acute airway obstruction secondary to inflammation and hyperresponsiveness. Oftentimes, COPD and asthma present simultaneously in adults and it is difficult to distinguish between the two entities. Specific preoperative preparations for COPD should be followed as mentioned above. It has been demonstrated for more than 50 years that surgical patients with asthma have an increased risk for perioperative complications and, when treated adequately before surgery, these patients have less postoperative complications.[30] Therefore, a thorough preoperative evaluation, including a physical examination, management of any electrolyte abnormalities secondary to medications such as B_2 agonists, an ECG to identify cardiac arrhythmias or abnormalities, continuation of asthma treatment, and treatment of other associated comorbidities, such as cor pulmonale, is essential. Identification of the usefulness of current medication, the number of medications needed, and precipitating factors are helpful to determine the severity of disease as well as managing avoidance of exposure during the perioperative period (ie, latex). The usefulness of spirometry and arterial blood gas analysis is questionable, as attacks are usually acute and resolve, and abnormalities may not be apparent. If, however, FEV_1 values during an exacerbation are less than 80% of the patient's personal best, corticosteroids should be prescribed.[31] Special attention should be given to these patients who receive steroids within 6 months of surgery, as they should receive systemic doses of steroids during the surgical period with a rapid wean within 24 hours postoperatively.[31]

Therapeutic considerations for optimization in the preoperative period include two categories: quick-acting and long-acting medications. The quick-acting medications for acute exacerbations include B_2 selective adrenergic agonists (metered-dose inhalers), such as albuterol, and an enantiomer, levalbuterol, with fewer side effects.[32] Corticosteroids can be used for more difficult to control attacks. Close monitoring of electrolytes with B_2 agonist treatment is essential. Long-acting medications include long-acting B_2 selective agonists, such as salmeterol, inhaled steroids, leukotriene modifier, inhaled anticholinergics, and IgE immunotherapy. To decrease the risk of postoperative complications, these patients should continue their medication regimen preoperatively and through the perioperative period.

RESTRICTIVE LUNG DISEASE

There are numerous pathophysiological states and disease processes that may be classified as restrictive lung disease. Causes are either pulmonary (parenchymal) or extrapulmonary (**Box 1**).

Restrictive pulmonary diseases are characterized by a reduction of lung volume and both total and vital capacity. Hence, patients with restrictive lung disease are at risk for exaggerated pulmonary dysfunction postoperatively.

Box 1
Restrictive lung disorders

Pulmonary causes

- Sarcoidosis
- Silicosis
- Tuberculosis
- Hypersensitivity pneumonitis
- Eosinophilic granulomatosis
- Pulmonary alveolar proteinosis
- Lung resection
- Atelectasis
- Acute respiratory distress syndrome
- Pulmonary edema

Extrapulmonary causes

- Obesity
- Skeletal/costovertebral deformities (eg, scoliosis)
- Sternal deformities (eg, pectus excavatum)
- Neuromuscular disorders
- Pneumothorax

The preoperative assessment of the patient with a restrictive lung disorder depends on the underlying cause. Exercise tolerance is important, and if impaired, the incidence of PPC may be increased. Chest radiographs are frequently obtained, but may only be helpful if comparison studies are available or if the study is being used to monitor the progression of the underlying disease. Similarly, CT studies are only indicated if tracheal compression or other associated pathologic condition is suspected. Preoperative arterial blood gases analysis may provide an estimate of baseline oxygenation and ventilation to be expected at the end of surgery.[33]

Unfortunately, there are very few evidence-based recommendations for the preoperative management of patients with restrictive lung disease. Some pulmonary conditions, such as hypersensitivity pneumonitis and sarcoidosis, may exhibit a degree of airway hyperreactivity and should be treated in a manner similar to COPD.[33] As with all pulmonary disease, preoperative management should be aimed at optimizing the patient's physiology with the goal of preventing PPC and additional morbidity and mortality.

OBSTRUCTIVE SLEEP APNEA

Obstructive sleep apnea (OSA) is an independent risk factor for mortality.[34,35] The prevalence of OSA in middle-aged men is 4% and 2% in women[35] and continues to increase. OSA is defined as multiple episodes of upper airway obstruction that occur during sleep, usually associated with oxygen desaturation.[36] It is secondary to anatomic features and pathologic abnormality resulting in decreased upper airway diameter and decreased patency during sleep. Risk factors are both anatomic and pathologic and OSA can present as acute, subacute, or chronic with severity of mild to severe (**Table 4**).

Table 4
Characterization and risk factors of OSA

	Characterization of OSA Severity	Risk Factors
Mild	Mild sleepiness	Male
	Mild insomnia	Obesity
	Minimal sleep disturbances	Nasopharyngeal abnormalities
	Mild oxygen desaturations	Hypertrophied tonsils and adenoids
	Benign cardiac arrhythmias	Severe upper respiratory tract
Moderate	Moderate sleepiness	infections
	Mild insomnia	Chronic allergic rhinitis
	Apneic episodes associated with	Craniofacial abnormalities
	moderate oxygen desaturation	
	Cardiac arrhythmias	
Severe	Severe sleepiness	
	Most sleep associated with respiratory	
	disturbances	
	Severe oxygen desaturations	
	Severe cardiac arrhythmias	
	Associated cardiopulmonary	
	dysfunction	

Data from American Academy of Sleep Medicine. International classification of sleep disorders, revised: Diagnostic and coding manual. Chicago: American Academy of Sleep Medicine; 2001.

In addition to the increase of risk of mortality with OSA, there are associated multi-organ diseases, including hypertension, congestive heart failure, coronary artery disease, arrhythmias, stroke, deep vein thrombosis, and renal disease.[37] Individuals with OSA have a decreased lifespan of 20 years and are at increased risk for perioperative complications, including reintubation, hypoxia, hypercapnia, sudden respiratory arrest, hemodynamic alterations, and myocardial infarction.[13] Moreover, more than 80% are undiagnosed,[37] making the surgical preoperative assessment critical to optimize morbidity and mortality in these patients. There have been a few preoperative questionnaires developed to assess the risk of OSA that have lacked sensitivity, leaving the overnight polysomnography the "gold standard" for diagnosis. However, in the preoperative setting, there are many limitations to overnight polysomnography, including scheduling, facility availability, cost, and convenience. Chung and colleagues[38] demonstrated the "STOP-Bang" questionnaire with an increased sensitivity of greater than 80% and improved negative predicted value in patients with moderate to severe OSA. This questionnaire allows for a practitioner to assess quickly for those at risk for OSA preoperatively with minimal training (**Table 5**).

A thorough preoperative assessment that identifies OSA as a possible risk can lead to investigation of other organ system insufficiency that should be addressed before elective surgeries. Patients with OSA or high risk for OSA should have routine chemistry and cell count analysis in conjunction with an ECG. If the patient's OSA is moderate to severe, preoperative arterial blood gas analysis and chest radiograph should be considered to establish baseline levels. An extended evaluation is needed for those treated with continuous positive airway pressure, including treatment settings and compliance, to aid in the anesthetic plan and perioperative management. Preoperative patient optimization is imperative to decrease perioperative complications, including morbidity, unplanned intensive care unit transfers, hospital length of stay, and mortality associated with OSA.[13]

Table 5
Components of the "STOP-Bang" questionnaire and scoring system

Components of the "STOP-Bang" Questionnaire	Scoring System
Snoring	High risk: >3 yes
Daytime Tiredness	Low risk <3 yes
Observed apnea	
Hypertension (Pressure)	
BMI >35 kg/m^2	
Age >50 y old	
Neck circumference >40 cm	
Male (Gender)	

Abbreviation: BMI, body mass index.
Data from Chung F, Yegneswaran B, Liao P, et al. STOP questionnaire: a tool to screen patients for obstructive sleep apnea. Anesthesiology 2008;108:812–21.

OBESITY

In 2010, about 35% of adults in the United States were obese, with obesity-related conditions leading the cause of preventable deaths.[39] This number has doubled since 1980 and continues to increase. Obesity is most often categorized by using the ratio of weight in kilograms to height in meters squared, otherwise known as body mass index (BMI). There are multiple associated comorbidities including coronary heart disease, hypertension, stroke, type 2 diabetes mellitus, cancer, and premature death, which are all beyond the scope of this article (**Table 6**). However, physiologic effects of

Table 6
Physiologic changes associated with obesity

Respiratory mechanics	Restrictive lung disease and decreased compliance (resulting in decreased FRC, ERV, FEV$_1$, FVC, TLC, RV), increased work of breathing, and increased atelectasis
Risk for OSA	5% of obese population
Anatomic changes	Increased upper airway adipose/soft tissue
Cardiovascular changes	Increased oxygen consumption Increased cardiac work and CO$_2$ production Increased blood volume Pulmonary hypertension Left ventricular hypertrophy Increased risk for arrhythmia
GERD	Increased intra-abdominal pressures Increased gastric acidic contents Increased risk for aspiration
Alterations in pharmacokinetics and pharmacodynamics	Affects volume of distribution Affects peak plasma concentrations, clearance, and elimination
Other comorbidities	Hypertension, hyperlipidemia, non-insulin-dependent diabetes mellitus and functional dependence
DVT	Doubled risk for DVT

Abbreviations: DVT, deep vein thrombosis; GERD, gastroesophageal reflux disease; RV, residual volume; TLC, total lung capacity.
Data from Refs.[40–44]

obesity on the pulmonary system and the preoperative assessments that need to be addressed before surgery are important to mention.

Although studies, to date, have not demonstrated any increased risk for postoperative complications,[13] the physiologic effect and changes must be acknowledged and optimization and treatment initiated, when possible, before surgical procedure. There are modifications for every medical sector that occur when an obese patient undergoes surgery. It may be these modifications that aid in the undifferentiated morbidity and mortality in this group perioperatively. A physical examination that incorporates a detailed pulmonary examination, assessment of OSA risk (as mentioned above), airway management, and functional status is critical.

SUMMARY

PPC are costly and a serious complication following surgery. Because PPC occur in more than 25% of patients requiring general anesthesia, preoperative diligence is imperative to reducing morbidity and mortality. This diligence is especially critical in patients with chronic pulmonary disease, including smokers, and patients with COPD, asthma, restrictive lung disease, OSA, and obesity. With a detailed preoperative assessment and appropriate preoperative testing, the risk of PPC, and subsequent sequelae, can be minimized in these challenging patients.

REFERENCES

1. Manku K, Bacchetti P, Leung JM. Prognostic significance of postoperative in-hospital complications in elderly patients. I. Long-term survival. Anesth Analg 2003;96:583–9 [table of contents].
2. Bruells CS, Rossaint R. Physiology of gas exchange during anaesthesia. Eur J Anaesthesiol 2011;28:570–9.
3. Coussa M, Roietti S, Schnyder P, et al. Prevention of atelectasis formation during the induction of general anesthesia in morbidly obese patients. Anesth Analg 2004;98:1491–5.
4. Wahba R. Perioperative functional residual capacity. Can J Anaesth 1991;38: 384–400.
5. Rock P, Rich PB. Postoperative pulmonary complications. Curr Opin Anaesthesiol 2003;16:123–31.
6. Canet J, Mazo V. Postoperative pulmonary complications. Minerva Anestesiol 2010;76:138–43.
7. Sweitzer BJ, Smetana GW. Identification and evaluation of the patient with lung disease. Anesthesiol Clin 2009;27:673–86.
8. Kearney D, Lee T, Reilly J, et al. Assessment of operative risk in patients undergoing lung resection. Chest 1994;105:753–9.
9. Dronkers JJ, Chorus AM, van Meeteren NL, et al. The association of pre-operative physical fitness and physical activity with outcome after scheduled major abdominal surgery. Anaesthesia 2013;68:67–73.
10. Arouzullah A, Khuri S, Henderson W, et al. Development and validation of a multi-factorial risk index for predicting postoperative pneumonia after major noncardiac surgery. Ann Intern Med 2001;135:847–57.
11. Blum JM, Stentz MJ, Dechert R, et al. Preoperative and intraoperative predictors of postoperative acute respiratory distress syndrome in a general surgical population. Anesthesiology 2013;118:19–29.

12. McAlister F, Bertsch K, Man J, et al. Incidence of and risk factors for pulmonary complications after noncardiothoracic surgery. Am J Respir Crit Care Med 2005; 171:514–7.
13. Smetana GW. Preoperative pulmonary evaluation: identifying and reducing risks for pulmonary complications. Cleve Clin J Med 2006;73(Suppl 1):S36–41.
14. Lawrence V, Dhanda R, Hislebeck S, et al. Risk of pulmonary complications after elective abdominal surgery. Chest 1996;110:744–50.
15. Barreiro TJ, Perillo I. An approach to interpreting spirometry. Am Fam Physician 2004;69:1107–14.
16. Bernstein W. Pulmonary function testing. Curr Opin Anaesthesiol 2012;25:11–6.
17. Brunelli A, Varela G, Rocco G, et al. A model to predict the immediate postoperative FEV1 following major lung resections. Eur J Cardiothorac Surg 2007;32: 783–6.
18. Miller M, Pedersen O. New concepts for expressing forced expiratory volume in 1 s arising from survival analysis. Eur Respir J 2010;35:873–82.
19. Arozullah A, Daley J, Henderson W, et al. Multifactorial risk index for predicting postoperative respiratory failure in men after major noncardiac surgery. The National Veterans Administration Surgical Quality Improvement Program. Ann Surg 2000;232:242–53.
20. Thomsen T, Villebro N, Moller AM. Interventions for preoperative smoking cessation. Cochrane Database Syst Rev 2010;(7):CD002294.
21. Quraishi SA, Orkin FK, Roizen MF. The anesthesia preoperative assessment: an opportunity for smoking cessation intervention. J Clin Anesth 2006;18:635–40.
22. Warner DO. Helping surgical patients quit smoking: why, when, and how. Anesth Analg 2005;101:481–7 [table of contents].
23. Wong J, Lam DP, Abrishami A, et al. Short-term preoperative smoking cessation and postoperative complications: a systematic review and meta-analysis. Can J Anaesth 2012;59:268–79.
24. Vestbo J, Hurd SS, Agusti AG, et al. Global strategy for the diagnosis, management, and prevention of chronic obstructive pulmonary disease: GOLD executive summary. Am J Respir Crit Care Med 2013;187:347–65.
25. Edrich T, Sadovnikoff N. Anesthesia for patients with severe chronic obstructive pulmonary disease. Curr Opin Anaesthesiol 2010;23:18–24.
26. Mandra A, Simic D, Stevanovic V, et al. Preoperative considerations for patients with chronic obstructive pulmonary disease. Acta Chir Iugosl 2011;58:71–5.
27. Spieth PM, Guldner A, de Abreu MG. Chronic obstructive pulmonary disease. Curr Opin Anaesthesiol 2012;25:24–9.
28. Lindenauer P, Pekow P, Lahti M, et al. Association of corticosteroid dose and route of administration with risk of treatment failure in acute exacerbation of chronic obstructive pulmonary disease. JAMA 2010;303:2359–67.
29. Masoli M, Fabian D, Holt S, et al. The global burden of asthma: executive summary of the GINA Dissemination Committee report. Allergy 2004;59:469–78.
30. Shnider S, Papper E. Anesthesia for the asthmatic patient. Anesthesiology 1961; 22:886–92.
31. Yamakage M, Iwasaki S, Namiki A. Guideline-oriented perioperative management of patients with bronchial asthma and chronic obstructive pulmonary disease. J Anesth 2008;22:412–28.
32. Woods BD, Sladen RN. Perioperative considerations for the patient with asthma and bronchospasm. Br J Anaesth 2009;103(Suppl 1)):i57–65.
33. Groeben H. Strategies in the patient with compromised respiratory function. Best Pract Res Clin Anaesthesiol 2004;18:579–94.

34. Marshall NS, Wong KK, Liu PY, et al. Sleep apnea as an independent risk factor for all-cause mortality: the Busselton Health Study. Sleep 2008;31:1079–85.
35. Young T, Palta M, Dempsey J, et al. The occurrence of sleep-disordered breathing among middle-aged adults. N Engl J Med 1993;328:1230–5.
36. American Academy of Sleep Medicine. The international classification of sleep disorders, revised. Diagnostic and coding manual. 2001. Available at: http://www.esst.org/adds/ICSD.pdf.
37. Young T, Evans L, Finn L, et al. Estimation of the clinically diagnosed proportion of sleep apnea syndrome in middle-aged men and women. Sleep 1997;20:705–6.
38. Chung F, Yegneswaran B, Liao P, et al. STOP questionnaire: a tool to screen patients for obstructive sleep apnea. Anesthesiology 2008;108:812–21.
39. Ogden CL, Carroll MD, Kit BK, et al. Prevalence of obesity in the United States, 2009-2010. NCHS Data Brief 2012;(82):1–8.
40. Salome CM, King GG, Berend N. Physiology of obesity and effects on lung function. J Appl Physiol 2010;108:206–11.
41. Pedoto A. Lung physiology and obesity: anesthetic implications for thoracic procedures. Anesthesiol Res Pract 2012;2012:154208.
42. Koenig SM. Pulmonary complications of obesity. Am J Med Sci 2001;321:249–79.
43. Catenacci VA, Hill JO, Wyatt HR. The obesity epidemic. Clin Chest Med 2009;30:415–44, vii.
44. Allman-Farinelli M. Obesity and venous thrombosis: a review. Semin Thromb Hemost 2011;37:903–7.

Pulmonary Rehabilitation at the Time of the COPD Exacerbation

Roger Goldstein, MB ChB, FRCP[a,b,c,d],*, Dina Brooks, PhD, PT[a,b,d]

KEYWORDS

- Pulmonary rehabilitation • COPD • Exercise • Physical therapy
- Acute exacerbation

KEY POINTS

- Pulmonary rehabilitation (PR) is associated with improvements in exercise capacity, health-related quality of life, psychological symptoms, and resource utilization.
- Acute exacerbations threaten these PR improvements.
- An awareness of the clinical sequelae of acute exacerbation of chronic obstructive pulmonary disease enables approaches, such as early post-exacerbation rehabilitation to mitigate its negative effects.

INTRODUCTION

In chronic obstructive pulmonary disease (COPD), severe exacerbations, especially when multiple, are an independent adverse prognostic variable[1] with an adjusted risk of death being 4 times higher than for those free of exacerbation. Therefore, a reduction in the number and the impact of exacerbations has become a priority in the management of COPD. There is growing evidence that pulmonary rehabilitation (PR) is an effective and safe intervention to improve health-related quality of life, peripheral muscle function, and exercise capacity as well as to reduce hospital admission and possibly mortality in patients with COPD post-exacerbation.[2] Despite this growing evidence, authoritative reviews of exacerbations in COPD make scant mention of non-pharmacologic approaches[3,4] such as rehabilitation. This article discusses the definition of an acute exacerbation (AE), the rationale, and evidence for post-exacerbation

This article originally appeared in *Clinics in Chest Medicine*, Volume 35, Issue 2, June 2014.
[a] Graduate Department of Rehabilitation Science, Faculty of Medicine, University of Toronto, Toronto, Ontario, Canada; [b] Department of Physical Therapy, University of Toronto, Toronto, Ontario, Canada; [c] Department of Medicine, Faculty of Medicine, University of Toronto, Toronto, Ontario, Canada; [d] Department of Respiratory Medicine, West Park Healthcare Centre, 82 Buttonwood Avenue, Toronto, Ontario, M6M 2J5, Canada
* Corresponding author. West Park Healthcare Centre, 82 Buttonwood Avenue, Toronto, Ontario, M6M 2J5, Canada.
E-mail address: rgoldstein@westpark.org

Clinics Collections 6 (2015) 147–158
http://dx.doi.org/10.1016/j.ccol.2015.05.036

PR and how the program might be modified to take into consideration the more frail state of such patients.

DEFINITION, CAUSE, AND PATHOPHYSIOLOGY OF ACUTE EXACERBATION
Definition

An AE was originally defined[5] based on symptoms and characterized by a change in purulence, viscosity, or volume of sputum production and/or an increase in dyspnea, which may be associated with nasal discharge, sore throat, fever, and increased cough or wheeze. Other experts have modified this definition or provided alternative definitions, for example, adding a duration for the symptoms of at least 2 consecutive days.[6] An international working group defined AE more broadly as "a sustained worsening of a patient's condition from stable state, and beyond the usual day-to-day variation, that is acute in onset and necessitates a change in regular medication in a patient with underlying COPD."[7] In the GOLD guidelines for treatment,[8] a definition of AE severity was developed based on the need for a therapeutic intervention (event-based definition). AEs were termed mild if they were managed at home by increased bronchodilator therapy without additional health care contact. Moderate exacerbations were also managed at home through unscheduled health care contact and/or the initiation of treatment with oral glucocorticosteroids, whereas severe exacerbations were managed in the emergency room and/or in hospital.[8]

The availability of multiple definitions, whether symptom or event-based, is problematic and has hampered the assessment of efficacy of treatment.[9] In fact, a systematic review found that less than 20% of trials used a symptom-based definition of AE, such as those mentioned earlier.[5,6] In half the trials, definition of AE was limited to those requiring new treatment with pharmacotherapy and/or hospitalization. The article concluded that clinical trials used varied definitions and analysis of AE, leading to biased estimates of treatment effects for new treatments for AEs.[10]

Cause and Incidence

The triggers of AEs are infections of the tracheobronchial tree, environmental exposures, or unidentified.[6,8,11–13] Infections account for up to 80% of acute exacerbation of COPD (AECOPD) and can be bacterial or viral.[12,14–17] The relative risk of hospital admissions for AECOPD increases with higher levels of air pollutants.[18,19] Although infections are the prime precipitating factors, a primary physiologic mechanism that contributes to the impact of an AE is dynamic hyperinflation. Dynamic hyperinflation refers to an acute increase in the retained air at the end of expiration that occurs during exercise in patients with airway obstruction such as COPD.[20] During AE, with increased airway obstruction, dynamic hyperinflation occurs as the respiratory rate increases and the expiratory flow rate decreases and can lead to increased mechanical disadvantage of the respiratory musculature, marked dyspnea, anxiety, and negative cardiovascular consequences.[20]

The frequency of AECOPD for severe COPD is 1 to 4 per year.[6,11,21] Hospitalization occurs in up to 16% of those with AE.[6,22] In those with severe AEs, mortality has been reported between 3% and 10%[23,24] and much higher (at 15%–24%) in those admitted to the intensive care unit.[25,26] In a 6-month longitudinal study of 1016 patients hospitalized for COPD, death during the AE was 11% and 2-year mortality was 49%. Hospital readmission rates were as high as 50% in the first 6 months after discharge.[24] In a study of 377 post-exacerbation COPD patients, the worst quality of life scores were associated with the highest readmission to hospital.[27] In a retrospective study of 551 post-exacerbation hospital discharges of whom 59% were readmitted within

12 months, dependency in self-care[28] was identified as an independent contributor to readmission.

ACUTE EXACERBATIONS—THE ENEMY OF REHABILITATION

In addition to the short- and long-term threat to mortality as a result of AECOPD, especially among those requiring hospitalization, the result of a single episode may threaten many of the gains achieved by PR. The positive impact of PR on exercise tolerance and health-related quality of life is well established, and as a result, PR is considered standard practice for COPD and recommended by professional societies around the world.[29] Much of this positive impact is the result of decreased dyspnea and improved peripheral muscle function.[30] In addition, functional activities of daily living and other secondary impairments such as anxiety and depression are improved by PR.[31] Health resource utilization in terms of unscheduled emergency room visits and reduced hospitalization is also reduced.[32,33]

Impact on Lung Function

To establish the impact of exacerbations on lung function, one study followed 109 patients with COPD over 4 years. The investigators noted that those with frequent exacerbations had a faster decline in FEV_1 (-40 mL/y) compared with those who experience fewer exacerbations (-32 mL/y),[34] even when adjusted for smoking status. Moreover, among 20 of 46 frequent exacerbators, the rate of hospitalization was 1.5 per annum in contrast to admissions on one occasion for only 7 of 63 infrequent exacerbators.

Impact on Muscle Strength

In addition to the consequences of bed rest, the multifactorial changes in metabolic and inflammatory states, as well as nutritional, oxidative, pharmacologic (eg, steroids), and gas exchange (eg, hypoxia) alterations associated with an AECOPD, all will affect peripheral muscle function. In 2003, investigators studied the impact of hospitalization for an AECOPD on muscle force[35] and reported that on admission the quadriceps peak torque (QPT) among hospitalized patients was 66% ($\pm$22%) of the values measured in healthy age-matched elderly subjects, declining by 5% between days 3 and 8 and partially recovering 3 months later (**Fig. 1**). There was an inverse correlation between QPT and levels of the inflammatory marker interleukin 8, which were increased in AECOPD patients compared with stable COPD and healthy elderly. These observations have led to interest in starting rehabilitation during the exacerbation, using resistance training to counterbalance the deterioration in quadriceps function during an AECOPD.[36] In fact, resistance training is feasible and effective. In 40 hospitalized patients with a COPD exacerbation, resistance training enhanced quadriceps force on discharge (+9% $\pm$ 16%) compared to untrained subjects (-1 ± 13%). The improvement was maintained at 1 month post-discharge (**Fig. 2**).

Impact on Health-related Quality of Life

In contrast to the gains made in PR, investigators[37] noted that among a group of COPD patients followed for 12 years, those labeled as frequent exacerbators (≥ 3 per annum) experienced a lower health-related quality of life as reflected by the total and component (symptoms, activities, and impact) scores on the disease-specific St George's Respiratory Questionnaire. Predictors of frequent exacerbations included daily cough, wheeze, and sputum production, as well as frequent exacerbations in the previous year. Subsequently, these same investigators described a prodromal preexacerbation period during which time subjective measurements of dyspnea

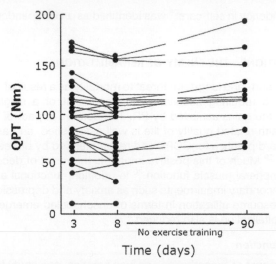

Fig. 1. QPT during hospitalization for AECOPD. (*Adapted from* Spruit MA, Gosselink R, Troosters T, et al. Muscle force during an acute exacerbation in hospitalized patients with COPD and its relationship with CXCL8 and IGF-I. Thorax 2003;58(9):752; with permission.)

increased. Subsequent to the AE, recovery of peak expiratory flow to baseline levels was complete after a week in only 75% of exacerbations, and in 7% of exacerbations, recovery to baseline had still not occurred at 3 months.[6] Although the investigators did not track activities during the period of observation, it is very likely that the increase in dyspnea and other symptoms would have reduced physical activities both during the prodromal period and subsequent to the exacerbation itself.

Impact on Physical Activity

A study looking at[38] the impact of exacerbations on the behavior of patients with COPD used diary card measures of time spent outside the home as a marker of physical activity. Of 147 patients followed for approximately 4 years, time indoors

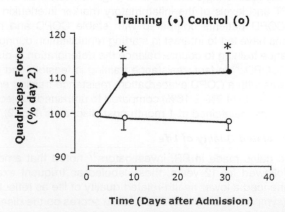

Fig. 2. Resistance training and quadriceps muscle function during AECOPD. * = $p < 0.05$. (*Data from* Troosters T, Probst VS, Crul T, et al. Resistance training prevents deterioration in quadriceps muscle function during acute exacerbations of chronic obstructive pulmonary disease. Am J Respir Crit Care Med 2010;181(10):1072.)

increased gradually. At baseline, patients spent all day at home for 2.1 days per week (34% of their days). After exacerbation they spent 2.5 days at home (44% of their days), decreasing gradually over the next few weeks. This study highlighted the negative impact of exacerbations on time spent outside the home, exactly the opposite of one of the goals of PR. In 2006, a group of investigators[39] studied whether the lower time spent in physical activity associated with bed rest during an AECOPD could contribute to the reductions in muscle force. Activity monitors were applied at the beginning and end of hospitalization for an AECOPD and again after 1 month. Compared to stable COPD patients who spent approximately one-third of their time during the day in weight bearing activities,[40] the time spent in physical activities such as walking and standing was low both on the second and seventh day of hospitalization (**Fig. 3**). Moreover, these activities were still reduced 1 month after discharge. These investigators further observed that the time spent in weight bearing activities after a week correlated positively with measurements of quadriceps force and that the reduction in quadriceps force correlated with a smaller improvement in walking time at 1 month. Although at the beginning of the exacerbation there were no differences in clinical characteristics, those hospitalized in the previous year walked for less time after 1 month compared with those who had not been hospitalized.

Impact on Hospital Readmission

Exacerbations that subsequently reduce physical activity not only reverse the gains made by PR but may also promote hospital readmission from further exacerbations. Of 340 patients recruited at the time of admission to hospital and followed for just over a year,[41] 63% of patients were readmitted at least once and 29% died. The investigators reported that more than 3 admissions for an AECOPD increased the risk of readmission (hazard ratio [HR] 1.66, 95% confidence interval [CI] 1.16–2.39). The investigators also showed for the first time that involvement in higher levels of usual physical activity was protective (HR 0.54, 95%CI 0.34–0.86). Physical activity was derived from a questionnaire, the results of which were converted to kcal/d. This strong association has important therapeutic implications, because the third of patients who reported activities equivalent to walking for more than 60 min/d had a reduction of almost 50% in risk of admission to hospital. Recent studies[42–44] are encouraging as to the impact of PR on domestic function and physical activity, especially when administered in a way that will promote longer-term adherence. A systematic review of the impact of exercise on physical activity noted the need

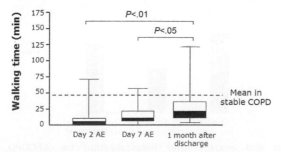

Fig. 3. Hospitalization and physical activity post-AECOPD. (*Adapted from* Pitta F, Troosters T, Probst VS, et al. Physical activity and hospitalization for exacerbation of COPD. Chest 2006;129(3):536; with permission.)

for larger randomized controlled trial in which activity is measured in absolute units such as steps or activity counts.[45]

PSYCHOLOGICAL IMPACT OF ACUTE EXACERBATION

AECOPDs have been associated with an increase in anxiety and depression.[46] In a series of home-based interviews and focus groups among 25 post-AECOPD patients, anxiety and depression was noted in 64% and 40%, respectively. Patients also expressed fear of another episode and uncertainty regarding the availability of social and medical care. In a Nordic study of the prevalence of psychological symptoms among 416 patients hospitalized with an AECOPD,[47] a high prevalence of anxiety and depression was noted (**Fig. 4**).

A recent interpretive meta-synthesis compiled the results of 8 qualitative studies exploring the perspectives of patients with COPD after an exacerbation.[48] AECOPD resulted in a "heightened patient arousal, vigilance and powerlessness". Breathlessness with an AE resulted in fear and anxiety and patients often perceived that their symptoms were dismissed by the medical team. Patients also felt that they lacked the knowledge on discharge from hospital to handle their medical condition. Concerns were also expressed about the impact of the AE on their caregiver's health and the strain of the illness on their relationship with the caregiver.[46,48] Of note, when asked to describe their experiences of an AE, in addition to the usual symptoms of dyspnea and cough, more than 80% of patients experienced fatigue and more than 40% experienced a change in mood.[49] These findings indicate that there is a need to address the psychological needs of the patients, design intervention to acknowledge their fears, and manage the high levels of anxiety and depression after AE. Such screening and intervention can occur during post-exacerbation rehabilitation.

REHABILITATION AFTER ACUTE EXACERBATION: THE EVIDENCE, PRACTICE, AND COMPONENTS

The gains of PR, especially dyspnea reduction, increased exercise capacity, and physical activities of daily living are diminished by AECOPD. Therefore, there is growing interest in the initiation of PR during or soon after an AECOPD to reverse the loss of peripheral muscle function, improve dyspnea and health-related quality

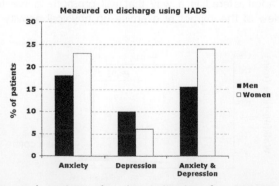

Fig. 4. Depression and anxiety after hospitalization for AECOPD. (*Adapted from* Gudmundsson G, Gislason T, Janson C, et al. Depression, anxiety and health status after hospitalisation for COPD: a multicentre study in the Nordic countries. Respir Med 2006;100(1):87; with permission.)

of life, decrease depression, and increase physical activity. PR post-exacerbation includes physical exercise in patients recently managed for an AE.[2]

Airway Clearance Techniques for Acute Exacerbation

The evidence for airway clearance techniques as a component of rehabilitation is unclear because of conflicting findings and poor methodological rigor.[50] Airway clearance techniques may include "postural drainage or gravity assisted positioning, breathing exercises, chest wall percussion and/or vibration, forced expiratory technique, coughing maneuvers and the use of devices such as positive expiratory pressure (PEP) masks."[51] Two systematic reviews examined the safety and effectiveness of airway clearance techniques in the management of AECOPD.[51,52] Both systematic reviews included studies with patients who were breathing spontaneously; although only one[51] reviewed randomized controlled trials or randomized cross over, the other[52] included cohort studies as well. Airway clearance techniques were found not to result in improvement in lung function or changes in measures of gas exchange or hospital length of stay.[51] In fact, chest wall percussion in gravity-assisted positions for approximately 5 minutes resulted in a reduction of forced expiratory volume in 1 second.[51] All other airway clearance techniques were reported to be safe.[51,52] In patients with copious secretions, mechanical vibration and PEP mask were beneficial in encouraging sputum expectoration.[51,52] There was insufficient evidence regarding effectiveness of breathing exercises.[52]

Consistent with the evidence, surveys of practice patterns on the management of patients with COPD hospitalized for AE have shown that treatment focuses on mobilization and much less on airway clearance techniques.[50,53] However, despite the lack of evidence to support their effectiveness techniques like purse lip breathing, active cycle breathing techniques and diaphragmatic breathing were used by most therapists.[50,53] These findings may indicate that patients hospitalized with an AECOPD require assistance to improve ventilation but not to clear secretions.

Pulmonary Rehabilitation

In a single-center randomized controlled trial evaluating early post-hospitalization community-based PR, investigators[54] reported on significant between-group improvements in the endurance shuttle walk (60 m 95% CI 27–93 m), the St. George's Respiratory Questionnaire (−12.7, −5 to −20), and all 4 components of the chronic respiratory questionnaire, noting that early PR is both feasible and effective (**Fig. 5**). Subsequently, a similar study by the same group[55] noted a reduction in hospital readmissions subsequent to PR with 33% of the control group and only 7% of the rehabilitation group being admitted during the subsequent 3 months. A Cochrane review[2] assessed the effects of PR after AE in individuals with COPD on future hospital admissions, exercise capacity, health-related quality of life, and mortality. PR was defined as any inpatient and/or outpatient PR program, started either immediately after initiation of AE treatment or up to 3 weeks after AE. PR resulted in a reduction in the odds of hospital readmission. There was also a favorable effect on health-related quality of life that exceeded the minimal clinically important difference. PR also resulted in improvement in 6-minute walk test and shuttle walk test, despite substantial differences between trials. There were no adverse effects in any of the studies. Although the pooled relative risk of death was decreased in the rehabilitation groups, this result requires confirmation because 2 of the 3 trials did not show an effect, and one study was reported only in abstract form. Although the limitation of this systematic review is the small total number of patients and methodological shortcomings of the study, the effect of PR after AE appears to be substantial.

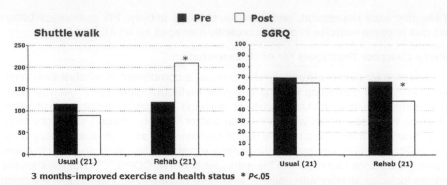

■ Pre   □ Post

3 months-improved exercise and health status * *P*<.05

Fig. 5. Early rehabilitation post-AECOPD. (*Data from* Man WD, Polkey MI, Donaldson N, et al. Community pulmonary rehabilitation after hospitalisation for acute exacerbations of chronic obstructive pulmonary disease: randomised controlled study. BMJ 2004;329(7476):1209.)

Despite the evidence in support of PR, less than 25% of patients are referred to PR on discharge from hospital.[50] This absence of referral may be the result of lack of availability of PR or lack of awareness of its effectiveness.[50] In a recent clinical audit in the UK,[56] of 448 post-exacerbation discharges, 286 were eligible for post-hospitalization PR, but only 31% were referred and of the 60 who began the course only 43 finished. Studies are required to investigate patient, staff, and organizational barriers to post-hospitalization PR. It is not clear what the optimal time or setting for initiation of PR is. In almost half the studies in the Cochrane systematic review, PR was initiated within 3 to 8 days of hospital admission and the setting included inpatient, outpatient, and home.

PROGRAM MODIFICATION POST-EXACERBATION

The extent to which the rehabilitation program will require modification post-AE depends on the severity of the exacerbation. For mild exacerbations little or no modifications are required. For moderate and severe exacerbations, dyspnea and fatigue will be markedly increased and exercise endurance will be decreased. It is advisable to encourage all patients to continue with their breathing exercises as they require only a modest effort and they improve flexibility, ventilation, and secretion clearance as well as promoting relaxation. For upper extremity strength training, the increased respiratory demands of the AE and the use of upper limbs as accessory muscles of respiration may require program modification with fewer sets, fewer repetitions, or longer rests in between. Similar adaptations may be required for lower-extremity resistance training. Self-paced leisure walking as a mechanism of increased physical activity should be encouraged and determined by patient tolerance, with eventual progression to more specific aerobic prescription using cycle or treadmill. The use of supplemental oxygen may be indicated for some patients, although oxygen has to be prescribed with care in those who are carbon dioxide retainers.

The multidisciplinary treatment team should be aware of the increase in anxiety, which stems from but may also increase dyspnea during and after an AE. For individuals with COPD who have received education on self-management, breathing control and energy conservation may be able to manage symptoms better that those without such education. For some, the combination of severe dyspnea and anxiety may result in panic that requires hospitalization. For patients with COPD who have previous experience of PR during stable periods, resuming activities post-exacerbation is important. However, getting back on track may be a slow process. Deconditioning occurs relatively quickly, and attempts by the patient to resume aerobic training at the same work rate as before will be met with frustration. Aerobic exercise may need to be resumed at a lower level of intensity. This information should be provided on completion of a PR program during stable periods so that subsequent patient expectations are realistic.

SUMMARY

PR is associated with improvements in exercise capacity, health-related quality of life, psychological symptoms, and resource utilization. AEs threaten each of these improvements. An awareness of the clinical sequelae of AECOPD enables approaches such as early post-exacerbation rehabilitation to mitigate the negative effects of the exacerbation. Such approaches should occur alongside pharmacologic management to maximize success and reduce the likelihood of repeat hospitalization.

REFERENCES

1. Soler-Cataluna JJ, Martinez-Garcia MA, Roman Sanchez P, et al. Severe acute exacerbations and mortality in patients with chronic obstructive pulmonary disease. Thorax 2005;60(11):925–31.
2. Puhan MA, Gimeno-Santos E, Scharplatz M, et al. Pulmonary rehabilitation following exacerbations of chronic obstructive pulmonary disease. Cochrane Database Syst Rev 2011;(10):CD005305.
3. Celli BR, Barnes PJ. Exacerbations of chronic obstructive pulmonary disease. Eur Respir J 2007;29(6):1224–38.
4. Bach PB, Brown C, Gelfand SE, et al, American College of Physicians-American Society of Internal Medicine, American College of Chest Physicians. Management of acute exacerbations of chronic obstructive pulmonary disease: a summary and appraisal of published evidence. Ann Intern Med 2001;134(7):600–20.
5. Anthonisen NR, Manfreda J, Warren CP, et al. Antibiotic therapy in exacerbations of chronic obstructive pulmonary disease. Ann Intern Med 1987;106(2):196–204.
6. Seemungal TA, Donaldson GC, Bhowmik A, et al. Time course and recovery of exacerbations in patients with chronic obstructive pulmonary disease. Am J Respir Crit Care Med 2000;161(5):1608–13.
7. Rodriguez-Roisin R. Toward a consensus definition for COPD exacerbations. Chest 2000;117(5 Suppl 2):398S–401S.
8. Global Strategy for the Diagnosis, Management and Prevention of COPD, Global Initiative for Chronic Obstructive Lung Disease (GOLD). 2013. Available at: http://www.goldcopd.org/. Accessed March 4, 2013.
9. Pauwels R, Calverley P, Buist AS, et al. COPD exacerbations: the importance of a standard definition. Respir Med 2004;98(2):99–107.
10. Aaron SD, Fergusson D, Marks GB, et al. Counting, analysing and reporting exacerbations of COPD in randomised controlled trials. Thorax 2008;63(2):122–8.
11. Wedzicha JA. Airway infection accelerates decline of lung function in chronic obstructive pulmonary disease. Am J Respir Crit Care Med 2001;164(10 Pt 1):1757–8.
12. Wedzicha JA. Exacerbations: etiology and pathophysiologic mechanisms. Chest 2002;121(5 Suppl):136S–41S.
13. Hogg JC. Role of latent viral infections in chronic obstructive pulmonary disease and asthma. Am J Respir Crit Care Med 2001;164(10 Pt 2):S71–5.

14. Sethi S. Infectious etiology of acute exacerbations of chronic bronchitis. Chest 2000;117(5 Suppl 2):380S–5S.
15. Sethi S, Murphy TF. Bacterial infection in chronic obstructive pulmonary disease in 2000: a state-of-the-art review. Clin Microbiol Rev 2001;14(2):336–63.
16. Sethi S, Evans N, Grant BJ, et al. New strains of bacteria and exacerbations of chronic obstructive pulmonary disease. N Engl J Med 2002;347(7):465–71.
17. Seemungal T, Harper-Owen R, Bhowmik A, et al. Respiratory viruses, symptoms, and inflammatory markers in acute exacerbations and stable chronic obstructive pulmonary disease. Am J Respir Crit Care Med 2001;164(9):1618–23.
18. Anderson HR, Spix C, Medina S, et al. Air pollution and daily admissions for chronic obstructive pulmonary disease in 6 European cities: results from the APHEA project. Eur Respir J 1997;10(5):1064–71.
19. Donaldson GC, Seemungal T, Jeffries DJ, et al. Effect of temperature on lung function and symptoms in chronic obstructive pulmonary disease. Eur Respir J 1999;13(4):844–9.
20. O'Donnell DE, Parker CM. COPD exacerbations. 3: pathophysiology. Thorax 2006;61(4):354–61.
21. Burge S, Wedzicha JA. COPD exacerbations: definitions and classifications. Eur Respir J Suppl 2003;41:46S–53S.
22. Miravitlles M, Espinosa C, Fernandez-Laso E, et al. Relationship between bacterial flora in sputum and functional impairment in patients with acute exacerbations of COPD. Study Group of Bacterial Infection in COPD. Chest 1999;116(1):40–6.
23. Mushlin AI, Black ER, Connolly CA, et al. The necessary length of hospital stay for chronic pulmonary disease. JAMA 1991;266(1):80–3.
24. Connors AF Jr, Dawson NV, Thomas C, et al. Outcomes following acute exacerbation of severe chronic obstructive lung disease. The SUPPORT investigators (Study to Understand Prognoses and Preferences for Outcomes and Risks of Treatments). Am J Respir Crit Care Med 1996;154(4 Pt 1):959–67.
25. Afessa B, Morales IJ, Scanlon PD, et al. Prognostic factors, clinical course, and hospital outcome of patients with chronic obstructive pulmonary disease admitted to an intensive care unit for acute respiratory failure. Crit Care Med 2002;30(7):1610–5.
26. Seneff MG, Wagner DP, Wagner RP, et al. Hospital and 1-year survival of patients admitted to intensive care units with acute exacerbation of chronic obstructive pulmonary disease. JAMA 1995;274(23):1852–7.
27. Osman IM, Godden DJ, Friend JA, et al. Quality of life and hospital re-admission in patients with chronic obstructive pulmonary disease. Thorax 1997;52(1):67–71.
28. Lau AC, Yam LY, Poon E. Hospital re-admission in patients with acute exacerbation of chronic obstructive pulmonary disease. Respir Med 2001;95(11):876–84.
29. Spruit MA, Singh SJ, Garvey C, et al. An official american thoracic society/european respiratory society statement: key concepts and advances in pulmonary rehabilitation. Am J Respir Crit Care Med 2013;188(8):e13–64.
30. Troosters T, Gosselink R, Decramer M. Short- and long-term effects of outpatient rehabilitation in patients with chronic obstructive pulmonary disease: a randomized trial. Am J Med 2000;109(3):207–12.
31. Emery CF, Leatherman NE, Burker EJ, et al. Psychological outcomes of a pulmonary rehabilitation program. Chest 1991;100(3):613–7.
32. Bourbeau J, Collet JP, Schwartzman K, et al. Economic benefits of self-management education in COPD. Chest 2006;130(6):1704–11.
33. Bourbeau J, Julien M, Maltais F, et al. Reduction of hospital utilization in patients with chronic obstructive pulmonary disease: a disease-specific self-management intervention. Arch Intern Med 2003;163(5):585–91.

34. Donaldson GC, Seemungal TA, Bhowmik A, et al. Relationship between exacerbation frequency and lung function decline in chronic obstructive pulmonary disease. Thorax 2002;57(10):847–52.
35. Spruit MA, Gosselink R, Troosters T, et al. Muscle force during an acute exacerbation in hospitalised patients with COPD and its relationship with CXCL8 and IGF-I. Thorax 2003;58(9):752–6.
36. Troosters T, Probst VS, Crul T, et al. Resistance training prevents deterioration in quadriceps muscle function during acute exacerbations of chronic obstructive pulmonary disease. Am J Respir Crit Care Med 2010;181(10):1072–7.
37. Seemungal TA, Donaldson GC, Paul EA, et al. Effect of exacerbation on quality of life in patients with chronic obstructive pulmonary disease. Am J Respir Crit Care Med 1998;157(5 Pt 1):1418–22.
38. Donaldson GC, Wilkinson TM, Hurst JR, et al. Exacerbations and time spent outdoors in chronic obstructive pulmonary disease. Am J Respir Crit Care Med 2005;171(5):446–52.
39. Pitta F, Troosters T, Probst VS, et al. Physical activity and hospitalization for exacerbation of COPD. Chest 2006;129(3):536–44.
40. Pitta F, Troosters T, Spruit MA, et al. Characteristics of physical activities in daily life in chronic obstructive pulmonary disease. Am J Respir Crit Care Med 2005;171(9):972–7
41. Garcia-Aymerich J, Farrero E, Felez MA, et al. Risk factors of readmission to hospital for a COPD exacerbation: a prospective study. Thorax 2003;58(2):100–5.
42. Sewell L, Singh SJ, Williams JE, et al. Can individualized rehabilitation improve functional independence in elderly patients with COPD? Chest 2005;128(3):1194–200.
43. de Blok BM, de Greef MH, ten Hacken NH, et al. The effects of a lifestyle physical activity counseling program with feedback of a pedometer during pulmonary rehabilitation in patients with COPD: a pilot study. Patient Educ Couns 2006;61(1):48–55.
44. Pitta F, Troosters T, Probst VS, et al. Are patients with COPD more active after pulmonary rehabilitation? Chest 2008;134(2):273–80.
45. Cindy Ng LW, Mackney J, Jenkins S, et al. Does exercise training change physical activity in people with COPD? A systematic review and meta-analysis. Chron Respir Dis 2012;9(1):17–26.
46. Gruffydd-Jones K, Langley-Johnson C, Dyer C, et al. What are the needs of patients following discharge from hospital after an acute exacerbation of chronic obstructive pulmonary disease (COPD)? Prim Care Respir J 2007;16(6):363–8.
47. Gudmundsson G, Gislason T, Janson C, et al. Depression, anxiety and health status after hospitalisation for COPD: a multicentre study in the Nordic countries. Respir Med 2006;100(1):87–93.
48. Harrison SL, Horton EJ, Smith R, et al. Physical activity monitoring: addressing the difficulties of accurately detecting slow walking speeds. Heart Lung 2013;42(5):361–4.e1.
49. Costi S, Brooks D, Goldstein RS. Perspectives that influence action plans for chronic obstructive pulmonary disease. Can Respir J 2006;13(7):362–8.
50. Harth L, Stuart J, Montgomery C, et al. Physical therapy practice patterns in acute exacerbations of chronic obstructive pulmonary disease. Can Respir J 2009;16(3):86–92.
51. Hill K, Patman S, Brooks D. Effect of airway clearance techniques in patients experiencing an acute exacerbation of chronic obstructive pulmonary disease: a systematic review. Chron Respir Dis 2010;7(1):9–17.

52. Tang CY, Taylor NF, Blackstock FC. Chest physiotherapy for patients admitted to hospital with an acute exacerbation of chronic obstructive pulmonary disease (COPD): a systematic review. Physiotherapy 2010;96(1):1–13.

53. Yohannes AM. Health status and quality of life after acute exacerbations of chronic obstructive pulmonary disease. Qual Life Res 2007;16(2):357–8.

54. Man WD, Polkey MI, Donaldson N, et al. Community pulmonary rehabilitation after hospitalisation for acute exacerbations of chronic obstructive pulmonary disease: randomised controlled study. BMJ 2004;329(7476):1209.

55. Seymour JM, Moore L, Jolley CJ, et al. Outpatient pulmonary rehabilitation following acute exacerbations of COPD. Thorax 2010;65(5):423–8.

56. Jones SE, Green SA, Clark AL, et al. Pulmonary rehabilitation following hospitalisation for acute exacerbation of COPD: referrals, uptake and adherence. Thorax 2014;69(2):181–2.

Acute COPD Exacerbations

Jadwiga A. Wedzicha, MD, FRCP*, Richa Singh, MRCP,
Alex J. Mackay, MRCP

KEYWORDS

• COPD • Exacerbations • Respiratory viral infections • Bacterial infections

KEY POINTS

- Chronic obstructive pulmonary disease (COPD) exacerbations are important events in COPD and are major determinants of health status in COPD.
- The natural course of COPD is interrupted by episodes of respiratory symptom worsening, termed *exacerbations*.
- Optimal management of acute exacerbations not only increases the rate of exacerbation recovery but also affects exacerbation rates and prevents hospital admissions.
- There is a need for the development of novel antiinflammatory agents that are effective at COPD exacerbations.

IMPACT OF COPD EXACERBATIONS

The natural course of COPD is interrupted by episodes of respiratory symptom worsening, termed exacerbations.[1] COPD exacerbations are important events in COPD and are major determinants of health status in COPD. COPD exacerbations are also independent predictors of mortality in COPD and also drive disease progression, with approximately 25% of the lung function decline attributed to exacerbations.[2]

COPD is the second largest cause of emergency admissions in the United Kingdom, with 1 in 8 hospital emergency admissions resulting from COPD, accounting for more than £800 million ($1.3 billion) in direct health care costs.[3] COPD exacerbations are also associated with cardiovascular events, especially myocardial infarction,[4,5] and patients hospitalized with exacerbations of COPD are a particularly vulnerable group for ischemic events. Every new severe exacerbation requiring hospitalization increases the risk of a subsequent exacerbation, and every new severe exacerbation

This article originally appeared in *Clinics in Chest Medicine*, Volume 35, Issue 1, March 2014.
Conflicts of Interest: J.A. Wedzicha has received honoraria for lectures and/or advisory boards from GSK, Novartis, Boehringer, Pfizer, Bayer, Takeda, and Vifor Pharma. She has received research grants from Novartis, Johnson and Johnson, Takeda, and Chiesi.
Centre for Respiratory Medicine, Royal Free Campus, University College London, Rowland Hill Street, London NW3 2PF, UK
* Corresponding author.
E-mail address: w.wedzicha@ucl.ac.uk

Clinics Collections 6 (2015) 159–168
http://dx.doi.org/10.1016/j.ccol.2015.05.037
2352-7986/15/$ – see front matter © 2015 Elsevier Inc. All rights reserved.

increases the risk of death, up to 5 times after the 10th compared with after a first COPD hospitalization.[6] COPD exacerbations are also more common and more severe in the winter months, when there are already pressures on numbers of admissions in hospitals.

Thus, the COPD strategy document developed by the Global Initiative for Chronic Obstructive Lung Disease (GOLD) highlights the importance of avoiding future risk in COPD by preventing exacerbations.[7] In view of the wide impact of COPD exacerbations, any therapy that prevents exacerbations will also improve health status and prevent forced expiratory volume in the first second of expiration (FEV_1) decline.

DEFINITION OF EXACERBATIONS

The common symptoms of a COPD exacerbation are increase in dyspnea, sputum purulence, and cough, but other symptoms may include increased wheezing, chest discomfort, and symptoms of an upper airway cold. Physiologic changes at COPD exacerbations (eg, falls in peak flow or FEV_1) are generally small and not useful in predicting or monitoring exacerbations.[1]

An exacerbation of COPD is defined in the GOLD strategy in terms of health care utilization as "an acute event characterised by a worsening of the patient's respiratory symptoms that is beyond normal day-to-day variations and leads to a change in medication." There is considerable evidence, however, that approximately half of all COPD exacerbations identified by symptom worsening are not reported to health care professionals for treatment.[8] Furthermore, these unreported exacerbations, although generally of lesser severity than reported or treated exacerbations, also have an impact on health status.[8]

For this reason, considerable interest exists in the potential of patient-reported outcomes in studies of exacerbation, and one of these is an instrument specifically designed for exacerbations, the Exacerbations of Chronic Pulmonary Disease Tool (EXACT). Although it may be useful in assessing the severity of exacerbations and the response to acute exacerbation therapy,[9] detection of an exacerbation probably still depends on patient report. Recently, a study in the London COPD cohort has shown that EXACT scores at the peak of the exacerbation were higher in treated than untreated events (**Fig. 1**), suggesting that the symptomatic burden of the exacerbation drives a patient's need for therapy. Further data from this study showed that the change in EXACT score to detect an exacerbation is smaller in severe COPD than in milder patients and highlights the difficulty in assigning scores to changes in exacerbations that occur across the disease spectrum. The scores on the COPD assessment test (CAT) also rise on exacerbation and reflect severity of the exacerbation, but the CAT has not been developed or validated for use at exacerbation.[10]

CAUSES AND PATHOGENESIS OF EXACERBATION

A majority of COPD exacerbations are triggered by respiratory viral infections, especially rhinovirus, the cause of the common cold. Using molecular techniques, respiratory viruses can be identified in up to 60% of exacerbations.[11] Exacerbations associated with viruses tend to have greater airway and systemic inflammatory effects than those without any evidence of viral infection and are more common in the winter months, with more chance of hospital admission. Airway pollutants may also be associated with precipitating exacerbations, especially by interacting with respiratory viruses, although significant effects of pollution are seen only in global areas of high urban pollution.[12]

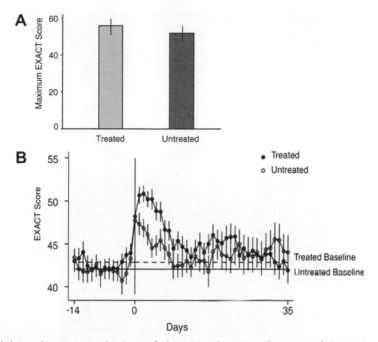

Fig. 1. (*A*) Maximum exacerbations of chronic pulmonary disease tool (EXACT) scores in chronic obstructive pulmonary disease patients treated and not treated with increased systemic therapy at exacerbation. Vertical lines represent standard errors. (*B*) Time course of EXACT scores during treated and untreated exacerbations. Vertical lines represent standard errors. (*From* Mackay AJ, Donaldson GC, Patel AR, et al. Detection and severity grading of COPD exacerbations using the exacerbations of Chronic Obstructive Pulmonary Disease Tool (EXACT). Eur Respir J 2013 Aug 29. [Epub ahead of print]).

Bacteria are present in the lower airway and are known to be present in the stable state and colonize the airway. Although airway bacterial load increases at exacerbation, it is now considered that bacteria are not often the primary infective cause of the exacerbation but are secondary invaders after a viral trigger. The effect of the infective triggers is to increase inflammation further in a chronically inflamed airway, leading to an increase in bronchoconstriction, edema, and mucus production, resulting in an increase in dynamic hyperinflation and symptoms of increased dyspnea characteristic of an exacerbation **Fig. 2.**[1] Thus, any intervention that reduces inflammation in COPD reduces the number and severity of exacerbation, whereas bronchodilators have an impact on exacerbation by their effects on reducing dynamic hyperinflation.

THE FREQUENT EXACERBATOR PHENOTYPE

Exacerbations become more frequent and severe as COPD severity increases. One distinct group of patients seems susceptible to exacerbations, irrespective of disease severity. This COPD phenotype of frequent exacerbations is stable over time and the major determinant of developing frequent exacerbations is a history of prior exacerbations.[13] This phenomenon is seen across all GOLD stages, including patients with stage 2 disease, of whom 22% had frequent exacerbations in the first year of the Evaluation of COPD Longitudinally to Identify Predictive Surrogate Endpoints (ECLIPSE) study.[14]

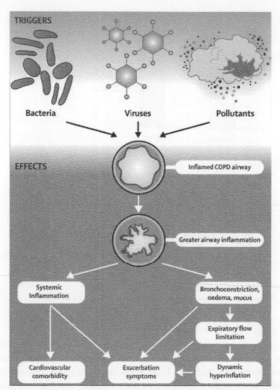

TRIGGERS

Bacteria   Viruses   Pollutants

EFFECTS   Inflamed COPD airway

                                  Greater airway inflammation

Systemic   Bronchoconstriction,
Inflammation   oedema, mucus

                                  Expiratory flow
                                  limitation

Cardiovascular   Exacerbation   Dynamic
comorbidity   symptoms   hyperinflation

Fig. 2. Triggers of COPD exacerbations and associated pathophysiologic changes leading to increased exacerbation symptoms. (*From* Wedzicha JA, Seemungal TA. COPD exacerbations: defining their cause and prevention. Lancet 2007;370:787; with permission.)

Patients with a history of frequent exacerbations are at particular future risk of further events and death **Fig. 3.**[15] Studies have shown that this group of patients has worse quality of life, increased risk of hospitalization, and a greater chance of recurrent exacerbations. Frequent exacerbators also exhibit faster decline in lung function and may have worse functional status. Thus, it is vital to identify patients at risk of frequent exacerbations and target this group for therapy (**Table 1**).

EXACERBATION PREVENTION
Vaccines

In retrospective cohort studies of community-dwelling elderly patients, influenza vaccination is associated with a 27% reduction in the risk of hospitalization for pneumonia or influenza and a 48% reduction in the risk of death.[16] Thus, influenza vaccines are recommended in a majority of patients with COPD. There is less evidence for the role of pneumococcal polysaccharide vaccine in preventing exacerbations and hospital admissions in COPD, but large studies are currently under way with vaccines with improved immunogenicity. Nevertheless, pneumococcal vaccines are commonly administered to COPD patients.

Inhaled Corticosteroids and Long-acting Bronchodilators

Both inhaled corticosteroids (ICSs) and long-acting β-agonists (LABAs) reduce exacerbation frequency. In the Towards a Revolution in COPD Health (TORCH) study,

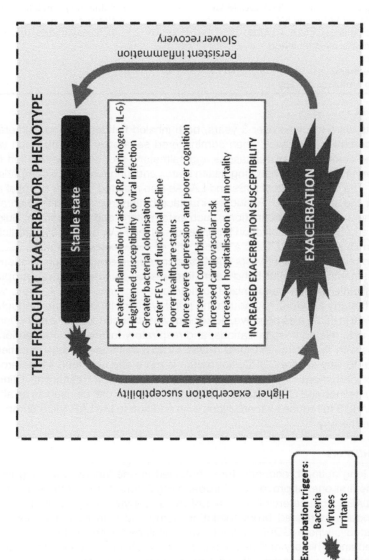

THE FREQUENT EXACERBATOR PHENOTYPE

Persistent inflammation
Slower recovery

Stable state

- Greater inflammation (raised CRP, fibrinogen, IL-6)
- Heightened susceptibility to viral infection
- Greater bacterial colonisation
- Faster FEV$_1$ and functional decline
- Poorer healthcare status
- More severe depression and poorer cognition
- Worsened comorbidity
- Increased cardiovascular risk
- Increased hospitalisation and mortality

INCREASED EXACERBATION SUSCEPTIBILITY

EXACERBATION

Higher exacerbation susceptibility

Exacerbation triggers:
Bacteria
Viruses
Irritants

Fig. 3. Effect of COPD exacerbations in the group with frequent exacerbations. CRP, C-reactive protein; IL, interleukin. (*Adapted from* Wedzicha JA, Brill SE, Allinson JP, et al. Mechanisms and impact of the frequent exacerbator phenotype in chronic obstructive pulmonary disease. BMC Medicine 2013;11:181; with permission.)

Table 1 Strategies to prevent exacerbations	
Pharmacologic Therapies for Exacerbation Prevention	**Nonpharmacologic Therapies**
• Antiviral therapy	• Smoking cessation
• Vaccines	• Pollution control
• Long-acting bronchodilators (LABAs/LAMAs)	○ Pulmonary rehabilitation
• Combinations of LABA and ICS	○ Home oxygen therapy
• Dual bronchodilators (LABA + LAMA)	○ Home ventilatory support
○ Phosphodiesterase-4 inhibitors	
○ Mucolytics	
○ Macrolide therapy	
• Long-acting antibiotic therapy	

where patients were followed over 3 years, both inhaled fluticasone and salmeterol reduced exacerbation frequency when administered separately in comparison with placebo.[17] The combination of fluticasone and salmeterol reduced exacerbation frequency further, in addition to improving health status and lung function in comparison with placebo. The combination of ICSs and LABAs also resulted in fewer hospital admissions over the study period. Reduction in exacerbation frequency has been also found with other LABA/ICS combinations, such as formoterol and budesonide. Guidelines indicate a LABA/ICS combination for patients with an FEV_1 below 50% predicted (groups C and D) and where there is a history of 2 or more exacerbations.

Long-acting *muscarinic antagonists* (LAMAs) also reduce exacerbation frequency. In the Understanding Potential Long-Term Impacts on Function with Tiotropium (UPLIFT) trial, patients were randomized to tiotropium or placebo for 4 years, with concomitant therapy allowed.[18] Although the primary endpoint of the trial (reduction in rate of decline in FEV_1) was negative, tiotropium was associated with a reduction in exacerbation risk, related hospitalizations, and respiratory failure. The Prevention of Exacerbations with Tiotropium in COPD (POET-COPD) trial showed that, in patients with moderate to very severe COPD, tiotropium is more effective than salmeterol in preventing exacerbations.[19] In both the National Institute for Health and Clinical Excellence guidelines and GOLD strategy document, LAMAs can be used as an alternative to LABA/ICS to reduce exacerbations or in addition to the LABA/ICS combination as a triple therapy.[3]

Dual Bronchodilators

Dual inhaled long-acting bronchodilators contained in one inhaler are being introduced and the first one, approved by European regulators, is QVA that is a combination of a LABA (indacaterolol) and a LAMA (glycopyrronium). QVA has been shown to produce increased bronchodilation compared with its components. In the SPARK study, where COPD patients were included with an FEV_1 of below 50% predicted and a history of COPD exacerbations, QVA reduced health care utilization exacerbation compared with glycopyrronium.[20] Diary cards were used in the SPARK study, however, to collect all exacerbation events and QVA was superior to both glycopyrronium and open-label tiotropium in the reduction of all exacerbations, that is, mild, moderate, and severe combined. Thus, future studies of dual bronchodilators must be designed to collect data on all exacerbation events as in the SPARK study. Availability of the new dual bronchodilators will change treatment algorithms because these therapies reduce both symptoms and prevent exacerbations.

Phosphodiesterase Inhibitors

Phosphodiesterase-4 inhibitors have broad antiinflammatory activity, inhibiting the airway inflammation associated with COPD, especially by reducing airway neutrophils that are key cells in COPD. Evidence from a pooled analysis of 2 large placebo-controlled, double-blind multicenter trials revealed a significant reduction of 17% in the frequency of moderate (glucocorticoid-treated) or severe (hospitalization/death) exacerbations with Roflumilast.[21] Only patients with an FEV_1 less than 50% (GOLD stages 3 and 4), presence of bronchitic symptoms, and a history of exacerbations, however, were enrolled. There currently are no comparator studies with ICSs. Weight loss was also noted in the roflumilast group, with a mean reduction of 2.1 kg after 1 year, and was highest in obese patients. Therefore, after treatment with roflumilast, weight needs to be monitored carefully. Recent evidence also suggests that roflumilast may reduce the number of patients in the frequent exacerbator group after 12 months of therapy.[22]

Long-term Antibiotics

At present there is insufficient evidence to recommend routine prophylactic antibiotic therapy in the management of stable COPD, but some studies have shown promise. Erythromycin reduced the frequency of moderate and/or severe exacerbations (treated with systemic steroids, treated with antibiotics, or hospitalized) and shortened exacerbation length when taken twice daily over 12 months by patients with moderate to severe COPD.[23] The macrolide azithromycin has been used as prophylaxis in patients with cystic fibrosis and when added to usual treatment azithromycin has also been shown to decrease exacerbation frequency and improve quality of life in COPD patients.[24] The benefits were most significant, however, in treatment-naive patients with mild disease (GOLD stage 2), and significant rates of hearing decrement (as measured by audiometry) and antibiotic resistance were found. Also, a recent large epidemiologic study has suggested a small increase in cardiovascular deaths in patients receiving azithromycin, particularly in those with a high baseline risk of cardiovascular disease.

Furthermore, intermittent pulsed moxifloxacin when given to stable patients has been shown to significantly reduce exacerbation frequency in a per protocol population and in a post hoc subgroup of patients with bronchitis at baseline.[25] This reduction did not meet statistical significance, however, in the intention-to-treat analysis, and further studies are required on nonmacrolide antibiotics, including assessment of safety.

Thus, before prescription of long-term antibiotics in COPD, patients should be treated with an optimum combination inhaled therapy, show evidence of ongoing frequent exacerbations, and be carefully assessed for risk of potential cardiovascular and auditory side effects.

Pulmonary Rehabilitation, Home Oxygen, and Ventilatory Support

There is some evidence from clinical trials that pulmonary rehabilitation programs reduce hospital stay. There is some evidence from epidemiologic studies in COPD patients that long-term oxygen therapy and noninvasive ventilatory support may reduce hospital admissions and prevent exacerbations,[26] but controlled trials have not yet addressed these issues. Although it is difficult to perform controlled trials of long-term oxygen therapy, there are ongoing studies of the role of home noninvasive ventilation in COPD patients who are hypercapnic and at risk of further events.

MANAGEMENT OF THE ACUTE EXACERBATION

After the earlier studies of Anthonisen and colleagues,[27] the standard management of an acute exacerbation consists of oral antibiotics, such as amoxicillin or doxycycline, if there is evidence of increased sputum purulence or increased sputum volume. Oral corticosteroids in short courses are also added depending on individual exacerbation severity, and there is recent evidence suggesting that shorter courses (5 days) may be as beneficial as longer ones, such as more conventional 14-day courses.[28] There is evidence that the earlier therapy is started at onset of exacerbation, the shorter the recovery of the event and less chance of hospital admission.[8] COPD exacerbations may show early recurrence, especially in patients who are frequent exacerbators. There is evidence that exacerbation therapy may prolong the time to subsequent events.[29] Thus, prompt and appropriate management of an exacerbation event not only will have an effect on optimizing recovery but also delay the time to the next event.

The use of oral corticosteroids at exacerbations is currently essential but it is possible that steroids may exacerbate bacterial infection at exacerbation in patients whose airways are colonized with bacteria, such as *Haemophilus influenzae* and *Streptococcus pneumoniae*. There is a high risk of recurrent exacerbations in COPD patients and this may be due to secondary infection.[30] Thus, there is a need for the development of novel antiinflammatory agents that are effective at COPD exacerbations. Optimal management of acute exacerbations not only will increase the rate of exacerbation recovery but also affect exacerbation rates and prevent hospital admissions.

REFERENCES

1. Wedzicha JA, Seemungal TA. COPD exacerbations: defining their cause and prevention. Lancet 2007;370:786–96.
2. Donaldson GC, Seemungal TA, Bhowmik A, et al. The relationship between exacerbation frequency and lung function decline in chronic obstructive pulmonary disease. Thorax 2002;57:847–52.
3. National Institute for Health and Clinical Excellence (NICE). Chronic obstructive pulmonary disease: management of chronic obstructive pulmonary disease in adults in primary and secondary care. Update 2010. Available at: http://guidance.nice.org.uk/CG101/Guidance/pdf/English. Accessed December 18, 2013.
4. Donaldson GC, Hurst JR, Smith CJ, et al. Increased risk of myocardial infarction and stroke following exacerbation of COPD. Chest 2010;137:1091–7.
5. McAllister DA, Maclay JD, Mills NL. Diagnosis of myocardial infarction following hospitalisation for exacerbation of COPD. Eur Respir J 2012;39:1097–103.
6. Suissa S, Dell'Aniello S, Ernst P. Long-term natural history of chronic obstructive pulmonary disease: severe exacerbations and mortality. Thorax 2012;67(11):957–63.
7. Global Initiative for Chronic Obstructive Lung Disease (GOLD). Global strategy for the diagnosis, management and prevention of COPD. GOLD. Am J Respir Crit Care Med 2013. Available at: www.goldcopd.org. Accessed December 18, 2013.
8. Wilkinson TM, Donaldson GC, Hurst JR, et al. Early therapy improves outcomes of exacerbations of chronic obstructive pulmonary disease. Am J Respir Crit Care Med 2004;169:1298–303.
9. Mackay AJ, Donaldson GC, Patel AR, et al. Detection and severity grading of COPD exacerbations using the exacerbations of Chronic Obstructive Pulmonary Disease Tool (EXACT). Eur Respir J 2013. http://dx.doi.org/10.1183/09031936.00110913.

10. Mackay AJ, Donaldson GC, Patel AR, et al. Usefulness of the Chronic Obstructive Pulmonary Disease assessment test to evaluate severity of COPD exacerbations. Am J Respir Crit Care Med 2012;185:1218–24.
11. Seemungal TA, Harper-Owen R, Bhowmik A, et al. Respiratory viruses, symptoms and inflammatory markers in acute exacerbations and stable chronic obstructive pulmonary disease. Am J Respir Crit Care Med 2001;164:1618–23.
12. Peacock JL, Anderson HR, Bremner SA, et al. Outdoor air pollution and respiratory health in patients with COPD. Thorax 2011;66:591–6.
13. Seemungal TA, Donaldson GC, Paul EA, et al. Effect of exacerbation on quality of life in patients with chronic obstructive pulmonary disease. Am J Respir Crit Care Med 1998;157:1418–22.
14. Hurst JR, Vestbo J, Anzueto A, et al. Susceptibility to exacerbation in chronic obstructive pulmonary disease. N Engl J Med 2010;63:1128–38.
15. Wedzicha JA, Brill SE, Allinson JP, et al. Mechanisms and impact of the frequent exacerbator phenotype in chronic obstructive pulmonary disease. BMC Medicine 2013;11:181.
16. Nichol KL, Nordin JD, Nelson DB, et al. Effectiveness of influenza vaccine in the community-dwelling elderly. N Engl J Med 2007;357:1373–81.
17. Calverley PM, Anderson JA, Celli B, et al. Salmeterol and fluticasone propionate and survival in chronic obstructive pulmonary disease. N Engl J Med 2007;356: 775–89.
18. Tashkin DP, Celli B, Senn S, et al. A 4-year trial of tiotropium in chronic obstructive pulmonary disease. N Engl J Med 2008;359:1543–54.
19. Vogelmeier C, Hederer B, Glaab T, et al. Tiotorpium versus salmeterol for the prevention of COPD exacerbations. N Engl J Med 2011;364(12):1093–103.
20. Wedzicha JA, Decramer M, Fucker JH, et al. Analysis of COPD exacerbations with the dual bronchodilator QVA149 compared with glycopyrronium and tiotropium (SPARK): a randomized, double-blind, parallel-group study. Lancet Respir Med 2013;1:199–209.
21. Calverley PM, Rabe KF, Goehring UM, et al. M2-124 and M2-125 study groups. Roflumilast in symptomatic chronic obstructive pulmonary disease: two randomised clinical trials. Lancet 2009;374(9691):685–94 [Erratum appears in Lancet 2010;376(9747):1146].
22. Wedzicha JA, Rabe KF, Martinez FJ, et al. Efficacy of roflumilast in the COPD frequent exacerbator phenotype. Chest 2013;143:1302–11.
23. Seemungal TA, Wilkinson T, Hurst JR, et al. Effect of erythromycin on exacerbations in COPD. Am J Respir Crit Care Med 2008;178:1139–47.
24. Albert RK, Connett J, Bailey WC, et al. Azithromycin for prevention of exacerbations of COPD. N Engl J Med 2011;365:689–98.
25. Sethi S, Jones PW, Theron MS, et al, PULSE Study group. Pulsed moxifloxacin for the prevention of exacerbations of chronic obstructive pulmonary disease: a randomized controlled trial. Respir Res 2010;11:10.
26. McEvoy RD, Pierce RJ, Hillman D, et al. Nocturnal non-invasive nasal ventilation in stable hypercapnic COPD: a randomised controlled trial. Thorax 2009;64: 561–6.
27. Anthonisen NR, Manfreda J, Warren CP, et al. Antibiotic therapy in exacerbations of chronic obstructive pulmonary disease. Ann Intern Med 1987;106: 196–204.
28. Leuppi JD, Schuetz P, Bingisser R. Short-term vs conventional glucocorticoid therapy in acute exacerbations of chronic obstructive pulmonary disease the REDUCE randomized clinical trial. JAMA 2013;309(21):2223–31.

168   Wedzicha et al

29. Roede BM, Bresser P, Bindels PJ, et al. Antibiotic treatment is associated with a reduced risk of a subsequent exacerbation in obstructive lung disease: a historical population-based cohort. Thorax 2008;63(11):968–73.
30. Hurst JR, Donaldson GC, Quint JK, et al. Temporal clustering of exacerbations in chronic obstructive pulmonary disease. Am J Respir Crit Care Med 2009;179: 369–74.

Evidence-Based Outcomes from Pulmonary Rehabilitation in the Chronic Obstructive Pulmonary Disease Patient

Milo A. Puhan, MD, PhD[a], Suzanne C. Lareau, RN, MS[b],*

KEYWORDS

- Chronic obstructive pulmonary disease • Pulmonary rehabilitation • Quality of life
- Self-management • Quality of evidence

KEY POINTS

- Pulmonary rehabilitation consists of exercise, education, and support in self-management behaviors.
- The quality of evidence is high for patient-centered outcomes such as health-related quality of life and exercise capacity in stable patients.
- Pulmonary rehabilitation after an exacerbation has strong effects, and the evidence for most outcomes at this time demonstrates moderate to high quality of evidence.

INTRODUCTION

Pulmonary rehabilitation consists of exercise, education, and support in self-management behaviors. Those completing pulmonary rehabilitation have shown measureable improvement in quality of life, symptoms, exercise performance, depression and anxiety, and health care utilization. Although it is obvious why an exercise program would improve the individual's exercise capacity, the reasons why improvement occurs in other outcome areas are not as clear.[1] The purpose of this article however, is not to provide details on the reasons for these improvements, but to describe the strength of the evidence demonstrating these changes in outcomes.

Historically, attempts were made to link rehabilitation outcomes with improvements in lung function, a common goal in many trials, in particular pharmaceutical trials.

This article originally appeared in Clinics in Chest Medicine, Volume 35, Issue 2, June 2014.
[a] Institute of Social and Preventive Medicine, University of Zurich, Hirschengraben 84, Zurich CH-8001, Switzerland; [b] College of Nursing, University of Colorado, Mail Stop C288, 13120 East 19th Avenue, Aurora, CO 80045, USA
* Corresponding author.
E-mail address: Suzanne.Lareau@ucdenver.edu

However, lung function has only occasionally been found to improve following pulmonary rehabilitation, suggesting that other changes resulting from pulmonary rehabilitation may underlie these beneficial effects. Any improvements in lung function, such as prolonged time to hyperinflation with exercise, is likely due to multiple factors, including physical deconditioning and reduction in anxiety related to dyspnea. However, given the body of evidence, one is able to make some conclusions about changes in outcomes based on the quality of evidence currently available.

Outcomes that will be the focus of this article include quality of life, symptoms, exercise capacity, hospitalizations, exacerbations, and mortality. Quality-of-life outcomes that have been consistently shown to improve have usually been measured with 2 common chronic obstructive pulmonary disease (COPD) instruments, the Chronic Respiratory Disease Questionnaire (CRQ)[2] and the Saint George's Respiratory Questionnaire (SGRQ).[3] Several symptoms have also been shown to improve with rehabilitation, with dyspnea, fatigue, depression, and anxiety being the most common and relevant to patients, and therefore most frequently measured and reported. Dyspnea and fatigue were among the earliest symptoms measured as outcomes in the rehabilitation setting, having been demonstrated to improve using the dyspnea and fatigue subscales on the CRQ. Symptoms relating to mood have also been responsive to rehabilitation, as measured by depression and anxiety scales such as the Hospital Anxiety and Depression Score (HADS),[4] the Center for Epidemiological Studies Depressions Scale (CES-D),[5] and the Revised Symptom Checklist (SCL-90-R).[6] Improvements in exercise capacity have been measured with field tests (the 6-minute walk distance [6MWD][7] and shuttle walk test [SWT])[8] or tests of maximal exercise capacity by either treadmill or bicycle. The latter tests of exercise capacity can determine peak exercise capacity or endurance exercise capacity. Although there are other measures that have been used to evaluate quality of life and symptoms, those noted were most frequently used in meta-analysis.[9] In the last decade, the capacity to expand areas of study has occurred, and more programs are delving into assessing other outcomes of rehabilitation. Consequently, outcome researchers now also assess the effects of pulmonary rehabilitation on exacerbations,[10] hospital utilization, and mortality.

The aim of this article is to systematically appraise the quality of evidence reported for important outcomes in pulmonary rehabilitation using the approach of the Grading of Recommendations Assessment, Development and Evaluation (GRADE) Working Group. This appraisal was carried out by identifying Cochrane systematic reviews and systematic reviews that have been subsequently reported since the last Cochrane report. The focus of this appraisal was to determine the effectiveness of pulmonary rehabilitation programs versus control therapy (usually otherwise standard care) in COPD patients. This analysis did not evaluate other aspects of the pulmonary rehabilitation intervention, such as which programs provided the most benefit (eg, inpatient vs outpatient) or how long the programs should be held (program duration).

METHODS

The approach of the GRADE Working Group[11,12] is one of several approaches to evaluate the quality of evidence in a systematic way. This approach has been adopted by over 70 organizations, including the World Health Organization (WHO), the Cochrane Collaboration, the National Institute of Health and Clinical Excellence in the UK (NICE), the American College of Physicians, and UpToDate. In brief, the GRADE approach evaluates the confidence in the estimates of effects for each outcome of interest as a function of the quality of the evidence. The result is the GRADE rating from high to low that can be used to gauge how well the estimates can be trusted. A rating of high means one can be confident that: (1) the true effect (eg, odds ratio for hospitalization in treated vs untreated patients or the difference in quality of life between treatment groups) lies close to the estimates from the available evidence, and (2) that additional evidence is unlikely to change the estimate. Very low means one should have very little confidence in the effect estimate and that the true effect estimate is likely to be substantially different when more data become available. Rating of the confidence in the effect estimates (if based on randomized trials) begins at the highest level and is rated down (if there are reasons to lose confidence in the effect estimates). For example, if there are serious concerns regarding risk of bias[13] (eg, failure to conceal random allocation or blind participants to the study intervention), then the quality of evidence is rated down from high to moderate. Other criteria that may lead to a downrating are inconsistency[14] of effect estimates across studies and indirectness[15] in cases where surrogate outcomes (such as inflammatory biomarkers) are used instead of patient-important outcomes (such as exacerbations). Another example is if patients are recruited from an intensive care setting, there is a good chance that the estimates of effect are unlikely to apply to a broader COPD population. Also, imprecision[16] (a wide confidence interval) may lead to down rating in that it makes decision making challenging. Other biases that may lead to a downgrading are publication bias[17] or outcome reporting bias, if, for example, only positive results were presented when clearly there must have been negative findings.

RESULTS
Health-Related Quality of Life

Health-related quality of life as measured by the SGRQ and the CRQ in stable COPD patients following pulmonary rehabilitation is shown in **Tables 1** and **2**. These tables identify

The subscales and total scores

The minimal important difference (MID) (defined as "the smallest difference in score in the domain of interest which patients perceive as beneficial and which would mandate, in the absence of troublesome side effects and excessive cost, a change in the patient's management"[18]) for the subscales (in order to understand if the 95% confidence interval meets the MID)

The number of participants in the studies upon which the review was based

The quality of evidence (GRADE)

As seen from these tables, there is a high quality of evidence that pulmonary rehabilitation improves the quality of life of COPD patients after pulmonary rehabilitation. The symptom subscale of the SGRQ was the only subscale on these quality-of-life instruments that was not rated with high confidence. The imprecision of the effect estimates led to downgrading of the quality of evidence to moderate for the symptom subscale, because it is possible that additional evidence might change the estimate of effect. The symptoms scale on the SGRQ is a composite score, evaluating 4 symptoms (cough, sputum, dyspnea, and wheezing), all of which may not be present in a patient with COPD and therefore may not be affected by an intervention such as rehabilitation. With the exception of this subscale, the 6 other scales and a total score provide high-quality evidence for a strong effect of rehabilitation on quality of life.

Table 1
Summary of findings in stable COPD patients following pulmonary rehabilitation

| | | | Pulmonary Rehabilitation in Patients with Stable COPD | | |
| | | | Participants: Patients with Stable COPD (No Exacerbations Within 4 wk of Enrollment) Intervention: Pulmonary Rehabilitation with At Least 4 wk of Exercise Training Setting: Out- or Inpatient | | |
Outcomes	Systematic Review	Minimal Important Difference	Effect (95% Confidence Interval), P-value Between Group Difference of Change	No of Participants (RCTs)	Quality of the Evidence (GRADE)
Total HRQL (SGRQ)	Lacasse	4	−6.11 (−8.98, −3.24), P = .00003	388 (6)	High ⊕⊕⊕⊕[a]
Symptoms (SGRQ)	Lacasse	4	−4.68 (−9.61, 0.25), P = .06	388 (6)	Moderate ⊕⊕⊕O[a,b]
Dyspnea (CRQ)	Lacasse	0.5	1.06 (0.85, 1.26), P<.00001	610 (11)	High ⊕⊕⊕⊕[a]
Fatigue (CRQ)	Lacasse	0.5	0.92 (0.71, 1.13), P<.00001	618 (11)	High ⊕⊕⊕⊕[a]
Depression	Coventry	0.2	−0.47 (−0.79, −0.16), P = .003	338 (5)	Low ⊕⊕OO[c,d]
Anxiety	Coventry	0.2	−0.38 (−0.60, −0.16), P = .006	338 (5)	Low ⊕⊕OO[c,d]
Emotional function (CRQ)	Lacasse	0.5	0.76 (0.52, 1.00), P<.00001	618 (11)	High ⊕⊕⊕⊕[a]
Activity (SGRQ)	Lacasse	4	−4.78 (−7.83, −1.72), P = .002	388 (6)	High ⊕⊕⊕⊕[a]
Physical activity	Ng	NA	No pooled estimate	472 (7)	Lack of evidence[e]
Mastery (CRQ)	Lacasse	0.5	0.97 (0.74, 1.20), P<.00001	618 (11)	High ⊕⊕⊕⊕[a]
Impacts (SGRQ)	Lacasse	4	−6.27 (−10.08, −2.47), P = .001	388 (6)	High ⊕⊕⊕⊕[a]
6-minute walk distance	Lacasse	30 m	48 m (32, 65), P<.00001	669 (16)	Moderate ⊕⊕⊕O[f]
Maximum exercise capacity	Lacasse	4 W	8.4 W (3.5, 13.4), P = .0009	511 (13)	Moderate ⊕⊕⊕O[f]

GRADE Working Group grades of evidence.
High quality: Further research is very unlikely to change one's confidence in the estimate of effect.
Moderate quality: Further research is likely to have an important impact on one's confidence in the estimate of effect and may change the estimate.
Low quality: Further research is very likely to have an important impact on one's confidence in the estimate of effect and is likely to change the estimate.
Very low quality: One should be very uncertain about the estimate.
[a] Blinding of outcome assessors not a reason for downgrading because not necessary for patient reported outcomes.
[b] Downgrade −1 for imprecision.
[c] Downgrade −1 for indirectness. Patients were enrolled based on their pulmonary status and not on their psychological status. There is uncertainty about the presence and type of depression and anxiety at baseline.
[d] Downgrade −1 for risk of bias. One of the 5 studies was likely not truly randomized, and groups were different in terms of the levels of symptoms of depression and anxiety at baseline. Method of randomization and concealment of random allocation not described in some trials.
[e] Downgrade −1 for risk of bias. In most studies outcome assessors were not blinded.
[f] Different activity monitors and questionnaires used, and MID not established for most measures of physical activity.

Symptoms

Symptoms were measured by the CRQ, SGRQ (previously described) and in a systematic review for depression and anxiety.[19] Dyspnea and fatigue have been consistently shown to improve with pulmonary rehabilitation. The dyspnea subscale of the CRQ, however, measures only 1 aspect of dyspnea (ie, the impact of pulmonary rehabilitation on dyspnea with specific activities). There are other aspects of dyspnea besides the impact of dyspnea (eg, intensity of dyspnea with activities), such as an affective component (distress with dyspnea) and sensory–perceptual impact (what breathing feels like).[20]

Mood-specific measures of depression and anxiety, as well as the more general emotional function subscale of the CRQ, have been reported to improve following pulmonary rehabilitation. The quality of evidence varies from low (for depression and anxiety) to high (on emotional function of CRQ) at this time. Reasons for downgrading the evidence are described in **Table 1**. For example, the quality of evidence was downgraded 1 point for the results in the systematic reviewed mentioned previously[18] because of indirectness (enrollment was based on the patients' lung function status, not their psychological status) and 1 point for risk of bias (one of the studies was likely not randomized; the groups were different in terms of the level of depression at baseline, and important features of a randomized clinical trial [RCT] were not reported for some studies).

Activity and Exercise Capacity

Activity following pulmonary rehabilitation measured by activity monitors or physical activity questionnaires has not, to date, been sufficiently evaluated. A recent meta-analysis of physical activity[21] is an example of the challenge that occurs when both objective and subjective measures are included. In this meta-analysis, one could not adequately evaluate activity due to the variation in measures of activity (activity monitors, questionnaires) and lack of established MID for many of these measures. There is, however, moderate quality of evidence (downgraded because of risk of bias) that pulmonary rehabilitation has a strong effect on exercise capacity as measured by the 6-minute walk distance (6MWD) or maximum exercise capacity.

Exacerbations

Meta-analyses are not currently available on the effect of pulmonary rehabilitation for stable outpatients with COPD on hospitalizations, exacerbations, or mortality. There is however, emerging evidence that pulmonary rehabilitation can successfully be provided to COPD patients following an exacerbation.

Exacerbations are a fairly common occurrence in COPD patients. Those experiencing an exacerbation run a high risk of morbidity, mortality, and increased health care utilization. One systematic review[10] evaluated studies for quality of life, symptoms, activity, hospitalization, and mortality among individuals undergoing pulmonary rehabilitation following an exacerbation of COPD. There is moderate quality evidence that pulmonary rehabilitation after an exacerbation substantially lowers the risk of both future exacerbations and mortality. There is also high quality of evidence that pulmonary rehabilitation improves health-related quality of life following an exacerbation. Improvement in symptoms showed moderate quality of evidence for improvement. Downrating was related to risk of bias and the heterogeneity of the estimates across studies but uprated to moderate quality of evidence due to the large effect size. Similarly, a disparity existed between field tests. The shuttle walk test (a field test) was rated as high quality of evidence, but the 6MWD was rated low for improvement

Table 2
Summary of findings in unstable COPD patients following pulmonary rehabilitation

Pulmonary Rehabilitation in Patients with Unstable COPD

Participants: Patients After Experiencing a COPD Exacerbations Intervention: Pulmonary Rehabilitation with At Least 4 wk of Exercise Training Setting: Outpatient or Inpatient

Outcomes	Systematic Review	Minimal Important Difference	Effect (95% Confidence Interval), P-value Between Group Difference of Change	No of Participants (RCTs)	Quality of the Evidence (GRADE)
Total HRQL (SGRQ)	Puhan	4	−9.9 (−14.4, −5.4), P<.00001	128 (3)	High ⊕⊕⊕⊕
Symptoms (SGRQ)	Puhan	4	0.9 (−6.8, 8.5), P = .83	128 (3)	Moderate ⊕⊕⊕O[a]
Dyspnea (CRQ)	Puhan	0.5	0.97 (0.35, 1.58), P = .002	259 (5)	Moderate ⊕⊕⊕O[b,c,d]
Fatigue (CRQ)	Puhan	0.5	0.81 (0.16, 1.45), P = .01	259 (5)	Moderate ⊕⊕⊕O[b,c,d]
Emotional function (CRQ)	Puhan	0.5	0.94 (0.46, 1.42), P = .0001	259 (5)	Moderate ⊕⊕⊕O[b,c,d]
Activity (SGRQ)	Puhan	4	−9.9 (−16.0, −3.9), P = .001	128 (3)	High ⊕⊕⊕⊕
Mastery (CRQ)	Puhan	0.5	0.93 (−0.13, 1.99), P = .09	259 (5)	Low ⊕⊕OO[a,b,c,d]
Impacts (SGRQ)	Puhan	4	−13.9 (−20.4, −7.5), P<.00001	128 (3)	High ⊕⊕⊕⊕
6-minute walk distance	Puhan	30 m	78 m (12, 143), P = .02	299 (6)	Low ⊕⊕OO[b,c]
Incremental shuttle walk test	Puhan	48 m	64 (41, 87), P<.00001	128 (3)	High ⊕⊕⊕⊕
Hospitalization	Puhan	NA	Odds ratio: 0.22 (0.08, 0.58), P = .002 In the control group 40 people out of 100 had hospital admission over 25 wk, compared with 13 (95% confidence interval 5–28) out of 100 for the active treatment group; this represents an NNT(B) of 4 (95% confidence interval 3–8) over 25 wk	250 (5)	Moderate ⊕⊕⊕O[c]

| Mortality | Puhan | NA | Odds ratio: 0.28 (0.10, 0.84), P = .02
In the control group 29 people out of 100 had mortality over 107 wk, compared to 10 (95% confidence interval 4–26) out of 100 for the active treatment group; this represents an NNT(B) of 6 (95% confidence interval: 5–30) over 107 wk | 111 (3) | Moderate ⊕ ⊕ ⊕ O[c] |

GRADE Working Group grades of evidence.

High quality: Further research is very unlikely to change one's confidence in the estimate of effect.

Moderate quality: Further research is likely to have an important impact on one's confidence in the estimate of effect and may change the estimate.

Low quality: Further research is very likely to have an important impact on one's confidence in the estimate of effect and is likely to change the estimate.

Very low quality: One should be very uncertain about the estimate.

Abbreviation: NNT(B), Number needed to treat for one patient to benefit.

[a] Downgraded −1 for imprecision.

[b] Downgraded −1 for risk of bias. Generation of the random sequence, concealment of random allocation, or blinding of outcome assessors in some studies not described.

[c] Downgraded −1 for heterogeneity.

[d] Upgraded +1 for large effect.

following rehabilitation. This may reflect the fact that the shuttle walk test is externally-paced, while the 6MWT is self-paced.

SUMMARY

Patients with both stable and unstable COPD demonstrate many important benefits following pulmonary rehabilitation. The quality of evidence is high for patient-centered outcomes such as health-related quality of life and exercise capacity in stable patients. Pulmonary rehabilitation after an exacerbation has strong effects too, and the evidence for most outcomes at this time demonstrates, moderate to high quality of evidence.

REFERENCES

1. Lareau S, Meek P, ZuWallack R. Chapter 14; the effect of pulmonary rehabilitation on dyspnea. In: Mahler D, O'Donnell D, editors. Dyspnea: mechanisms, measurement, and management, third edition. Boca Raton, FL: CRC Press, Taylor & Francis; 2014. p. 196.
2. Guyatt GH, Berman LB, Townsend M, et al. A measure of quality of life for clinical trials in chronic lung disease. Thorax 1987;42:773-8.
3. Jones PW, Quirk FH, Baveystock CM, et al. A self-complete measure of health status for chronic airflow limitation: the St. George's Respiratory Questionnaire. Am Rev Respir Dis 1992;145:1321-7.
4. Zigmond AS, Snaith RP. The Hospital anxiety and depression scale. Acta Psychiatr Scand 1983;67:361-70.
5. Radloff LS. The CES-D scale: a self-report depression scale for research in the general population. Appl Psychol Meas 1977;1:385-401.
6. Derogatis LR, Lipman RS, Covi L. SCL-90: an outpatient psychiatric rating scale—preliminary report. Psychopharmacol Bull 1973;9:13-28.
7. Butland RJ, Pang J, Gross ER, et al. Two-, six-, and 12-minute walking tests in respiratory disease. Br Med J (Clin Res Ed) 1982;284:1607-8.
8. Singh SJ, Morgan MD, Scott S, et al. Development of a shuttle walking test of disability in patients with chronic airways obstruction. Thorax 1992;47:1019-24.
9. Lacasse Y, Goldstein R, Lasserson TJ, et al. Pulmonary rehabilitation for chronic obstructive pulmonary disease. Cochrane Database Syst Rev 2006;(4):CD003793.
10. Puhan MA, Gimeno-Santos E, Scharplatz M, et al. Pulmonary rehabilitation following exacerbations of chronic obstructive pulmonary disease. Cochrane Database Syst Rev 2011;(10):CD005305.
11. Guyatt GH, Oxman AD, Kunz R, et al. GRADE: going from evidence to recommendations. BMJ 2008;336:1049-51.
12. Schünemann HJ, Jaeschke R, Cook DJ, et al. An official ATS statement: grading the quality of evidence and strength of recommendations in ATS guidelines and recommendations. Am J Respir Crit Care Med 2006;174:605-14.
13. Guyatt GH, Oxman AD, Vist G, et al. GRADE guidelines: 4. Rating the quality of evidence–study limitations (risk of bias). J Clin Epidemiol 2011;64:407-15.
14. Guyatt GH, Oxman AD, Kunz R, et al. GRADE guidelines: 7. Rating the quality of evidence–inconsistency. J Clin Epidemiol 2011;64:1294-302.
15. Guyatt GH, Oxman AD, Kunz R, et al. GRADE guidelines: 8. Rating the quality of evidence–indirectness. J Clin Epidemiol 2011;64:1303-10.
16. Guyatt GH, Oxman AD, Kunz R, et al. GRADE guidelines 6. Rating the quality of evidence–imprecision. J Clin Epidemiol 2011;64:1283-93.

17. Guyatt GH, Oxman AD, Montori V, et al. GRADE guidelines: 5. Rating the quality of evidence–publication bias. J Clin Epidemiol 2011;64:1277–82.
18. Jaeschke R, Singer J, Guyatt GH. Measurement of health status. Ascertaining the minimal clinically important difference. Control Clin Trials 1989;10:407–15.
19. Coventry PA. Does pulmonary rehabilitation reduce anxiety and depression in chronic obstructive pulmonary disease? Curr Opin Pulm Med 2009;15:143–9.
20. Parshall MB, Schwartzstein RM, Adams L, et al. An official American Thoracic Society statement: update on the mechanisms, assessment, and management of dyspnea. Am J Respir Crit Care Med 2012;185:435–52.
21. Ng KW, Mackney J, Jenkins S, et al. Does exercise training change physical activity in people with COPD? A systematic review and meta-analysis. Chron Respir Dis 2012;9:17–26.

Role of Infections

Kamen Rangelov, MD[a], Sanjay Sethi, MD[b],*

KEYWORDS

- Infection in COPD • Airway colonization • Chronic infection
- New strain exacerbations • Pneumonia and COPD • Innate immunity in COPD
- Virulence factors • Vicious-circle hypothesis

KEY POINTS

- Infection and chronic obstructive pulmonary disease (COPD) can be regarded as comorbid conditions, because infections contribute the progression of COPD, and COPD alters the susceptibility and manifestations of lung infections.
- The underlying mechanism of acute exacerbations of COPD is acquisition of new strains of bacteria and viruses. A complex host-pathogen interaction then determines the clinical manifestations and outcomes of such acquisition.
- COPD predisposes to community-acquired pneumonia and alters its cause, treatment, and outcomes.
- Several lines of evidence now suggest that chronic airway infection by bacteria is prevalent in COPD, and by triggering a chronic inflammatory response contributes to progression of disease.
- Lung innate immune defenses are impaired in COPD, making these patients more susceptible to infection. Respiratory pathogens prevalent in COPD use various mechanisms to evade host responses and thereby cause acute and persistent infections.

INTRODUCTION

The role of infection in chronic obstructive pulmonary disease (COPD) was first postulated in 1953 by Stuart-Harris and colleagues[1] in what is now known as the British hypothesis. They speculated that the decline in the lung function in COPD was the result of mucus hypersecretion and recurrent bacterial infections. In the next 2 decades, several studies were performed to confirm the hypothesis. In some of these studies,

This article originally appeared in *Clinics in Chest Medicine*, Volume 35, Issue 1, March 2014.
Funding Sources: S. Sethi, supported by VA Merit Review and NHLBI. K. Rangelov, Nil.
Conflict of Interest: The authors declare no conflict of interest.
[a] Pulmonary and Critical Care Medicine, University at Buffalo, SUNY, 3435 Main Street, Buffalo, NY 14214, USA; [b] Pulmonary, Critical Care, and Sleep Medicine, VA Western New York Healthcare System, University at Buffalo, The State University of New York, 3495 Bailey Avenue, Buffalo, NY 14215, USA
* Corresponding author.
E-mail address: ssethi@buffalo.edu

Clinics Collections 6 (2015) 179–198
http://dx.doi.org/10.1016/j.ccol.2015.05.039

sputum microbiology was used to compare the rate of bacterial infection in patients with chronic bronchitis at baseline and during exacerbations, as well as in comparison with individuals without COPD.[2-7] Some differences in bacterial infection related to disease state were found; for example, Smith and colleagues[2,3,8] found increased colonization with *Haemophilus influenzae* in patients with severe COPD compared with mild COPD. However, for the most part, differences in the rate of bacterial isolation from sputum at stable state (ie, colonization) versus at acute exacerbation (ie, infection) were not seen in these studies. Advanced molecular biology techniques to differentiate bacterial strains within species had not been developed and were therefore not available to these investigators. Other investigators examined this hypothesis by using serologic studies to determine levels of antibacterial antibodies in patients with chronic bronchitis. These results were also confusing and contradictory and were confounded by the use of laboratory strains as an antigen (discussed in Ref.[9]). In 1977, Fletcher and colleagues[10] published a landmark study that showed that frequency of exacerbations and mucus hypersecretion did not result in faster decline of lung function in patients with COPD. By the early 1980s, because of these observations and the appreciation of the importance of tobacco smoke in COPD pathogenesis, the British hypothesis was rejected, and bacterial infection was relegated to an epiphenomenon in this disease.[7]

The role of viral infection in COPD exacerbations was also extensively investigated in the 1960s and 1970s with viral cultures and serology at exacerbation.[3,5,8] Because of the lack of confounding by chronic colonization and serologic cross reactivity, about 30% of exacerbations were confirmed to be of viral origin. Following 20 to –30 years of scant investigation, the role of infection has been revisited in the last 2 decades with new molecular biology, immunology, and microbiology techniques.[11] Understanding of infection in COPD, both in the acute and chronic settings, has consequently developed substantially, as discussed later (**Fig. 1**).

ACUTE INFECTION

Acute infections in COPD are clinically recognized either as exacerbations or as episodes of pneumonia. The differentiation between the two presentations is based on the presence (pneumonia) or absence (exacerbation) of lung parenchymal

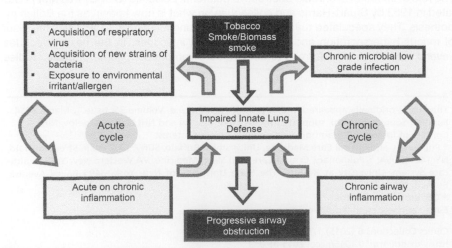

Fig. 1. Acute and chronic infection cycles in the pathogenesis of COPD.

involvement, which presents as an infiltrate on chest radiology. Although pneumonia has been always considered to be a more significant acute infection, exacerbations occur with much greater frequency and also have serious consequences in COPD. As the British hypothesis was being largely discredited, the importance of exacerbations in COPD was also minimized. They came to be regarded as self-resolving viral illness of little consequence (chest colds) for which no specific therapy was available and that were part of the natural course of the disease. The last 2 decades have seen considerable revision in this point of view, because data have emerged that exacerbations do contribute to the loss of quality of life and lung function in COPD and account for as much as half the cost of care of COPD. Furthermore, bacterial infection contributes to exacerbations, specific therapies are of benefit, and prevention of exacerbations is possible and is an important therapeutic goal in COPD.

Causes of Exacerbations

Exacerbations of COPD are airway inflammatory events that are induced by infection in most instances. The aggravating infection can be viral, bacterial, or a combination of viral and bacterial infections. Although there are episodes that are induced by poorly understood noninfectious factors, infections likely account for about 80% of exacerbations (**Table 1**).

Virus

The role of viruses in exacerbation was established in older studies (as discussed earlier) by viral culture and serology. Understanding of viral exacerbations has recently been expanded by the use of molecular diagnostic techniques and with the development of a human experimental model of rhinoviral exacerbations. The most common viruses detected in airway secretions at exacerbation are rhinovirus, influenza, respiratory syncytial virus (RSV), parainfluenza, and adenovirus. A recent systematic review found that viruses were detected in 34.1% of exacerbations.[12] More recent studies using molecular detection of virus by polymerase chain reaction (PCR) techniques have found viruses in up to half of all exacerbations.[13] The human experimental model of rhinoviral exacerbations was described in a study in which 13 subjects with COPD and 13 control subjects were nasally inoculated with a low dose of rhinovirus.[14] An increased neutrophilic inflammatory response in the lower airway, and more prominent lower respiratory symptoms and airway obstruction, were found in COPD compared with controls. An impaired interferon response to the infection was seen in patients with COPD. This work confirms the viral causation of exacerbations and has provided insights into susceptibility and pathogenic mechanisms involved in viral exacerbations.

Bacteria

In contrast with the role of viruses, the role of bacteria as a cause of exacerbations has been controversial and was not fully appreciated until recently. At present, pathogens clearly implicated in COPD exacerbations are nontypeable *H influenzae*, *Streptococcus pneumoniae*, *Moraxella catarrhalis*, and *Pseudomonas aeruginosa*. Whether *Staphylococcus aureus* and gram-negative enteric bacteria (Enterobacteriaceae), which are frequently isolated from sputum in COPD, are causative for exacerbations or are only capable of airway colonization is unclear at present.

Previous studies that defined bacterial pathogens isolated from sputum only at a species level were unable to fully appreciate the dynamic nature of bacterial infection in COPD. In a longitudinal prospective cohort study in patients with COPD, when bacterial strains in sputum were characterized by molecular techniques, combined with a

Table 1
Microbial pathogens in COPD

Microbe	Role in Exacerbations	Role in Stable Disease
Bacteria		
H influenzae	20%–30% of exacerbations	Major pathogen
Streptococcus pneumoniae	10%–15% of exacerbations	Minor role
Moraxella catarrhalis	10%–15% of exacerbations	Minor role
Pseudomonas aeruginosa	5%–10% of exacerbations, prevalent in advanced disease	Likely important in advanced disease
Enterobacteriaceae	Isolated in advanced disease, pathogenic significance undefined	Undefined
Haemophilus haemolyticus	Isolated frequently, unlikely cause	Unlikely
Haemophilus parainfluenzae	Isolated frequently, unlikely cause	Unlikely
Staphylococcus aureus	Isolated infrequently, unlikely cause	Unlikely
Viruses		
Rhinovirus	20%–25% of exacerbations	Unlikely
Parainfluenza	5%–10% of exacerbations	Unlikely
Influenza	5%–10% of exacerbations	Unlikely
Respiratory syncytial virus	5%–10% of exacerbations	Controversial
Coronavirus	5%–10% of exacerbations	Unlikely
Adenovirus	3%–5% of exacerbations	Latent infection seen, pathogenic significance undefined
Human metapneumovirus	3%–5% of exacerbations	Unlikely
Atypical Bacteria		
Chlamydophila pneumoniae	3%–5% of exacerbations	Commonly detected, pathogenic significance undefined
Mycoplasma pneumoniae	1%–2%	Unlikely
Fungi		
Pneumocystis jiroveci	Undefined	Commonly detected, pathogenic significance undefined

From Sethi S, Murphy TF. Infection in the pathogenesis and course of chronic obstructive pulmonary disease. N Engl J Med 2008;359:2356; with permission.

careful analysis of host immune and immunologic responses, an important mechanism that likely underlies exacerbations caused by the 4 major pathogens listed earlier was found (**Fig. 2**).[15] The risk of having an exacerbation was increased by more than 2-fold with respiratory tract acquisition of strains of these bacterial pathogens that were new to the patient. In this initial study, 33% of the visits within a month of new strain acquisition were associated with an exacerbation compared with 15.4% without a new strain.[16] Subsequent analyses from this study have now shown that the incidence of exacerbations at a visit with a new strain isolated from sputum is 40% to 50%, and that this holds true for each of the 4 major pathogens (nontypeable *H influenzae*, *S pneumoniae*, *M catarrhalis*, and *P aeruginosa*).[17–19] Additional support for this mechanism for exacerbations comes from various observations. Exacerbation-associated strains of *H influenzae* are more inflammatory in in vitro and animal models than strains associated with colonization, showing that clinical implications of bacterial acquisition correlate with strain virulence.[20] Strain-specific host immune response and a vigorous neutrophilic inflammatory response distinguish new strain exacerbations from those without new strains.[21]

Whether an increase in bacterial concentration (load) in the airway of a preexisting (colonizing) strain can be an additional independent mechanism of exacerbations is controversial. When bacterial sputum concentrations from our longitudinal cohort study were analyzed, either no differences or small differences were found between stable disease and exacerbation, and the small differences were no longer seen

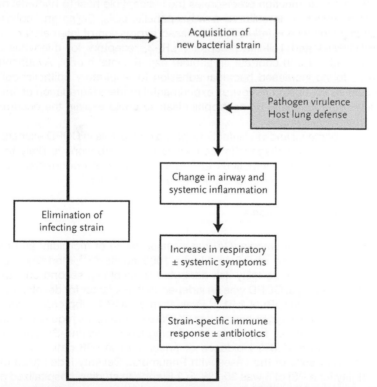

Fig. 2. Proposed mechanism of bacterial exacerbations in COPD. (*From* Sethi S, Murphy TF. Infection in the pathogenesis and course of chronic obstructive pulmonary disease. N Engl J Med 2008;359:2357; with permission.)

once new strain acquisition was taken into account.[21] In contrast, Rosell and colleagues[22] showed in pooled analysis of their data from bronchoscopic protected brush specimens that 54% of the patients with COPD exacerbation had pathogenic bacteria present in their airway secretions at significant concentrations compared with 29% of the patients with stable COPD. Intracellular *H influenzae* was found in bronchial mucosal biopsies in 87% of intubated patients with COPD exacerbation, compared with 33% of the patients with stable COPD.[23] Garcha and colleagues,[24] using quantitative PCR, found higher sputum bacterial loads at exacerbation than at stable state. However, these studies that have shown higher bacterial loads in sputum at exacerbation have not taken into account bacterial strain variation in their specimens.

Coinfection with virus and bacteria

A few recent studies have examined the impact of simultaneous or sequential bacterial and viral infection at exacerbation. Papi and colleagues[25] examined 64 patients with COPD exacerbation requiring hospital admission; 25% had combined bacterial and viral infections, and these patients had more severe symptoms and longer hospitalization. Presence of cold symptoms and *H influenzae* in sputum has also been associated with more symptoms and a larger decrease in lung function than when either is present alone.[26] In the rhinoviral human experimental model discussed earlier, as many as 60% of patients with COPD developed a secondary bacterial infection with a greater inflammatory response and duration of symptoms.[27] However, the severity of the exacerbations was mild and none of the patients required steroids or antibiotics.

It is likely that viral infection predisposes the susceptible host to bacterial coinfection and vice versa.[28,29] In cultured airway epithelial cells, Sajjan and colleagues[29] found that infection with *H influenzae* increased expression of intercellular adhesion molecule (ICAM)-1 and Toll-like receptor (TLR)-3, receptors for rhinovirus and its double-stranded RNA. In contrast, in another experimental model, Avadhanula and colleagues[28] found increased bacterial adhesion to respiratory epithelial cells after viral infection. In the human rhinovirus experimental model, degradation of antimicrobial peptides such as elafin by neutrophil elastase could explain the occurrence of secondary bacterial infection.[27]

In summary, bacterial and viral infections play a critical role in COPD exacerbations. Application of molecular diagnostic techniques to exacerbations is likely to further enhance understanding of infectious episodes. The role of opportunistic bacterial pathogens in causing exacerbations still needs to be defined.

Community-acquired Pneumonia

Epidemiology

Community-acquired pneumonia (CAP) is a major cause of morbidity and mortality worldwide, with incidence of 2.6 to 11 per 1000 adults.[30,31] Mortality can reach 20%, with 14.9% of the mortality risk attributed to smoking, second only to age.[32] In a multivariate analysis, COPD was an independent risk factor for developing severe CAP, with an odds ratio (OR) of 1.91.[33] Evaluation of COPD subgroups revealed that severe COPD on home oxygen and severe COPD exacerbations requiring hospitalization were independent risk factors for developing CAP.[34] Merino-Sanchez and colleagues[35] observed a 12.6% incidence of pneumonia in 596 patients with COPD over 3 years, with 55% of the cases with Pneumonia Severity Index (PSI) of 4 and 5. The mortality for a PSI of 5 was 35.7%. In 2 European studies, hospitalized patients with CAP with and without COPD were compared. Although mortality differences between the groups were not seen, patients with COPD experienced more severe pneumonia, higher rates of readmission, and recurrent pneumonia. Lower serum tumor necrosis factor alpha (TNF-α) and interleukin-6 levels were seen in the COPD group, suggesting an impaired inflammatory response in these patients.[36,37] Higher mortality with CAP in COPD has been observed in other studies, reiterating the importance of early recognition and appropriate management in this high-risk population.[38–40]

Causes of CAP in COPD

S pneumoniae remains the most common cause of CAP in COPD. However, because of alterations in the lung microbiome in COPD, pathogens such as H influenzae, M catarrhalis, and P aeruginosa may play a larger role in the development of CAP in these patients. Moreover, patients with COPD are exposed to frequent antibiotic courses and they are more likely to be infected with antibiotic-resistant pathogens, making empiric antibiotic choices challenging.[41] In a study of hospitalized patients with COPD with CAP, more infections attributable to P aeruginosa were observed.[42] However, the use of respiratory specimens to determine the microbiological cause of CAP in COPD is challenging, because chronic colonization with CAP-associated pathogens is common in COPD.

Role of inhaled corticosteroids

Inhaled corticosteroids (ICS), in combination with long acting beta agonists (LABA), are widely used in COPD, and reduce the frequency of exacerbations and daily symptoms in these patients.[43] However, the benefits come at a cost of increased risk of pneumonia. This increased risk was originally observed in the TORCH (Toward a Revolution in COPD Health) study, in which the ICS/LABA group had a higher probability (19.6%) of developing pneumonia over the course of 3 years.[43] A recent meta-analysis of 24 randomized controlled trials of ICS in COPD confirmed these results with a calculated relative risk of developing pneumonia at 1.56, and a number needed to harm of 60.[44–46] However, mortality was no different from the use of a LABA alone. The association between ICS use and pneumonia should be interpreted with caution. None of these trials were specifically designed to assess the risk of pneumonia, most episodes lack radiological confirmation, and COPD exacerbations may have been misdiagnosed as pneumonia. Mechanisms underlying this association have not been examined, but corticosteroid-induced impairment of local immune response to microbial pathogens is likely responsible.

Antimicrobial therapy in COPD and CAP

In outpatients with CAP, the presence of COPD as a comorbid condition places them in a high-risk group, and treatment with a respiratory fluoroquinolone or a β-lactam plus a macrolide is recommended.[47] Monotherapy with a macrolide or doxycycline is not appropriate in these patients. Because antibiotic use is common in these patients, a review of antibiotic use in the previous 3 months should guide empiric choice, and antibiotic classes used in the previous 3 months should be avoided. Among inpatients with CAP and COPD, the same choices are applicable. However, in patients requiring intensive care admission, combination therapy is always recommended, with a β-lactam and a respiratory fluoroquinolone or a macrolide. If Pseudomonas is suspected (previous Pseudomonas isolation, bronchiectasis, malnutrition, recent broad-spectrum antibiotic exposure), an antipseudomonal regimen is recommended.

CHRONIC INFECTION

In contrast with the (almost) sterile airways of a healthy lung, the lower airway of patients with COPD is frequently colonized with bacteria.[48,49] Although a wide variety of pathogens can be isolated, the two most common are H influenzae and

P aeruginosa (see **Table 1**). Until recently, the presence of these bacteria was regarded as colonization, implying an innocuous process in the airway without sequelae. A growing body of evidence now suggests that this colonization in stable COPD, via complex interactions with the host immune-inflammatory system, could contribute to COPD pathogenesis and progression.

Vicious-circle Hypothesis

Similar to bronchiectasis and cystic fibrosis, the host-pathogen interaction in stable COPD is well described by the vicious-circle hypothesis (**Fig. 3**). Repeated insults to the lung, such as smoking and environmental exposures, lead to impairment of the host immune defenses, thus allowing bacterial colonization. The bacteria cause subclinical inflammatory response in the airway, resulting in further damage to the innate lung defense and persistence of chronic bacterial infection. This process accelerates during acute exacerbations.

Evidence to Support Chronic Infection

Colonization is defined by the absence of damaging effects to the host related to the presence of a pathogen and the absence of a specific immune response. There are several parts of the body where such colonization is seen (eg, skin, colon) and is essential for health. The microbial pathogens that colonize these surfaces constitute a microbiome. Recent advances in research technologies, especially high-throughput genomic characterization, have made it possible to characterize the microbiome. The healthy lung is sterile by standard culture techniques. Even with molecular techniques, the microbiome of the healthy lung is sparse and transient, composed primarily of oral flora that are microaspirated and cleared.[50] In contrast, in a third of patients with COPD, potential respiratory pathogens can be retrieved by culture of lower airway samples.[49,51] An abundant microbiome can be found by molecular techniques in COPD lungs.[52] Unlike other body surfaces, like the skin and gut mucosa, the lung is not well equipped to handle a microbiome. Therefore, microbial presence in the lower airways in COPD is harmful.

Several studies have described excess inflammation in stable patients with COPD when colonized with bacterial pathogens.[51,53–56] The airway inflammation associated with bacterial colonization is predominantly neutrophilic. Studies comparing sputum samples from colonized and noncolonized patients have found higher levels of TNF-α, interleukin-8, interleukin-6, leukotriene B4, neutrophil myeloperoxidase, and elastase, and lower levels of the antiprotease secretory leukocyte protease inhibitor.[53,54,56,57] Bronchoscopic sampling of the lower airway with bronchoalveolar lavage showed increased levels of neutrophils, TNF-α, interleukin-8, matrix metalloproteinase 9, and endotoxin in association with bacterial colonization.[49,51,58] Although several mediators contribute to COPD pathogenesis, interleukin-8 in particular has been associated with increased exacerbation frequency, longer recovery periods, worsening airway obstruction, and development of bronchiectasis.[58,59] Bacterial (*M catarrhalis*) acquisition, even without an increase in symptoms of an exacerbation, has been associated with increases in proteolytic activity and a reduction in antiproteolytic defense, resulting in worsening of the protease/antiprotease imbalance that is thought to cause progressive lung damage in COPD.[56] The inflammatory profile seen with bacterial colonization is similar to that seen with bacterial exacerbations, implying that colonization is a low-grade infection.

Following exacerbations of COPD, specific immune responses, both systemic and mucosal, to the infecting strain are often observed. Similar observations have now been described following colonization.[18,19] This active immune response supports

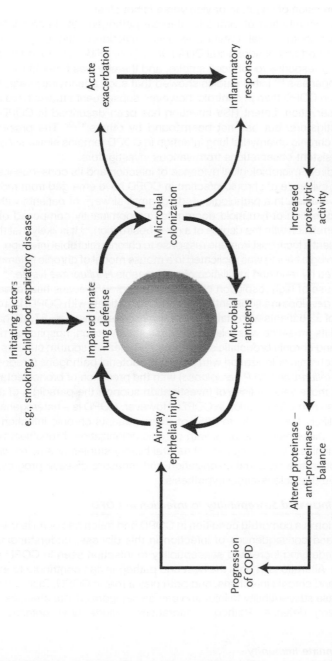

Fig. 3. The vicious-circle hypothesis of infection and inflammation in the pathogenesis and course of chronic obstructive pulmonary disease. N Engl J Med 2008;359:2361; with permission.)

the presence of chronic infection in COPD. Furthermore, with *M catarrhalis*, a differential immune response is seen with colonization, which is accompanied by a stronger mucosal immune response, compared with a stronger systemic immune response accompanying exacerbations.[18] Whether the nature of the immune response dictates the clinical expression of infection or vice versa is not clear.

The potential contribution of viral and atypical pathogens to chronic infection in COPD has been controversial. Latent adenoviral infection of the lungs, in the form of integration of portions of adenoviral DNA into cellular DNA, was found to enhance the inflammatory response to tobacco smoke, and thereby was thought to contribute to COPD pathogenesis.[60] Initial studies showed that such adenoviral integration was more common in COPD than in controls; however, subsequent studies have not supported this observation. Latent RSV infection has been described in COPD by one group of investigators, but has not been found by others.[61,62] The presence and contribution of chronic chlamydial lung infection in COPD remains similarly controversial, with inconsistent observations from various investigators.

Besides the direct microbiological evidence of infection and its consequences, other indirect lines of evidence of chronic infection in COPD have emerged from radiological and pathologic studies. In a pathologic study of small airways of patients with COPD, the extent of formation of lymphoid aggregates predominantly composed of B cells had the best correlation with the degree of airflow obstruction.[63] It is likely that these aggregates represent a local host immune response to chronic microbial infection. Furthermore, this pathologic finding was replicated in a mouse model of chronic inflammation in the lungs induced by repeated instillation of nontypeable *H influenzae* lysate.[64]

Widespread use of high resolution computed tomography scans has revealed that bronchiectasis develops in a substantial proportion of patients with COPD. In a comprehensive study of 92 patients with stable moderate or severe disease, 57.5% had bronchiectasis, and its presence was related to worse lung function, hospital admission in the past year, and chronic bronchitic symptoms.[65] Repeated sputum cultures in these patients linked chronic colonization with potential bacterial pathogens (predominantly nontypeable *H influenzae* and *P aeruginosa*) with the presence of bronchiectasis.[65]

In summary, these various lines of investigation support the paradigm of a vicious circle of infection and inflammation in COPD. However, COPD is a heterogeneous disease and it is likely that in 30% to 50% of these patients chronic infection plays a prominent role, these being the ones with chronic colonization, bronchiectasis, and/or chronic bronchitis. Future longitudinal natural history studies or studies with interventions that decrease bacterial colonization and measure disease progression are needed to prove the vicious-circle hypothesis.

Mechanism of Increased Susceptibility to Infection in COPD

Although infection is a comorbid condition in COPD and much has been learned about the incidence and consequences of infection in this disease, understanding of the mechanisms underlying increased susceptibility to infection seen in COPD is still in its early stages. Alterations in both the host and pathogen can contribute to establishment of acute and chronic infections, and both play a role in COPD. Disruptions in the host that increase susceptibility to infection can be categorized into changes in innate or adaptive lung defense. Pathogen alterations include host defense evasion mechanisms.

Host Defects: Innate Immunity

The healthy lung possesses a multilayered, redundant, and highly efficient innate defense system that allows it to maintain an almost pathogen-free environment in spite of being constantly exposed to a variety of microbes through inhalation and microaspiration. This innate immune system of the lung has 3 components: mechanical barrier, humoral, and cellular response systems. This nonspecific immunity is the first line of defense against viruses, bacteria, and other particulates. It recognizes antigenic ligands entering the airway via pattern-recognition receptors and triggers series of responses resulting in complement activation and phagocytosis. The end result is elimination of the antigen or its presentation on the surface of the macrophages and activation of the adaptive immunity. In patients with COPD, several innate responses are impaired, leading to increased susceptibility to infection.

Mucociliary clearance

The mucociliary clearance is the first barrier to noxious agents, by effectively trapping and clearing inhaled and microaspirated microbial pathogens. Both normal mucus and a normal ciliary apparatus are required for effective mucociliary clearance. Abnormal mucus (such as in cystic fibrosis) and a dysfunctional ciliary apparatus (such as in ciliary dyskinesia) are associated with acute and chronic bronchial infection. Augmented mucus production can be regarded as a defensive response to particulate or microbial exposure. However, when the exposure is chronic, and inflammation and ciliary dysfunction are also present, it could worsen mucociliary clearance.

Smoking disrupts mucociliary clearance, not only by augmenting mucus production but also by inducing structural abnormalities in the ciliary apparatus.[66] Studies in moderate to heavy smokers have shown longer lung clearance times, although the degree of impairment is variable.[67,68] Further deterioration in mucociliary clearance is seen with development of chronic bronchitis and airway obstruction in smokers.[69–71] Patients with COPD have hypertrophy and hyperplasia of their airway goblet cells and increased mucus stores.[72,73] In tissue and animal models, exposure to *S pneumoniae* and *H influenzae* results in further upregulation of mucin production.[74,75] Neutrophilic inflammation also worsens mucociliary function, mediated by increased mucus production, reduced ciliary beating, and altered viscoelastic properties of mucus.

Immunoglobulin A

Immunoglobulin (Ig) A, especially polymeric secretory IgA, plays an important role in innate defense by coating the bacterial pathogen, thereby interfering with its ability to interact with the mucosal surface (immune exclusion). IgA can also neutralize infectious agents and could act as an opsonin assisting in pathogen elimination. Localized areas of IgA deficiency in the large and small airways are seen in COPD that were associated with squamous metaplasia. Polymeric IgG receptor expression, a receptor required for transcytosis of the IgA molecule from the basolateral to the apical surface of the epithelial cell, was reduced in these areas.[76] These changes in IgA could be an important mechanism of infection susceptibility in COPD.

Antimicrobial peptides

Antimicrobial polypeptides abundant in the airway surface lining fluid have antimicrobial and immunoregulatory functions. One major group, the cationic polypeptides, includes lysozyme, lactoferrin, defensins, the cathelicidins (LL-37), and secretory leukocyte protease inhibitor (SLPI).[77–82] Another important group, the collectins, include surfactant protein-A (SP-A), surfactant protein-D (SP-D), and mannose-binding lectin.[83] Complex and dynamic alterations in various antimicrobial polypeptides have been described in COPD, both in the stable state and during exacerbations.

Deficiencies of SLPI and lysozyme in the stable state have been associated with more frequent exacerbations.[84,85] Decreased serum mannose-binding lectin has been linked with exacerbation frequency in COPD, but this has not been a consistent observation.[86] Lower airway concentrations of SP-A and SP-D are seen in smokers, with further decreases in association with emphysema.[87,88] Lower levels of beta-defensin 2 and Clara Cell Protein 16 (CC16) and increased levels of elafin and SLPI in sputum supernatants in stable COPD have been observed.[89] Decreased levels of beta-defensin 2 in the central airways, but not in the distal airways, of smokers with COPD were found in a study of resected lung specimens.[90]

Dynamic changes in antimicrobial peptides have also been described with exacerbations of COPD. SLPI levels decrease significantly at the time of such exacerbations, which return to baseline after resolution.[78] Lysozyme and lactoferrin levels decrease and LL-37 levels increase with both colonization and infective exacerbations with H influenzae and M catarrhalis.[78] In a human model of rhinoviral infection, impaired elafin and SLPI responses following rhinoviral infection were associated with secondary bacterial infection.[27]

Macrophage function

Key cellular components on innate lung defense are alveolar macrophages and airway epithelial cells. Phagocytic and cytokine responses of alveolar macrophages to bacterial pathogens are crucial for dealing with small pathogen inocula, without invoking potentially damaging inflammatory and adaptive immune responses. Alveolar macrophages from patients with COPD show impaired ability to phagocytose H influenzae and M catarrhalis, but not S pneumoniae or inert microspheres. This impairment is correlated with worsening lung function (**Fig. 4**).[91] Alveolar macrophages from patients with COPD also have a less robust cytokine response to bacterial proteins, specifically outer membrane protein P6 and lipo-oligosaccharide (endotoxin) of H influenzae.[92–94] Following exposure to rhinovirus, alveolar macrophages showed decreased cytokine responses to bacterial lipopolysaccharide and lipoteichoic acid,[95] which could explain the increased susceptibility to bacterial infection after viral infection in COPD.

These decrements in macrophage function are likely secondary to several mechanisms, including reduction in pattern-recognition receptors such as Toll-like receptors TLR2 and TLR4, reduction in scavenger receptors such as macrophage receptor with collagenous structure (MARCO), or alteration in subpopulations of macrophages in the airway.[96–98] TLR2 has been found to be downregulated in smokers, patients with COPD, and farmers exposed to organic dust.[96,99,100] TLR4 downregulation is associated with the development of emphysema and worse airflow limitation in smokers.[101] Polymorphism T399I of the TLR4 gene has been associated with development of COPD phenotype in smokers.[102]

Pathogen Mechanisms

Tissue invasion

H influenzae was traditionally regarded as an extracellular pathogen. However, molecular detection techniques have shown this pathogen in the bronchial epithelium and inside subepithelial macrophages in COPD.[23,48] These tissue bacteria could be shielded from the actions of antibiotics and antibodies, and therefore could be more resistant to eradication. Molecular detection often detects H influenzae in airway secretions and lung samples when cultures are negative, which could be explained by such tissue invasion.

Biofilm formation

Biofilms are bacteria encased with an extracellular matrix, which is usually composed of polysaccharides produced and secreted by bacteria. Bacteria in the core of the film, which is predominantly anaerobic, are in a low metabolic state. Antibiotic penetration

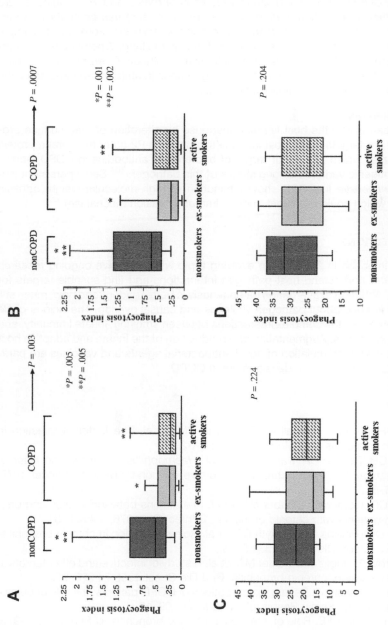

Fig. 4. Comparison of phagocytosis of nontypeable *H influenzae* (*A*), *Moraxella catarrhalis* (*B*), *Streptococcus pneumoniae* (*C*), and latex microspheres (*D*) by human alveolar macrophages from healthy controls, current smokers with COPD, and ex-smokers with COPD. (*Modified from* Berenson CS, Kruzel RL, Eberhardt E, et al. Phagocytic dysfunction of human alveolar macrophages and severity of chronic obstructive pulmonary disease. J Infect Dis 2013; with permission.)

into biofilms is limited, requiring up to 1000 times higher concentrations to achieve eradication.[103] Parts of the biofilm can detach and cause distant infection. Pathogens common in COPD, including *H influenzae*, *M catarrhalis*, and *P aeruginosa*, are capable of biofilm formation. Furthermore, smoke exposure has been shown to increase biofilm formation.[104] *P aeruginosa* in cystic fibrosis is the prototypical example of biofilm formation as a mechanism of persistence in the lung. Whether bacterial biofilms are present in COPD airways is not yet known.[105] Mucoid *P aeruginosa* and some strains of *H influenzae* persist clinically for long periods in spite of repeated antibiotic exposure, which is reminiscent of cystic fibrosis.

Antigenic alteration

Pathogens can evade the host immune response by alteration of their surface proteins, which are targets of the host immune system. The P2 outer membrane protein of *H influenzae*, which is a major target of bactericidal antibodies in COPD, shows extensive antigenic variation among strains of this pathogen.[106] Serial persistent isolates of *H influenzae* in COPD show diminution of high-molecular-weight adhesin expression, which could represent another immune evasion mechanism.[107]

FUTURE DIRECTIONS

The role of infection in COPD is an evolving topic with extensive ongoing research trying to better understand host-pathogen interactions and find suitable targets for intervention. Although exacerbation pathogenesis is better understood now, much still needs to be learned about pathogen virulence and causal overlap. The vicious-circle hypothesis exposes the complex interactions between smoking, innate immunity, and respiratory pathogens. Augmentation and modulation of the innate and adaptive host immunity as well as formulation of novel antibacterial agents and vaccines are paramount in future research and development in COPD.

REFERENCES

1. Stuart-Harris CH, Pownall M, Scothorne CM, et al. The factor of infection in chronic bronchitis. Q J Med 1953;22:121–32.
2. Smith CB, Golden CA, Kanner RE, et al. *Haemophilus influenzae* and *Haemophilus parainfluenzae* in chronic obstructive pulmonary disease. Lancet 1976; 1:1253–5.
3. Smith CB, Golden C, Klauber MR, et al. Interactions between viruses and bacteria in patients with chronic bronchitis. J Infect Dis 1976;134:552–61.
4. Gump DW, Phillips CA, Forsyth BR, et al. Role of infection in chronic bronchitis. Am Rev Respir Dis 1976;113:465–73.
5. McHardy VU, Inglis JM, Calder MA, et al. A study of infective and other factors in exacerbations of chronic bronchitis. Br J Dis Chest 1980;74:228–38.
6. Fagon JY, Chastre J. Severe exacerbations of COPD patients: the role of pulmonary infections. Semin Respir Infect 1996;11:109–18.
7. Tager I, Speizer FE. Role of infection in chronic bronchitis. N Engl J Med 1975; 292:563–71.
8. Smith CB, Golden C, Kanner R, et al. Association of viral and *Mycoplasma pneumoniae* infections with acute respiratory illness in patients with chronic obstructive pulmonary diseases. Am Rev Respir Dis 1980;121:225–32.
9. Murphy TF, Sethi S. Bacterial infection in chronic obstructive pulmonary disease. Am Rev Respir Dis 1992;146:1067–83.

10. Fletcher F, Peto R. The natural history of chronic airflow obstruction. Br Med J 1977;1:1645–8.
11. Sethi S, Murphy TF. Infection in the pathogenesis and course of chronic obstructive pulmonary disease. N Engl J Med 2008;359:2355–65.
12. Mohan A, Chandra S, Agarwal D, et al. Prevalence of viral infection detected by PCR and RT-PCR in patients with acute exacerbation of COPD: a systematic review. Respirology 2010;15:536–42.
13. Kherad O, Kaiser L, Bridevaux PO, et al. Upper-respiratory viral infection, biomarkers, and COPD exacerbations. Chest 2010;138:896–904.
14. Mallia P, Message SD, Gielen V, et al. Experimental rhinovirus infection as a human model of chronic obstructive pulmonary disease exacerbation. Am J Respir Crit Care Med 2011;183:734–42.
15. Sethi S, Sethi R, Eschberger K, et al. Airway bacterial concentrations and exacerbations of chronic obstructive pulmonary disease. Am J Respir Crit Care Med 2007;176(4):356–61.
16. Sethi S, Evans N, Grant BJ, et al. New strains of bacteria and exacerbations of chronic obstructive pulmonary disease. N Engl J Med 2002;347:465–71.
17. Murphy TF, Brauer AL, Sethi S, et al. Haemophilus haemolyticus: a human respiratory tract commensal to be distinguished from Haemophilus influenzae. J Infect Dis 2007;195:81–9.
18. Murphy TF, Brauer AL, Grant BJ, et al. Moraxella catarrhalis in chronic obstructive pulmonary disease: burden of disease and immune response. Am J Respir Crit Care Med 2005;172:195–9.
19. Murphy TF, Brauer AL, Eschberger K, et al. Pseudomonas aeruginosa in chronic obstructive pulmonary disease. Am J Respir Crit Care Med 2008;177:853–60.
20. Chin CL, Manzel LJ, Lehman EE, et al. Haemophilus influenzae from patients with chronic obstructive pulmonary disease exacerbation induce more inflammation than colonizers. Am J Respir Crit Care Med 2005;172:85–91.
21. Sethi S, Wrona C, Eschberger K, et al. Inflammatory profile of new bacterial strain exacerbations of chronic obstructive pulmonary disease. Am J Respir Crit Care Med 2008;177:491–7.
22. Rosell A, Monso E, Soler N, et al. Microbiologic determinants of exacerbation in chronic obstructive pulmonary disease. Arch Intern Med 2005;165:891–7.
23. Bandi V, Apicella MA, Mason E, et al. Nontypeable Haemophilus influenzae in the lower respiratory tract of patients with chronic bronchitis. Am J Respir Crit Care Med 2001;164:2114–9.
24. Garcha DS, Thurston SJ, Patel AR, et al. Changes in prevalence and load of airway bacteria using quantitative PCR in stable and exacerbated COPD. Thorax 2012;67:1075–80.
25. Papi A, Bellettato CM, Braccioni F, et al. Infections and airway inflammation in chronic obstructive pulmonary disease severe exacerbations. Am J Respir Crit Care Med 2006;173:1114–21.
26. Wilkinson TM, Hurst JR, Perera WR, et al. Effect of interactions between lower airway bacterial and rhinoviral infection in exacerbations of COPD. Chest 2006;129:317–24.
27. Mallia P, Footitt J, Sotero R, et al. Rhinovirus infection induces degradation of antimicrobial peptides and secondary bacterial infection in chronic obstructive pulmonary disease. Am J Respir Crit Care Med 2012;186:1117–24.
28. Avadhanula V, Rodriguez CA, Devincenzo JP, et al. Respiratory viruses augment the adhesion of bacterial pathogens to respiratory epithelium in a viral species- and cell type-dependent manner. J Virol 2006;80:1629–36.

29. Sajjan US, Jia Y, Newcomb DC, et al. *H. influenzae* potentiates airway epithelial cell responses to rhinovirus by increasing ICAM-1 and TLR3 expression. FASEB J 2006;20:2121–3.

30. Marston BJ, Plouffe JF, File TM Jr, et al. Incidence of community-acquired pneumonia requiring hospitalization. Results of a population-based active surveillance Study in Ohio. The Community-Based Pneumonia Incidence Study Group. Arch Intern Med 1997;157:1709–18.

31. Vinogradova Y, Hippisley-Cox J, Coupland C. Identification of new risk factors for pneumonia: population-based case-control study. Br J Gen Pract 2009;59: e329–38.

32. Naucler P, Darenberg J, Morfeldt E, et al. Contribution of host, bacterial factors and antibiotic treatment to mortality in adult patients with bacteraemic pneumococcal pneumonia. Thorax 2013;68:571–9.

33. Ishiguro T, Takayanagi N, Yamaguchi S, et al. Etiology and factors contributing to the severity and mortality of community-acquired pneumonia. Intern Med 2013;52:317–24.

34. Mullerova H, Chigbo C, Hagan GW, et al. The natural history of community-acquired pneumonia in COPD patients: a population database analysis. Respir Med 2012;106:1124–33.

35. Merino-Sanchez M, Alfageme-Michavila I, Reyes-Nunez N, et al. Prognosis in patients with pneumonia and chronic obstructive pulmonary disease. Arch Bronconeumol 2005;41:607–11 [in Spanish].

36. Crisafulli E, Menendez R, Huerta A, et al. Systemic inflammatory pattern of patients with community-acquired pneumonia with and without COPD. Chest 2013; 143:1009–17.

37. Liapikou A, Polverino E, Ewig S, et al. Severity and outcomes of hospitalised community-acquired pneumonia in COPD patients. Eur Respir J 2012;39:855–61.

38. Arancibia F, Bauer TT, Ewig S, et al. Community-acquired pneumonia due to gram-negative bacteria and *Pseudomonas aeruginosa*: incidence, risk, and prognosis. Arch Intern Med 2002;162:1849–58.

39. Torres A, Dorca J, Zalacain R, et al. Community-acquired pneumonia in chronic obstructive pulmonary disease: a Spanish multicenter study. Am J Respir Crit Care Med 1996;154:1456–61.

40. Rello J, Rodriguez A, Torres A, et al. Implications of COPD in patients admitted to the intensive care unit by community-acquired pneumonia. Eur Respir J 2006; 27:1210–6.

41. Desai H, Richter S, Doern G, et al. Antibiotic resistance in sputum isolates of *Streptococcus pneumoniae* in chronic obstructive pulmonary disease is related to antibiotic exposure. COPD 2010;7:337–44.

42. Restrepo MI, Mortensen EM, Pugh JA, et al. COPD is associated with increased mortality in patients with community-acquired pneumonia. Eur Respir J 2006;28: 346–51.

43. Calverley PM, Anderson JA, Celli B, et al. Salmeterol and fluticasone propionate and survival in chronic obstructive pulmonary disease. N Engl J Med 2007;356: 775–89.

44. Singh S, Loke YK. An overview of the benefits and drawbacks of inhaled corticosteroids in chronic obstructive pulmonary disease. Int J Chron Obstruct Pulmon Dis 2010;5:189–95.

45. Singh S, Amin AV, Loke YK. Long-term use of inhaled corticosteroids and the risk of pneumonia in chronic obstructive pulmonary disease: a meta-analysis. Arch Intern Med 2009;169:219–29.

46. Spencer S, Karner C, Cates CJ, et al. Inhaled corticosteroids versus long-acting beta(2)-agonists for chronic obstructive pulmonary disease. Cochrane Database Syst Rev 2011;(12):CD007033.
47. Mandell LA, Wunderink RG, Anzueto A, et al. Infectious Diseases Society of America/American Thoracic Society consensus guidelines on the management of community-acquired pneumonia in adults. Clin Infect Dis 2007;44(Suppl 2): S27–72.
48. Murphy TF, Brauer AL, Schiffmacher AT, et al. Persistent colonization by *Haemophilus influenzae* in chronic obstructive pulmonary disease. Am J Respir Crit Care Med 2004;170:266–72.
49. Sethi S, Maloney J, Grove L, et al. Airway inflammation and bronchial bacterial colonization in chronic obstructive pulmonary disease. Am J Respir Crit Care Med 2006;173:991–8.
50. Charlson ES, Bittinger K, Haas AR, et al. Topographical continuity of bacterial populations in the healthy human respiratory tract. Am J Respir Crit Care Med 2011;184:957–63.
51. Soler N, Ewig S, Torres A, et al. Airway inflammation and bronchial microbial patterns in patients with stable chronic obstructive pulmonary disease. Eur Respir J 1999;14:1015–22.
52. Cabrera-Rubio R, Garcia-Nunez M, Seto L, et al. Microbiome diversity in the bronchial tracts of patients with chronic obstructive pulmonary disease. J Clin Microbiol 2012;50:3562–8.
53. Bresser P, Out TA, van Alphen L, et al. Airway inflammation in nonobstructive and obstructive chronic bronchitis with chronic *Haemophilus influenzae* airway infection. Comparison with noninfected patients with chronic obstructive pulmonary disease. Am J Respir Crit Care Med 2000;162:947–52.
54. Banerjee D, Khair OA, Honeybourne D. Impact of sputum bacteria on airway inflammation and health status in clinical stable COPD. Eur Respir J 2004;23: 685–91.
55. Hill AT, Campbell EJ, Hill SL, et al. Association between airway bacterial load and markers of airway inflammation in patients with stable chronic bronchitis. Am J Med 2000;109:288–95.
56. Parameswaran GI, Wrona CT, Murphy TF, et al. *Moraxella catarrhalis* acquisition, airway inflammation and protease-antiprotease balance in chronic obstructive pulmonary disease. BMC Infect Dis 2009;9:178.
57. Zhang M, Li Q, Zhang XY, et al. Relevance of lower airway bacterial colonization, airway inflammation, and pulmonary function in the stable stage of chronic obstructive pulmonary disease. Eur J Clin Microbiol Infect Dis 2010;29: 1487–93.
58. Tumkaya M, Atis S, Ozge C, et al. Relationship between airway colonization, inflammation and exacerbation frequency in COPD. Respir Med 2007;101: 729–37.
59. Patel IS, Vlahos I, Wilkinson TM, et al. Bronchiectasis, exacerbation indices, and inflammation in chronic obstructive pulmonary disease. Am J Respir Crit Care Med 2004;170:400–7.
60. Retamales I, Elliott WM, Meshi B, et al. Amplification of inflammation in emphysema and its association with latent adenoviral infection. Am J Respir Crit Care Med 2001;164:469–73.
61. Falsey AR, Formica MA, Hennessey PA, et al. Detection of respiratory syncytial virus in adults with chronic obstructive pulmonary disease. Am J Respir Crit Care Med 2006;173:639–43.

62. Wilkinson TM, Donaldson GC, Johnston SL, et al. Respiratory syncytial virus, airway inflammation, and FEV1 decline in patients with chronic obstructive pulmonary disease. Am J Respir Crit Care Med 2006;173:871–6.

63. Hogg JC, Chu F, Utokaparch S, et al. The nature of small-airway obstruction in chronic obstructive pulmonary disease. N Engl J Med 2004;350:2645–53.

64. Moghaddam SJ, Clement CG, De la Garza MM, et al. Haemophilus influenzae lysate induces aspects of the chronic obstructive pulmonary disease phenotype. Am J Respir Cell Mol Biol 2008;38:629–38.

65. Martinez-Garcia MA, Soler-Cataluna JJ, Donat-Sanz Y, et al. Factors associated with bronchiectasis in chronic obstructive pulmonary disease patients. Chest 2011;140(5):1130–7.

66. Verra F, Escudier E, Lebargy F, et al. Ciliary abnormalities in bronchial epithelium of smokers, ex-smokers, and nonsmokers. Am J Respir Crit Care Med 1995;151: 630–4.

67. Foster WM, Langenback EG, Bergofsky EH. Disassociation in the mucociliary function of central and peripheral airways of asymptomatic smokers. Am Rev Respir Dis 1985;132:633–9.

68. Koblizek V, Tomsova M, Cermakova E, et al. Impairment of nasal mucociliary clearance in former smokers with stable chronic obstructive pulmonary disease relates to the presence of a chronic bronchitis phenotype. Rhinology 2011;49: 397–406.

69. Smaldone GC, Foster WM, O'Riordan TG, et al. Regional impairment of mucociliary clearance in chronic obstructive pulmonary disease. Chest 1993;103: 1390–6.

70. Vastag E, Matthys H, Zsamboki G, et al. Mucociliary clearance in smokers. Eur J Respir Dis 1986;68:107–13.

71. Wanner A, Salathe M, O'Riordan TG. Mucociliary clearance in the airways. Am J Respir Crit Care Med 1996;154:1868–902.

72. Innes AL, Woodruff PG, Ferrando RE, et al. Epithelial mucin stores are increased in the large airways of smokers with airflow obstruction. Chest 2006;130:1102–8.

73. Ma R, Wang Y, Cheng G, et al. MUC5AC expression up-regulation goblet cell hyperplasia in the airway of patients with chronic obstructive pulmonary disease. Chin Med Sci J 2005;20:181–4.

74. Ha U, Lim JH, Jono H, et al. A novel role for IkappaB kinase (IKK) alpha and IKKbeta in ERK-dependent up-regulation of MUC5AC mucin transcription by Streptococcus pneumoniae. J Immunol 2007;178:1736–47.

75. Chen R, Lim JH, Jono H, et al. Nontypeable Haemophilus influenzae lipoprotein P6 induces MUC5AC mucin transcription via TLR2-TAK1-dependent p38 MAPK-AP1 and IKKbeta-IkappaBalpha-NF-kappaB signaling pathways. Biochem Biophys Res Commun 2004;324:1087–94.

76. Polosukhin VV, Cates JM, Lawson WE, et al. Bronchial secretory immunoglobulin a deficiency correlates with airway inflammation and progression of chronic obstructive pulmonary disease. Am J Respir Crit Care Med 2011;184:317–27.

77. Ganz T. Defensins: antimicrobial peptides of vertebrates. C R Biol 2004;327: 539–49.

78. Parameswaran GI, Sethi S, Murphy TF. Effects of bacterial infection on airway antimicrobial peptides and proteins in chronic obstructive pulmonary disease. Chest 2011;140(3):611–7.

79. Tjabringa GS, Rabe KF, Hiemstra PS. The human cathelicidin LL-37: a multifunctional peptide involved in infection and inflammation in the lung. Pulm Pharmacol Ther 2005;18:321–7.

80. Dajani R, Zhang Y, Taft PJ, et al. Lysozyme secretion by submucosal glands protects the airway from bacterial infection. Am J Respir Cell Mol Biol 2005;32:548–52.
81. Ellison RT 3rd, Giehl TJ. Killing of gram-negative bacteria by lactoferrin and lysozyme. J Clin Invest 1991;88:1080–91.
82. Fitch PM, Roghanian A, Howie SE, et al. Human neutrophil elastase inhibitors in innate and adaptive immunity. Biochem Soc Trans 2006;34:279–82.
83. Crouch EC. Structure, biologic properties, and expression of surfactant protein D (SP-D). Biochim Biophys Acta 1998;1408:278–89.
84. Taylor D, Cripps A, Clancy R. A possible role for lysozyme in determining acute exacerbation in chronic bronchitis. Clin Exp Immunol 1995;102:406–16.
85. Gompertz S, Bayley DL, Hill SL, et al. Relationship between airway inflammation and the frequency of exacerbations in patients with smoking related COPD. Thorax 2001;56:36–41.
86. Yang IA, Seeney SL, Wolter JM, et al. Mannose-binding lectin gene polymorphism predicts hospital admissions for COPD infections. Genes Immun 2003; 4:269–74.
87. Betsuyaku T, Kuroki Y, Nagai K, et al. Effects of ageing and smoking on SP-A and SP-D levels in bronchoalveolar lavage fluid. Eur Respir J 2004;24:964–70.
88. Honda Y, Takahashi H, Kuroki Y, et al. Decreased contents of surfactant proteins A and D in BAL fluids of healthy smokers. Chest 1996;109:1006–9.
89. Tsoumakidou M, Bouloukaki I, Thimaki K, et al. Innate immunity proteins in chronic obstructive pulmonary disease and idiopathic pulmonary fibrosis. Exp Lung Res 2010;36:373–80.
90. Pace F, Ferraro M, Minervini MI, et al. Beta defensin-2 is reduced in central but not in distal airways of smoker COPD patients. PLoS One 2012;7:e33601.
91. Berenson CS, Kruzel RL, Eberhardt E, et al. Phagocytic dysfunction of human alveolar macrophages and severity of chronic obstructive pulmonary disease. J Infect Dis 2013. [Epub ahead of print].
92. Hodge S, Hodge G, Ahern J, et al. Smoking alters alveolar macrophage recognition and phagocytic ability: implications in chronic obstructive pulmonary disease. Am J Respir Cell Mol Biol 2007;37:748–55.
93. Berenson CS, Garlipp MA, Grove LJ, et al. Impaired phagocytosis of nontypeable *Haemophilus influenzae* by human alveolar macrophages in chronic obstructive pulmonary disease. J Infect Dis 2006;194:1375–84.
94. Berenson CS, Wrona CT, Grove LJ, et al. Impaired alveolar macrophage response to *Haemophilus* antigens in chronic obstructive lung disease. Am J Respir Crit Care Med 2006;174:31–40.
95. Oliver BG, Lim S, Wark P, et al. Rhinovirus exposure impairs immune responses to bacterial products in human alveolar macrophages. Thorax 2008;63:519–25.
96. Droemann D, Goldmann T, Tiedje T, et al. Toll-like receptor 2 expression is decreased on alveolar macrophages in cigarette smokers and COPD patients. Respir Res 2005;6:68.
97. Harvey CJ, Thimmulappa RK, Sethi S, et al. Targeting Nrf2 signaling improves bacterial clearance by alveolar macrophages in patients with COPD and in a mouse model. Sci Transl Med 2011;3:78ra32.
98. Kunz LI, Lapperre TS, Snoeck-Stroband JB, et al. Smoking status and anti-inflammatory macrophages in bronchoalveolar lavage and induced sputum in COPD. Respir Res 2011;12:34.
99. Macredmond RE, Greene CM, Dorscheid DR, et al. Epithelial expression of TLR4 is modulated in COPD and by steroids, salmeterol and cigarette smoke. Respir Res 2007;8:84.

100. Sahlander K, Larsson K, Palmberg L. Daily exposure to dust alters innate immunity. PLoS One 2012;7:e31646.
101. Lee SW, Kim DR, Kim TJ, et al. The association of down-regulated toll-like receptor 4 expression with airflow limitation and emphysema in smokers. Respir Res 2012;13:106.
102. Speletas M, Merentiti V, Kostikas K, et al. Association of TLR4-T399I polymorphism with chronic obstructive pulmonary disease in smokers. Clin Dev Immunol 2009;2009:260286.
103. Hoiby N, Ciofu O, Johansen HK, et al. The clinical impact of bacterial biofilms. Int J Oral Sci 2011;3:55–65.
104. Goldstein-Daruech N, Cope EK, Zhao KQ, et al. Tobacco smoke mediated induction of sinonasal microbial biofilms. PLoS One 2011;6:e15700.
105. Starner TD, Zhang N, Kim G, et al. *Haemophilus influenzae* forms biofilms on airway epithelia: implications in cystic fibrosis. Am J Respir Crit Care Med 2006;174:213–20.
106. Hiltke TJ, Sethi S, Murphy TF. Sequence stability of the gene encoding outer membrane protein P2 of nontypeable *Haemophilus influenzae* in the human respiratory tract. J Infect Dis 2002;185:627–31.
107. Cholon DM, Cutter D, Richardson SK, et al. Serial isolates of persistent *Haemophilus influenzae* in patients with chronic obstructive pulmonary disease express diminishing quantities of the HMW1 and HMW2 adhesins. Infect Immun 2008;76(10):4463–8.

Multidetector Computed Tomographic Imaging in Chronic Obstructive Pulmonary Disease

Emphysema and Airways Assessment

Diana E. Litmanovich, MD[a],*, Kirsten Hartwick[a],
Mario Silva, MD[a,b], Alexander A. Bankier, MD, PhD[a]

KEYWORDS

- COPD - Emphysema - Airway imaging - CT - Phenotyping

KEY POINTS

- Computed tomography (CT) imaging is crucial for both subjective and objective assessment of severity of emphysema and airway disease in chronic obstructive pulmonary disease (COPD).
- Standardization of the CT acquisition and reconstruction parameters is crucial for both subjective and objective assessment of COPD.
- Substantial correlation between imaging findings and clinical severity of emphysema and airway disease has been established.
- Investigation of the role of CT in phenotyping COPD and its contribution to large-scale studies is under way.

INTRODUCTION

Chronic obstructive pulmonary disease (COPD) is defined as incompletely reversible expiratory airflow obstruction, likely caused by exposure to noxious inhaled particles.[1] The airflow limitation that underlies functional obstruction is usually progressive and

This article originally appeared in *Radiologic Clinics*, Volume 52, Issue 1, January 2014.

Disclosures: D.E. Litmanovich discloses being employed by Beth Israel Deaconess Medical Center and Harvard Medical Faculty Physicians and receiving research grants from Society of Thoracic Radiology and Radiological Society of North America. A.A. Bankier discloses being employed by Beth Israel Deaconess Medical Center and Harvard Medical Faculty Physicians. Dr A.A. Bankier is a consultant to Spiration and receives royalties from Amisrsys and Elsevier. K. Hartwick and M. Silva, MD have nothing to disclose.

[a] Department of Radiology, Beth Israel Deaconess Medical Center, 330 Brookline Avenue-Shapiro 4, Boston, MA 02215, USA; [b] Section of Diagnostic Imaging, Department of Surgical Sciences, University of Parma, Parma, Italy

* Corresponding author.

E-mail address: dlitmano@bidmc.harvard.edu

associated with an abnormal inflammatory response of the lung.[2] Clinically, the severity of COPD is graded based on the Global Initiative for Chronic Obstructive Lung Disease (GOLD) classification, which relies on the spirometric parameters forced expiratory volume in 1 second (FEV_1) and the ratio of FEV_1 to forced vital capacity (FEV_1/FVC). Because the GOLD classification was designed as an epidemiologic instrument rather than as a tool for assessing severity in individual patients, it has weaknesses, notably in the evaluation of patients with early disease and in patients with complex or complicated disease.[2] These weaknesses can be explained by the complex nature of COPD itself, which seems to have evaded any sustainable evaluation by 1 classification system alone.

What is clinically called COPD reflects a complex syndrome encompassing potentially overlapping diseases such as pulmonary emphysema, chronic bronchitis, and small airways disease. In addition, there is increasing evidence of nonpulmonary contributors to (or consequences of) COPD, such as cardiac disease, neurologic and cognitive dysfunction, and musculoskeletal disorders. COPD seems to be related by unknown ties to generalized inflammation and metabolic syndrome. Diagnostic imaging is well established in the individual assessment of these disorders. This situation and the wide availability of imaging, combined with the growing expertise that radiologists have acquired with these diseases, have revived interest in the imaging of COPD in general. Thus, the current expectation of imaging is to complement the assessment of COPD using the GOLD classification with a more sophisticated definition of COPD subtypes, according to the prevailing underlying disease or diseases. This process, often referred to as phenotyping, could identify clinically meaningful subcategories of disease for a more tailored approach to both diagnosis and treatment.

In this article, the role of imaging in COPD is discussed as related to the most prevalent subtypes of the disease. Given the importance of computed tomography (CT) in the assessment of the individual diseases contributing to COPD, most of the text is limited to this modality. The role of CT in phenotyping COPD and its contribution to large-scale studies under way that aim to establish potential links between the imaging, clinical, and genetic manifestations of COPD are also discussed. Areas in which imaging could play a vital role in the discussion of COPD are highlighted.

CT Imaging in COPD

CT technique

Because chest radiography has shown little sensitivity in detecting COPD-related changes, and high costs and cumbersome technical procedures can restrict access to magnetic resonance imaging, CT has become the primary imaging modality in patients with suspected COPD, in both clinical and research contexts. The establishment of CT in this role was determined by rigorous validation and confirmation studies, as well as by recent large epidemiologically oriented studies. However, important questions related to the overall impact of CT in the workup of COPD remain to be answered. This section summarizes established knowledge of CT in patients with COPD and concludes with newly emerging areas of research.

Technical CT parameters recommended by the COPD Gene study[3] reflect the necessity to obtain image acquisition with high signal-to-noise ratio to secure both subjective and objective assessment of the images. Thin sections (0.5-mm–1-mm reconstructions) are generally recommended for assessing patients with COPD.[4] Because intravenous iodinated contrast material influences the attenuation values of the organs imaged, non–contrast-enhanced volumetric CT acquisition is a standard technique for COPD imaging. Although a high-resolution reconstruction algorithm is appropriate for visual assessment of the lungs, a high-resolution reconstruction algorithm has been shown to increase the percentage of emphysema measured by the density mask method.[5] Thus, the standard reconstruction algorithm is required for computerized analysis, implying that 2 separate sets of reconstructions are essential for CT assessment.[2] Acquisition at full inspiration is required for quantification of pulmonary emphysema, because submaximal inspiration can cause underestimation of emphysema severity.[6] Hence, appropriate breathing instructions during the scanning are of paramount importance.[7] The solution would be spirometric gating in CT acquisitions for quantitative emphysema assessment.[6]

The CT radiation dose level used for evaluation of COPD is driven by the balance between radiation dose and image noise, although radiation exposure may be of secondary importance in this specific group, given their age profile. Because excessive image noise simulates emphysema, particularly on quantitative evaluation,[8,9] standard kVp and mAs parameters are recommended. A proposed technique is shown in **Table 1**. Dr Madani has also shown that radiation dose does not substantially influence the strength of correlations between histopathologic indexes and relative areas or percentiles. Therefore, reducing the dose might be appropriate for CT quantification of pulmonary emphysema, especially in patients who undergo repeated follow-up examinations. However, because radiation dose does affect relative areas of lung with attenuation coefficients lower than −960 and −970 HU (RA_{960} and RA_{970}) it should be kept constant in comparative and follow-up examinations.[9]

Although iterative reconstruction (IR) techniques have been proved to be a valuable tool in image noise reduction in chest imaging,[1] IR may also substantially alter the quantitative assessment of emphysema and air trapping; therefore, researchers should pay careful attention to the protocols used for CT data acquisition and image reconstruction/analysis.[10] Expiratory/inspiratory ratio of mean lung density (E/I-ratio$_{MLD}$) might be the preferred method for assessment of air trapping, given its insensitivity to differences in the evaluated reconstruction algorithms.[10] If IR is applied in combination with low kVp and mA setup, the effect on parameters such as threshold or percentile cutoff in quantitative emphysema measurements is substantial.[11]

CT acquisition and reconstruction parameters are similar for assessment of emphysema and airways,[2] and recent algorithms were developed to optimize quantitative airway assessment.[12–18] The major challenge for quantitative analysis of the airway tree is the partial volume effect that blurs the inner lumen and bronchial wall into an

Table 1
Proposed technique for emphysema and airway imaging

Tube potential (kVp)	120
Tube current (mAs)	
Inspiratory acquisition	<200
End-expiratory acquisition	<50
Pitch	0.9–1.1
Detector configuration (mm)	16–128 × 0.6–0.75 Depending on the scanner manufacturer
Reconstruction algorithms	High-resolution, standard
Section thickness (mm)	0.625–1.0

Data from Regan EA, Hokanson JE, Murphy JR, et al. Genetic epidemiology of COPD (COPDGene) study design. COPD 2010;7(1):32–43.

indistinguishable mass, with a CT density similar to lung parenchyma, particularly crucial at the level of distal generations. The advent of multidetector row CT (MDCT) scanning allows users to acquire thin-slice contiguous images of the lung using a Z dimension approaching that of the X-Y dimensions, with near isotropic voxel resolution and within a single breath hold.[19,20] A CT scanner with a minimum of 64 detectors is preferable to achieve 0.5-mm slice thickness; although most studies still use CT slices with 1-mm to 1.25-mm slice thickness. If the CT images are acquired using 1 mm or less slice thickness, it is now possible for investigators to segment the airway tree in 3 dimensions, starting in the trachea and projecting out to the fifth or sixth generation (**Fig. 1**).[21,22] CT slices used to create this three-dimensional (3D) reconstruction are contiguous, and thus, it is possible in airway reformation to create a single long tube of the central axis that is segmented in true cross-section. Then, bronchial segments can be labeled by applying advanced knowledge to the branching pattern of the airway tree.[23]

Studies using low-dose algorithms to measure airway dimensions have shown acceptable measurement errors,[6,20] but no studies investigating the consistency of measurements obtained with commonly available algorithms under low-dose conditions have yet been published. Although IR has been shown to cause no effect on the delineation of segmental airway structures,[10] more research on that topic is required. Consistent measurements from available algorithms with low-dose CT are crucial for future longitudinal studies, especially on young individuals. The influence of intravenous contrast material on measurements of airway dimensions should also be investigated to avoid additional acquisitions in certain clinical scenarios.

As with quantification of emphysema, lung volumes are known to affect airway caliber,[24] as well as the attenuation of tissue surrounding the airway,[6] thus potentially affecting the measurements. 3D segmentation of the lung, and subsequent measurements of lung volume from the voxel count, can be used to adjust airway dimensions to lung volume,[25,26] However, as with emphysema assessment, careful breathing instructions are needed and in the future would be used in conjunction with spirometric gating.

CT images should be viewed at window level settings suitable for lung evaluation (typically, a window level of −700 and window width of 1500). A narrower window (1000 or 800) may be useful for detecting or excluding early emphysema. In addition, the assessment of mild emphysema might benefit from minimum intensity projection technique.[27]

Ongoing research is focusing on standardization of the CT acquisition and reconstruction parameters, including low-dose image acquisition, role of spirometric gating, and appropriate use of IRs. Most appropriate uniform methods for quantifying emphysema and airways in clinical practice and research trials should be established, with emphasis on reproducibility in longitudinal trials. The Quantitative Imaging Biomarkers Alliance (QIBA) was organized by the Radiological Society of North America (RSNA) in 2007 to unite researchers, health care professionals, and industry stakeholders in the advancement of quantitative imaging and the use of biomarkers in clinical trials and practice, including standardization of multimodality COPD imaging.

CT in Emphysema

Definitions

Emphysema is defined as a "condition of the lung characterized by abnormal, permanent enlargement of the air spaces distal to the terminal bronchiole, accompanied by destruction of alveolar walls."[28] Because emphysema decreases the elastic recoil force that drives air out of the lung and thereby reduces maximal expiratory airflow,

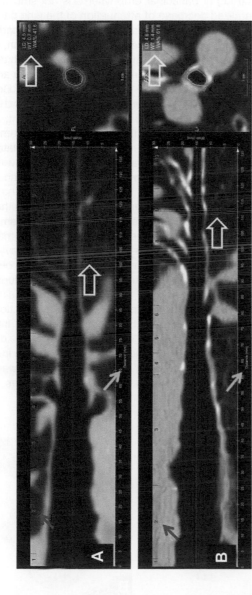

Fig. 1. CT quantification of normal and abnormal airway dimensions. The airway is segmented, reconstructed, and artificially stretched into a straight structure, to facilitate quantification. Red arrow indicates the bronchial generation and the green arrow indicates distance from anatomic landmarks. A vertical marker (*open arrow*) can be placed at any location along the airway image. The computer then shows predetermined dimensional metrics, such as lumen diameter (LD), wall thickness (WT), and wall area percent (WA%) (*right images, open arrows*). Compared with the normal airway (*A*), the airway of a patient with chronic bronchitis (*B*) shows a substantially more irregular wall as well as a substantially increased wall thickness and wall area percent.

the disease is clinically classified as a COPD.[29] Morphologically, 3 main types of emphysema exist.

(1) Centrilobular emphysema (CLE) or the centriacinar form of emphysema results from dilatation or destruction of the respiratory bronchioles and is the type of emphysema most closely associated with cigarette smoking.[28]

(2) Panlobular emphysema (PLE) or panacinar emphysema is not smoking related and it is manifested as a generalized decrease of attenuation of the lung parenchyma without focal lucencies (**Fig. 2**).[30] Interlobular septa are often preserved and splayed, facilitating identification of pulmonary lobular hyperexpansion. In addition, the more central pulmonary vessels are often distorted, splayed, and narrowed with decreased branching (architectural distortion). The terms centrilobular and panlobular are derived from their gross distributions within the secondary pulmonary lobule.[31,32] Because of the central location of the terminal bronchioles, the terms centroacinar and centrilobular, and panacinar and panlobular, respectively, are roughly equivalent, and both terms are used interchangeably.[33] The panlobular (or panacinar) form of emphysema is associated with α_1-antitrypsin deficiency and results in an even dilatation and destruction of the entire acinus.[28] A similar pattern may be seen with severe smoking-related emphysema,[34] and emphysema related to intravenous drug abuse.[35–37]

It has been suggested that when both are present in severe disease, either CLE or PLE predominates, and the CLE subtype is associated with more severe small airway obstruction.[34] There is a relationship between the severity of emphysema and the pack-years of cigarette smoking, but this relation is weak. Only 40% of heavy smokers develop substantial lung destruction resulting from emphysema. On the other hand, emphysema can occasionally be found in individuals with normal lung function and who have never smoked.[38,39]

(3) Paraseptal emphysema (PSE) reflects an emphysematous destruction pattern located in the periphery of the lung adjacent to the pleura or along the interlobular septa (**Fig. 3**). It is thus subpleural in location, and characterized by single or multiple bullae (ie, sharply demarcated, air-containing spaces measuring ≥ 1 cm in diameter and possessing a smooth wall ≤ 1 mm thick). It may occasionally occur as an isolated finding. PSE is one of the many causes for spontaneous pneumothoraces. Although

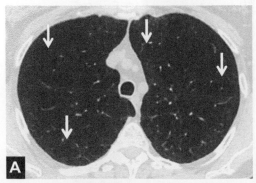 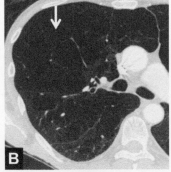

Fig. 2. Transverse CT sections at the level of the upper and mid lung zones in 2 patients with PLE. In both the upper (*A*) and mid (*B*) lung zones, CT shows the extensive destructive nature of PLE (*arrows*), which, unlike CLE, destroys the structure of the secondary pulmonary lobule; Therefore, the destructive pattern of PLE appears more homogeneous on CT than CLE.

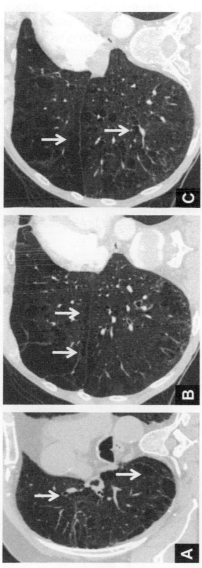

Fig. 3. Transverse CT sections at the level of the mid and lower lung zones in 2 patients with PSE. CT shows the distribution of emphysema along interstitial structures, including the subpleural areas (A), the perifissural areas (B, C), and along the peribronchovascular interstitium (C).

the pathogenesis is unclear, the relationship between PSE and a thin and tall body habitus has led to the suggestion that this subtype of emphysema is caused by the effects of gravitational pull on the lungs, with a greater negative pleural pressure at the lung apices.[33,40,41]

Bullae can be seen in all types of emphysema,[42] but are most commonly associated with PSE.[42] Bullae are seen as avascular low attenuation areas that are larger than 1 cm in diameter, with a thin but perceptible wall, often located in the upper lobes in both CLE and PSE, but are more evenly distributed in the lungs of patients with PLE.[43] Occasionally, large bullae can cause some reduced expansion of adjacent lung parenchyma, resulting in atelectasis. The term giant bullous emphysema refers to the presence of bullae occupying one-third or more of the hemithorax.[37]

CT findings in emphysema On CT, emphysema is characterized by the presence of areas of low attenuation that contrast with the surrounding lung parenchyma with normal attenuation (**Fig. 4**).[31,44] Mild to moderate CLE is characterized by the presence of multiple rounded and small areas of low attenuation with diameters of several millimeters and generally upper lobe predominance. The lesions have no walls, because they are limited by the surrounding lung parenchyma. Sometimes, the lesions may seem to be grouped around the center of secondary pulmonary lobules (see **Fig. 4**A).[45] PLE is characterized by uniform destruction of the secondary pulmonary lobule, leading to widespread and relatively homogeneous patterns of low attenuation.[32,46] PLE can involve the entire lung in a homogeneous manner or it may show lower lobe predominance.

CT and qualitative (subjective) assessment of emphysema The accuracy of MDCT in assessing the presence and extent of emphysema has been documented in numerous studies,[45–49] with excellent in vitro and in vivo correlation between CT emphysema

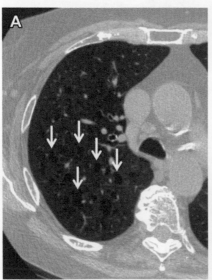 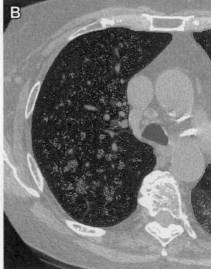

Fig. 4. Transverse CT section (*detail*) and corresponding density map at the level of the right upper lobe in a patient with CLE. CT (*A*) shows the well-defined emphysematous lesions in the lung parenchyma (*arrows*), and the density map (*B*) shows the profusion of disease throughout the anatomic area covered by the CT section (*orange highlights*).

score and the pathologic grade of emphysema, although very mild emphysema could be missed in vivo (**Fig. 5**).[27] Visual qualitative (subjective) assessment of emphysema is usually based on a 0-point to 4-point grading system, on a lobe or lung zone basis.[50] This grading has shown statistically significant correlation between visual scores and panel of standards.[51] Since its introduction, subjective grading of emphysema has been used for assessment of severity of emphysema as well as assessment for potential surgical/endobronchial emphysema treatment.[52] A validation study comparing objective and subjective quantification was performed, in which the objective quantification of horizontal paper-mounted lung sections by a computer-assisted method of densitometric evaluation of mean lung attenuation was used as a standard of reference, and subjective visual assessments were performed by 3 readers.[50] The study found that subjective grading of emphysema was significantly less accurate than objective CT densitometric results when correlated with pathologic scores. There was a systematic overestimation of emphysema by all 3 readers. However, most studies have shown reasonably good correlations between CT emphysema scores and pathologic specimen, good agreement between expert readers for the assessment of presence and extent of emphysema, and good correlations between subjective and objective assessment of emphysema.[53–55]

CT and quantitative (objective) assessment of emphysema The inherent limitations of subjective visual scoring, the characteristic CT morphology of emphysema, and the digital nature of the CT dataset have fostered considerable interest in the use of CT as an objective quantification tool for pulmonary emphysema.[56] Three main approaches have been used to objectively quantify emphysema with CT. First is the

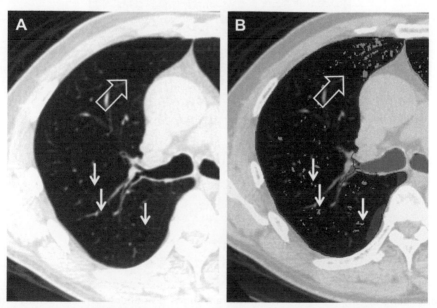

Fig. 5. Transverse CT section (*detail*) and density map at the level of the right upper lobe in a patient with mild CLE. The CT image (*A*) shows subtle dorsal areas of emphysema (*arrows*); however, more ventral emphysema is barely seen (*open arrow*). The density map (*B*) shows emphysematous lesions (*orange highlights*) in both the dorsal (*arrows*) and ventral lung (*open arrow*), complementing the diagnostic information provided by CT.

use of a threshold density value lower than which emphysema is considered to be present (threshold technique). Second is the assessment of a range of densities present in a CT section that is shown as a distribution curve (histogram technique) **(Fig. 6)**. Third is the measurement of the overall CT density of the lung parenchyma.

With the threshold technique, the CT image can be seen as a densitometric map of the lung; thus, it is ideally suited to quantitative assessments of emphysema **(Fig. 7A, B)**.[57] In an attempt to determine the best attenuation threshold for recognition of emphysema, Gevenois and colleagues[48,58] applied to 1-mm-thick CT sections a program that automatically recognizes the lungs, traces the lung contours, determines histograms of attenuation values, and measures the lung area occupied by pixels included in the predetermined range of attenuation value.[59] These investigators showed that the only threshold for which there was no statistically significant difference between the distribution of the CT measurements and the distribution of macroscopic measurements was –950 HU. Thresholds lower than –950 HU underestimated emphysema, and thresholds higher than –950 HU overestimated emphysema.[49]

In order to predict the lung surface/volume ratio from CT attenuation values, Coxson and colleagues[19] considered a threshold of –910 HU and compared CT measurements with histologic estimates of surface area. Lung volume was calculated by summing the voxel dimensions in each slice, and lung weight was estimated by multiplying the mean lung attenuation value by the lung volume. This method appeared more accurate than the histologic surface area occupied by emphysema, because these investigators observed a reduced surface/volume ratio in mild emphysema, whereas

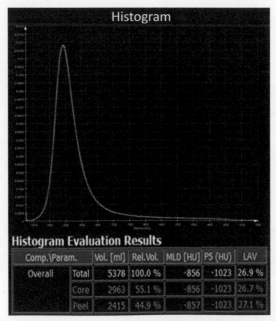

Histogram Evaluation Results

Comp.\Param.		Vol. [ml]	Rel.Vol.	MLD [HU]	P5 (HU)	LAV
Overall	Total	5378	100.0 %	-856	-1023	26.9 %
	Core	2963	55.1 %	-856	-1023	26.7 %
	Peel	2415	44.9 %	-857	-1023	27.1 %

Fig. 6. Lung density histogram. The histogram shows distribution of voxel density with respect to the whole lung volume: x-axis represents density range expressed in HU, whereas y-axis scales the relative amount of voxels as a percentage of total lung volume. Evaluation of the histogram allows quantification of parameters relating to the severity of emphysema such as mean lung density (MLD), lowest fifth percentile value (P5), and relative volume of parenchyma with density lower than –950 HU. LAV, low attenuation volume.

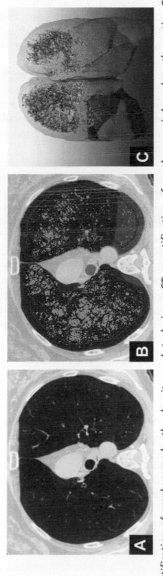

Fig. 7. CT quantification of emphysema by the density mask technique. CT quantification of emphysema is based on the native CT image (A). After computer processing, voxels reflecting emphysema are highlighted (B, *orange highlights*). This image can be superimposed on the source image (B), or shown for the entire lung volume (C).

surface area and tissue weight were decreased only in severe disease. Desai and colleagues[60] recommended using a combined morphologic and functional (composite) score to assess emphysema.

Percentile technique is based on assessment of different densities in the lungs (represented by voxels). Each density is represented by a percentile on a percentage scale. The cumulative percentage of densities lower than a certain threshold (preselected percentile) corresponds to the severity of emphysema and functional impairment. This representation is called a histogram (see **Fig. 6**). The lowest fifth percentile value correlated with the extent of emphysema[57] and surface area/volume ratio.[61] The 15th percentile value serves as a best measurement of lung destruction.[62,63]

In practice, the cutoff values of −950 HU and 15th percentile values are widely used.[64] Although the term % emphysema is commonly used to refer to percentage of lung voxels with CT attenuation lower than a given threshold on inspiratory CT, more precise descriptors such as %LAA−950insp are preferred: percentage of voxels with density of less than −950 HU or RA950 − relative area occupied by attenuation values lower than −950 HU.

Texture-based methods rely on analysis of detailed morphologic patterns on high-resolution CT (eg, shape, skewness, kurtosis gradient, contrast, correlation, circularity, aspect ratio, area, number of clusters).[65,66] Although offering more information, texture-based analysis involves greater computational complexity and higher cost. Based on this methodology, Yilmaz and colleagues have shown that lobar air volume increases substantially in emphysema, sparing only the right middle lobe; whereas lobar tissue volume, which increases slightly at the beginning of the process, decreases in advanced stages. Fractional tissue volume has been shown to decline in severe cases in all lobes in correlation with pulmonary function.

Volumetric measurements of emphysema is based on measurements of abnormally low attenuation lung parenchyma, and can be performed using 3D reconstructions of volumetric CT performed in inspiration (see **Fig. 7**C) and expiration, with good correlation of airflow obstruction and air trapping.[67,68]

Factors influencing CT densitometry Quantitative assessment of emphysema can be influenced by multiple parameters: intrinsic (related to the patient) as well as extrinsic (related to the scanner).

With intrinsic parameters, airspace size correlates with age according to morphometric data.[69,70] Thus, increase of airspace size associated with advanced age could influence the CT density parameters and should be taken into account in longitudinal study designs.[71,72] Madani and colleagues[6] have shown the importance of optimal inspiration on quantification of pulmonary emphysema, because submaximal inspiration causes underestimation of pulmonary emphysema, leading to the necessity for spirometric gating for CT acquisitions focused on quantitative emphysema assessment. Race, gender, and weight also play an important role.[73,74] Independent of the lung volume at which CT is obtained (depth of inspiration), the lung size itself could influence CT parameters.[71,75]

With intrinsic parameters, scanner type, CT acquisition and reconstruction technique (see earlier discussion), number of representative slices assessed,[76] and current smoking status all play an important role in assessment of CT densitometry.[77]

End-inspiratory and end-expiratory CT acquisition in emphysema Comprehensive assessment of emphysema is based on end-inspiration acquisitions. With end-inspiratory acquisition, in addition to the quantitative assessment discussed earlier, dedicated programs can reconstruct a 3D model of the lungs, calculate lung volume, and provide a frequency distribution curve of attenuation values within the target lung volume, which can be applied to spiral CT data.[78,79] Quantification of the lung surface area in emphysema can also be obtained.[19] Other potential measures that can be derived from inspiratory quantitative CT include total inspiratory lung volume, mean lung attenuation, Hounsfield unit values at each percentile cutoff, ratio of emphysema in the upper and lower lungs and lobes.[80,81] In addition to the density histogram, the α value (the negative slope from the log-log relationship of hole size vs frequency of holes, with hole membership defined as contiguous voxels at −950 HU, −910 HU, or −856 HU) can be evaluated (**Fig. 8**).[76,81–83] Comparison between lung volumes measured by end-inspiration volumetric CT and plethysmography showed significant correlations between both measurements and an underestimation of total lung capacity by 12%, measured by CT, likely because of the supine posture of the subject in the CT gantry compared with the seated posture in the plethysmograph.[67]

Clinical importance of CT emphysema assessment and quantification Qualitative and quantitative emphysema assessment methods have helped in the clinical assessment of patients' morbidity status and prognosis. Martinez and colleagues[84] have shown a correlation between the presence of lower lobe emphysema and worse prognosis. Strong correlation between CT measures of emphysema and mortality has been shown in patients with %LAA−950insp greater than 10.[85] Lobar distribution of emphysema has a substantial implication on pulmonary function tests, with lower lobe emphysema correlating strongly with functional impairment.[86,87] In addition, central rather than peripheral emphysema affects more substantially diffusion lung capacity.[81,88] Assessment of patients with COPD with MDCT and micro-CT shows that narrowing and disappearance of small conducting airways before the onset of emphysematous destruction can explain the increased peripheral airway resistance reported in COPD.[89]

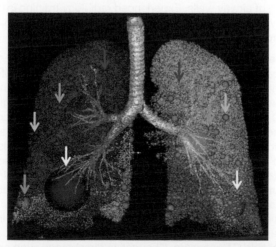

Fig. 8. Cluster analysis of pulmonary emphysema. Dedicated software platform allows quantification of the size of emphysema clusters in the lungs. Larger clusters are reflected by larger circles (*white, green, and orange arrows*) and smaller clusters are reflected by smaller circles (*red and blue arrows*).

Airway Imaging in COPD

Definition and pathologic changes

A normal airway has a treelike structure with almost cylindrical branches of decreasing radius. Small airways, defined as having an internal diameter of less than 2 mm,[90–92] reflect the fourth to the 14th generations of branching.[93] Exposure to tobacco smoke and toxic particles leads to rapid immune response of the small airways, including mucociliary clearance, which removes the particles deposited on the airway walls.[94] This response triggers cough and sputum production, on which the definition of chronic bronchitis is based.[38,95] Abnormal response can consist of increased production of mucus, defective mucociliary clearance, disruption of the epithelial barrier, and infiltration of the airway walls by inflammatory immune cells forming lymphoid follicles.[96,97] Accumulation of inflammatory mucous exudates within the airway lumen and thickening of the airway wall in part caused by airway smooth muscle hypertrophy and contraction result in airway obstruction and airflow limitation.[2]

Compared with control samples, CT samples from patients with COPD showed that the number of airways measuring 2.0 to 2.5 mm in diameter was reduced in patients with all GOLD stages.[89] Comparison of the number of terminal bronchioles and dimensions at different levels of emphysematous destruction (ie, an increasing value for the mean linear intercept) showed that the narrowing and loss of terminal bronchioles preceded emphysematous destruction in COPD.[89] More pronounced thickening of the large airways in patients with signs and symptoms of chronic bronchitis and the presence of a significant familial concordance of airway wall thickening with COPD encourage further research of airway wall parameters (see **Fig. 1**).[98,99]

Qualitative (subjective) assessment of airways Bronchial wall thickening has been considered the main clinically relevant parameter for subjective assessment of the airways, relying on the judgment of the individual reader. There are limited data in qualitative assessment of airways, mainly because of lack of reproducibility and standardization. Bankier and colleagues[100] have shown the importance of specific window setting for bronchial wall thickness assessment, when deviation from predetermined window setup, notably window width greater than 1000 HU, can result in substantial artificial thickening of airway walls. Experienced radiology training is of limited value in improving sensitivity and specificity in the subjective differentiation between normal and pathologic bronchi.[101]

Quantitative (objective) assessment of airways With the development of highly accurate MDCT and quantification methods, an objective assessment of airway obstruction in patients with COPD has predominated in recent literature. There are a variety of methods to assess the distal airways in order to quantify physiologic changes associated with COPD, but there is no universal parameter that can describe morphologic changes and clinical symptoms. Furthermore, there is the classic paradigm between minimizing radiation dose and maintaining an adequate signal-to-noise ratio. The next sections describe currently available methods of airway quantification.

Small airways (<2 mm in diameter) are the known site of major airflow limitation in COPD,[38,39,102] but cannot be reliably measured with currently available CT scanners. CT measurements are consistently accurate and reproducible, showing good correlation with pathologic examination[103] in airways 2 mm or more in internal diameter.[103–110] For larger airways (≥fifth generation), wall thickness can be measured with currently available CT scanners. Changes in dimensions such as luminal narrowing and wall thickening can be assessed, providing noninvasive quantification of potentially reversible changes and regional assessment throughout the lungs, which require only 1 inspiratory CT acquisition, with the obtained measurements strongly correlating with airflow obstruction.[2] A study by Hasegawa and colleagues[23] showed that airway wall dimensions in the smallest airways measurable had the strongest correlation with FEV_1 compared with larger segmental (third-generation) airways. Large airway thickening or narrowing has been shown as a potential method for estimating the degree of small airway disease[103] through quantitative assessment of the bronchial diameter, luminal diameter (**Fig. 9**A), airway lumen area, area of the bronchial wall as a percentage of the total bronchial cross-sectional area: wall area percentage (WA%) (see **Fig. 9**B) and mean (standard deviation) standardized airway wall thickness (AWT) at an internal perimeter of 10 mm (AWT–Pi10).[111]

Measuring the airway lumen originally was based on attenuation values. These algorithms include quantification of (1) attenuation values based on a predetermined threshold such as –500HU or more specifically –577HU,[107,112] (2) the perimeter of the lumen through a combination of manual tracing and computer-generated attenuation,[113] and (3) voxels regardless of airway orientation.[114] Such methods are limited, because they describe neither the differences in wall thickness nor the relationship between wall thickness and lumen size.

Measuring the airway lumen and wall dimensions simultaneously answers the critical need for visualization of both the airway lumen and the wall dimensions in order to better understand the clinical implications. One of the earliest methods for quantification is the fill width at half maximum (FWHM).[110,115] This technique is based on the assumption that the image gray level at the true airway wall is halfway between the minimum and maximum gray levels. Although this method results in CT measurements that are standardized and unbiased, it is prone to overestimating wall dimensions and underestimating lumen dimensions, especially in small airways.[115] Because of this known flaw, other algorithms have been created to modify FWHM to provide better analysis of airways by adjusting for airway angle,[116] creating 3D airway trees,[104,117,118] measuring phase congruency,[13] placing a seed point in the center of the lumen,[107] and using second-derivative filters.[105] More recent algorithms abandon FWHM altogether, and instead reformat segments of the airway trees orthogonally using mathematical

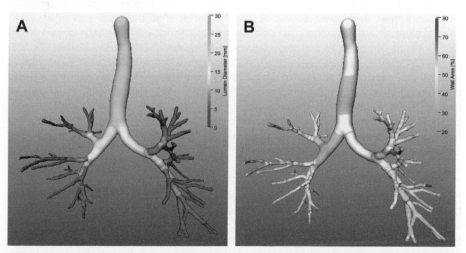

Fig. 9. CT quantification of airway dimensions. CT map of segmented and reconstructed airway tree shows airway dimensions such as lumen diameter (*A*) and wall area percent (*B*). The airway tree is color-coded according to dimensional thresholds, as indicated on the scale (*upper right*).

algorithms and compare a variety of different factors such as attenuation value, distance from other pixels, and parameters of neighboring pixels.[12,14–18]

Small airway obstruction is measured through assessment of air trapping: retention of air in the lung distal to an obstruction that can be seen on expiratory CT scans, as lung areas with a less-than-normal increase in attenuation, usually less than –856 HU.[2] Pulmonary densitometry parameters are calculated by dedicated software, similar to that used in quantification of emphysema by expiratory CT scans or paired inspiratory and expiratory CT scans, allowing the indirect evaluation of airway obstruction in patients with COPD. This method is used as an alternative, or in some studies, supplemental method for assessment of morphologic changes in lung structure.[2] Change in relative lung volume with attenuation values from –860 HU to –950 HU (RVC$_{-860\ to\ -950}$) between paired inspiratory and expiratory examinations,[119] and expiratory/inspiratory ratio of mean lung density (E/I-ratio$_{MLD}$)[10,120] can be assessed.

To minimize the confounding influence of emphysema in the quantification of air trapping, a range of low attenuation values has been proposed.[26] In patients with minimal to mild and moderate to severe emphysema, strongest correlations with the obstructive deficit were found with changes in attenuation values between –860 HU and –950 HU in portions of lung with little emphysema, suggesting limited influence of emphysema on the indirect assessment of airways changes.[26] These findings suggest that the exclusion of voxels with attenuation of –950 HU or less from both inspiratory and expiratory CT data sets is desirable for quantifying air trapping.[119] Such indirect quantification allows assessment without considering airway generations, better correlation with airflow limitation compared with those obtained by measuring bronchial dimensions, and the possibility for regional assessment of the disease.[23,26] The major drawbacks of this technique are inability to compare the results with pathologic assessment, obligatory 2 CT acquisitions, and overlap between air trapping caused by small airway disease and that caused by emphysema.

Measurements of airway wall changes focus on both changes in the wall thickness and wall composition (resulting in wall density changes). When a small object such as the airway is scanned, mean attenuation value underestimates the density.[121,122] The peak attenuation value, on the other hand, is a function of size, density, and reconstruction kernel. Thus, with a fixed reconstruction kernel, the peak wall attenuation value reflects wall changes in both thickness and composition observed in COPD.[123,124] Although this method allows regional assessment and correlates with airflow limitations, it indirectly reflects only changes within the wall, with no validation against independent references.[2] Automatic rays spread from the manually placed centroid point can be further assessed with the FWHM technique, providing attenuation profiles along each ray.[115] Mean lumen area, mean wall area, WA%, and the mean peak wall attenuation value can then be calculated.[123] Correlation with pulmonary function test results suggests that peak wall attenuation was comparable with WA % for predicting obstructive deficit.[123]

Trachea and COPD

Recently, the potential association between COPD and tracheobronchomalacia has been investigated (**Fig. 10**).[125,126] Excessive expiratory tracheal collapse was observed in a subset of patients with COPD, but the magnitude of collapse was independent of disease severity and did not correlate significantly with physiologic parameters. Thus, the incidental identification of excessive expiratory tracheal collapse in a general COPD population may not necessarily be clinically significant.[126] In patients with COPD, the tracheal morphologic change showed clinically significant correlation with severity of emphysema.[127] Expiratory collapse was significantly associated with

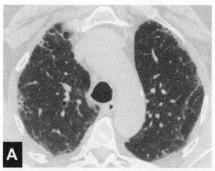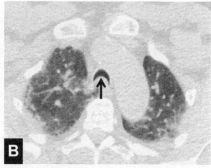

Fig. 10. Transverse CT sections at breath-hold inspiration and dynamic expiration in a patient with tracheobronchomalacia. Inspiratory CT scan (*A*) shows a normal oval shape of the tracheal lumen. Dynamic expiratory CT scan (*B*) shows excessive expiratory collapse (>70% of inspiratory lumen area) (*arrow*), consistent with tracheomalacia. Collapse of posterior membranous wall is also known as the frown sign on CT imaging. Patchy areas of peripheral ground-glass attenuation and septal thickening are seen in apical regions of inspiratory scan (*A*). These limited alterations can be referred to mild fibrosis from nonspecific interstitial pneumonia.

body mass index (BMI, calculated as weight in kilograms divided by the square of height in meters) among morbidly obese patients with BMI of 35 km/m² or greater, thus suggesting evaluating for excessive expiratory tracheal collapse if confronted with a morbidly obese patient with COPD with greater quality-of-life impairment and worse exercise performance than expected based on functional measures.[125]

Imaging in classification of COPD

MDCT plays an important role in phenotype classification of COPD based on the presence or absence of apparent emphysema and bronchial wall thickening.[119] Fujimoto and colleagues[128,129] have shown the complex relationship between morphologic phenotypes and airflow limitation: airflow limitation in COPD results from a combination of small airway remodeling and a loss of lung elastic recoil; and the relative contributions of these pathologic abnormalities may vary among patients with the same degree of airflow limitation.[130–132] Three COPD phenotypes were identified based on morphologic CT changes and clinical features of COPD: phenotype A, characterized by no or minimal emphysema with or without bronchial wall thickening; phenotype E, characterized by emphysema without bronchial wall thickening; and phenotype M, characterized by emphysema with bronchial wall thickening.[128] Phenotype M disease showed the best response to bronchodilators expressed as an increase in the percentage of predicted FEV_1 when compared with phenotype E, most likely because of intrinsic airway remodeling and not decreased elastic recoil as in phenotype E. This study along with many additional investigations has shown that COPD should be classified based on the extent of emphysema in combination with others parameters, including airway dimensions.[2,62,89,133] Also, the extent of small airway remodeling was greater in patients with CLE than in those with PLE, and no association was found between small airway wall thickening and the severity of emphysema in patients with PLE.[130] The cumulative knowledge of COPD phenotyping shows that identifying the main cause(s) of airflow limitation in patients with COPD is crucial for determining the appropriate therapeutic strategy.[119,134]

COPD and systemic inflammation

Recent findings have credited the heterogeneity of COPD to systemic inflammation. Although pathophysiologic explanations are still developing, it is evident that the link between systemic inflammation and COPD will become clearer only as investigations continue. Numerous studies have showing correlations between COPD and pulmonary hypertension, coronary calcifications, osteoporosis, and perhaps most telling of all, the onset of systemic inflammation.[135–138] Various comorbidities associated with COPD such as increases in atherosclerosis, inflammatory markers, endothelial permeability, thromboembolism, and myocardial infarction may now be considered multimorbidities of COPD instigated by common risk factors (eg, smoking, alcohol, poor diet) rather than 1 chronic disease (eg, COPD) causing another (eg, osteoporosis).[139] As part of the COPD Gene study, Wells and colleagues[140] assessed the association between the lumen size of the main pulmonary artery (PA) at the level of its bifurcation to ascending aorta (AA) at the same level (PA/AA ratio) in patients with COPD and concluded that a PA/AA ratio of more than 1 correlates with acute exacerbations within 3 years in patients with COPD. Matsuoka and colleagues[136] investigated the relation between aortic calcifications as measured from CT and pulmonary vascular alteration. These investigators concluded that based on this and previous studies these calcifications were most likely caused by endothelial dysfunction and systemic inflammation.[141–143] In addition, there is continuing evaluation of the effective use of nongated CT to determine pulmonary calcinosis.[144] As part of the longitudinal Evaluation of COPD Longitudinally to Identify Predictive Surrogate Endpoints (ECLIPSE) study, Romme and colleagues[138] determined that lower bone attenuation was associated with higher exacerbations and hospitalization, but had little connection with mortality in patients with COPD.

SUMMARY

COPD refers to incompletely reversible expiratory airflow obstruction, likely caused by exposure to noxious inhaled particles, leading to airway remodeling and emphysema. This disorder is heterogeneous, reflecting a complex syndrome of overlapping diseases such as pulmonary emphysema, chronic bronchitis, and small airways disease, as well as systemic inflammation. Advances in MDCT and postprocessing technology allow for noninvasive qualitative and quantitative assessment of relative contribution and severity of each of those pathologic changes, with accuracy similar to histopathologic assessment. Together with quantification of emphysema, quantification of airway disease at CT can allow clinically meaningful phenotyping of COPD. Because both qualitative and even more, quantitative, assessment of COPD can be affected by variations in image acquisition parameters, adherence to a standard CT protocol is necessary for precise evaluation of the image data. Future research in COPD should focus on standardizing to MDCT acquisition and postprocessing parameters as well as defining the most appropriate method for quantifying airway disease and emphysema in clinical practice.

    As evident in this review and several others, both subjective quantification imaging and phenotyping of COPD have increased in popularity and accuracy. However, it is imperative for researchers and clinicians to realize that even with the creation of a magic bullet diagnostic tool, the implementation of such a tool to treat the 24 million Americans afflicted with COPD would result in cost and collaboration challenges. Therefore, longitudinal studies should be undertaken to determine the contributions of CT quantification of airway disease and emphysema for predicting outcomes in patients with COPD to determine their cost-effectiveness.

ACKNOWLEDGMENTS

We would like to acknowledge Donna Wolfe, MFA and Meredith Cunningham for their outstanding editorial assistance.

REFERENCES

1. Rabe KF, Hurd S, Anzueto A, et al. Global strategy for the diagnosis, management, and prevention of chronic obstructive pulmonary disease: GOLD executive summary. Am J Respir Crit Care Med 2007;176:532–55.
2. Hackx M, Bankier AA, Gevenois PA. Chronic obstructive pulmonary disease: CT quantification of airways disease. Radiology 2012;265:34–48.
3. Regan EA, Hokanson JE, Murphy JR, et al. Genetic epidemiology of COPD (COPDGene) study design. COPD 2010;7:32–43.
4. Mayo JR. CT evaluation of diffuse infiltrative lung disease: dose considerations and optimal technique. J Thorac Imaging 2009;24:252–9.
5. Boedeker KL, McNitt-Gray MF, Rogers SR, et al. Emphysema: effect of reconstruction algorithm on CT imaging measures. Radiology 2004;232:295–301.
6. Madani A, Van Muylem A, Gevenois PA. Pulmonary emphysema: effect of lung volume on objective quantification at thin-section CT. Radiology 2010;257: 260–8.
7. Bankier AA, O'Donnell CR, Boiselle PM. Quality initiatives. Respiratory instructions for CT examinations of the lungs: a hands-on guide. Radiographics 2008;28:919–31.
8. Zaporozhan J, Ley S, Weinheimer O, et al. Multi-detector CT of the chest: influence of dose onto quantitative evaluation of severe emphysema: a simulation study. J Comput Assist Tomogr 2006;30:460–8.
9. Madani A, De Maertelaer V, Zanen J, et al. Pulmonary emphysema: radiation dose and section thickness at multidetector CT quantification–comparison with macroscopic and microscopic morphometry. Radiology 2007;243:250–7.
10. Mets OM, Willemink MJ, de Kort FP, et al. The effect of iterative reconstruction on computed tomography assessment of emphysema, air trapping and airway dimensions. Eur Radiol 2012;22:2103–9.
11. Krowchuk N, Hague C, Leipsic J, et al. The effects of iterative reconstruction algorithms on the measurement of emphysema using low radiation dose computed tomography scans [abstract]. Am J Respir Crit Care Med 2011; 183:A5205.
12. Brillet PY, Fetita CI, Beigelman-Aubry C, et al. Quantification of bronchial dimensions at MDCT using dedicated software. Eur Radiol 2007;17:1483–9.
13. Estepar RS, Washko GG, Silverman EK, et al. Accurate airway wall estimation using phase congruency. Med Image Comput Comput Assist Interv 2006;9: 125–34.
14. Kiraly AP, Odry BL, Naidich DP, et al. Boundary-specific cost functions for quantitative airway analysis. Med Image Comput Comput Assist Interv 2007;10: 784–91.
15. Odry B, Kiraly A, Novak C, et al. Automated airway evaluation system for multi-slice computed tomography using airway lumen diameter, airway wall thickness, and broncho-arterial ratio. SPIE Proceedings 2006;6143. http://dx.doi.org/10.1117/12.653796.
16. Saraglia A, Fetita C, Preteux F, et al. Accurate 3D quantification of the bronchial parameters in MDCT. SPIE Proceedings 2005;5916. http://dx.doi.org/10.1117/12.617669.

17. Sonka M, Reddy GK, Winniford MD, et al. Adaptive approach to accurate analysis of small-diameter vessels in cineangiograms. IEEE Trans Med Imaging 1997;16:87–95.
18. Tschirren J, Hoffman EA, McLennan G, et al. Segmentation and quantitative analysis of intrathoracic airway trees from computed tomography images. Proc Am Thorac Soc 2005;2:484–7, 503–4.
19. Coxson HO, Whittall RM, D'yachkova KP, et al. A quantification of the lung surface area in emphysema using computed tomography. Am J Respir Crit Care Med 1999;159:851–6.
20. Tschirren J, Hoffman EA, McLennan G, et al. Intrathoracic airway trees: segmentation and airway morphology analysis from low-dose CT scans. IEEE Trans Med Imaging 2005;24:1529–39.
21. Coxson HO. Quantitative computed tomography assessment of airway wall dimensions: current status and potential applications for phenotyping chronic obstructive pulmonary disease. Proc Am Thorac Soc 2008;5:940–5.
22. Coxson HO. Quantitative chest tomography in COPD research: chairman's summary. Proc Am Thorac Soc 2008;5:874–7.
23. Hasegawa M, Nasuhara Y, Onodera Y, et al. Airflow limitation and airway dimensions in chronic obstructive pulmonary disease. Am J Respir Crit Care Med 2006;173:1309–15.
24. Brown RH, Scichilone N, Mudge B, et al. High-resolution computed tomographic evaluation of airway distensibility and the effects of lung inflation on airway caliber in healthy subjects and individuals with asthma. Am J Respir Crit Care Med 2001;163:994–1001.
25. Akira M, Toyokawa K, Inoue Y, et al. Quantitative CT in chronic obstructive pulmonary disease: inspiratory and expiratory assessment. AJR Am J Roentgenol 2009;192:267–72.
26. Matsuoka S, Kurihara Y, Yagihashi K, et al. Quantitative assessment of air trapping in chronic obstructive pulmonary disease using inspiratory and expiratory volumetric MDCT. AJR Am J Roentgenol 2008;190:762–9.
27. Remy-Jardin MR. Sliding thin slab, minimum intensity projection technique in the diagnosis of emphysema: histopathologic-CT correlation. Radiology 1996;200:665–71.
28. Snider GL, Kleinerman JL, Thurlbeck WM, et al. The definition of emphysema: report of a National Heart, Lung, and Blood Institute, Division of Lung Disease Workshop. Am Rev Respir Dis 1985;132:182–3.
29. MacNee W. Pathogenesis of chronic obstructive pulmonary disease. Proc Am Thorac Soc 2005;2:258–66 [discussion: 290–1].
30. Spouge D, Mayo JR, Cardoso W, et al. Panacinar emphysema: CT and pathologic findings. J Comput Assist Tomogr 1993;17:710–3.
31. Webb WR. Thin-section CT of the secondary pulmonary lobule: anatomy and the image–the 2004 Fleischner lecture. Radiology 2006;239:322–38.
32. Webb WR, Stein MG, Finkbeiner WE, et al. Normal and diseased isolated lungs: high-resolution CT. Radiology 1988;166:81–7.
33. Wright JL, Churg A. Advances in the pathology of COPD. Histopathology 2006;49:1–9.
34. Kim WD, Eidelman DH, Izquierdo JL, et al. Centrilobular and panlobular emphysema in smokers. Two distinct morphologic and functional entities. Am Rev Respir Dis 1991;144:1385–90.
35. Stern EJ, Frank MS. CT of the lung in patients with pulmonary emphysema: diagnosis, quantification, and correlation with pathologic and physiologic findings. AJR Am J Roentgenol 1994;162:791–8.

36. Stern EJ, Song JK, Frank MS. CT of the lungs in patients with pulmonary emphysema. Semin Ultrasound CT MR 1995;16:345–52.
37. Stern EJ, Webb WR, Weinacker A, et al. Idiopathic giant bullous emphysema (vanishing lung syndrome): imaging findings in nine patients. AJR Am J Roentgenol 1994;162:279–82.
38. Hogg JC. Pathophysiology of airflow limitation in chronic obstructive pulmonary disease. Lancet 2004;364:709–21.
39. Hogg JC, Chu F, Utokaparch S, et al. The nature of small-airway obstruction in chronic obstructive pulmonary disease. N Engl J Med 2004;350:2645–53.
40. Churg A, Wright JL. Proteases and emphysema. Curr Opin Pulm Med 2005;11: 153–9.
41. Wright JL, Churg A. Animal models of cigarette smoke-induced COPD. Chest 2002;122:301S–6S.
42. Hansell DM, Bankier AA, MacMahon H, et al. Fleischner Society: glossary of terms for thoracic imaging. Radiology 2008;246:697–722.
43. Guest PJ, Hansell DM. High resolution computed tomography (HRCT) in emphysema associated with alpha-1-antitrypsin deficiency. Clin Radiol 1992; 45:260–6.
44. Hruban RH, Meziane MA, Zerhouni EA, et al. High resolution computed tomography of inflation-fixed lungs. Pathologic-radiologic correlation of centrilobular emphysema. Am Rev Respir Dis 1987;136:935–40.
45. Murata K, Khan A, Herman PG. Pulmonary parenchymal disease: evaluation with high-resolution CT. Radiology 1989;170:629–35.
46. Murata K, Itoh H, Todo G, et al. Centrilobular lesions of the lung: demonstration by high-resolution CT and pathologic correlation. Radiology 1986;161:641–5.
47. Kuwano K, Matsuba K, Ikeda T, et al. The diagnosis of mild emphysema. Correlation of computed tomography and pathology scores. Am Rev Respir Dis 1990; 141:169–78.
48. Gevenois PA, De Vuyst P, de Maertelaer V, et al. Comparison of computed density and microscopic morphometry in pulmonary emphysema. Am J Respir Crit Care Med 1996;154:187–92.
49. Gevenois PA, de Maertelaer V, De Vuyst P, et al. Comparison of computed density and macroscopic morphometry in pulmonary emphysema. Am J Respir Crit Care Med 1995;152:653–7.
50. Bankier AA, De Maertelaer V, Keyzer C, et al. Pulmonary emphysema: subjective visual grading versus objective quantification with macroscopic morphometry and thin-section CT densitometry. Radiology 1999;211:851–8.
51. Thurlbeck WM, Dunnill MS, Hartung W, et al. A comparison of three methods of measuring emphysema. Hum Pathol 1970;1:215–26.
52. Akuthota P, Litmanovich D, Zutler M, et al. An evidence-based estimate on the size of the potential patient pool for lung volume reduction surgery. Ann Thorac Surg 2012;94:205–11.
53. Müller NL, Coxson H. Chronic obstructive pulmonary disease. 4: imaging the lungs in patients with chronic obstructive pulmonary disease. Thorax 2002;57: 982–5.
54. Müller NL, Staples CA, Miller RR, et al. "Density mask". An objective method to quantitate emphysema using computed tomography. Chest 1988;94:782–7.
55. Gelb AF, Zamel N, Hogg JC, et al. Pseudophysiologic emphysema resulting from severe small-airways disease. Am J Respir Crit Care Med 1998;158:815–9.
56. Gevenois PA, Yernault JC. Can computed tomography quantify pulmonary emphysema? Eur Respir J 1995;8:843–8.

57. Hayhurst MD, MacNee W, Flenley DC, et al. Diagnosis of pulmonary emphysema by computerised tomography. Lancet 1984;2:320–2.
58. Gevenois PA, De Vuyst P, Sy M, et al. Pulmonary emphysema: quantitative CT during expiration. Radiology 1996;199:825–9.
59. Madani A, Zanen J, de Maertelaer V, et al. Pulmonary emphysema: objective quantification at multi-detector row CT–comparison with macroscopic and microscopic morphometry. Radiology 2006;238:1036–43.
60. Desai SR, Hansell DM, Walker A, et al. Quantification of emphysema: a composite physiologic index derived from CT estimation of disease extent. Eur Radiol 2007;17:911–8.
61. Gould GA, MacNee W, McLean A, et al. CT measurements of lung density in life can quantitate distal airspace enlargement–an essential defining feature of human emphysema. Am Rev Respir Dis 1988;137:380–92.
62. Washko GR, Parraga G, Coxson HO. Quantitative pulmonary imaging using computed tomography and magnetic resonance imaging. Respirology 2012; 17:432–44.
63. Dirksen A, Piitulainen E, Parr DG, et al. Exploring the role of CT densitometry: a randomised study of augmentation therapy in alpha1-antitrypsin deficiency. Eur Respir J 2009;33:1345–53.
64. Schroeder JD, McKenzie AS, Zach JA, et al. Relationships between airflow obstruction and quantitative CT measurements of emphysema, air trapping and airways in subjects with and without COPD. AJR Am J Roentgenol 2013; 201(3):W460–70.
65. Bakker ME, Putter H, Stolk J, et al. Assessment of regional progression of pulmonary emphysema with CT densitometry. Chest 2008;134:931–7.
66. Yilmaz C, Dane DM, Patel NC, et al. Quantifying heterogeneity in emphysema from high-resolution computed tomography: a lung tissue research consortium study. Acad Radiol 2013;20:181–93.
67. Kauczor HU, Heussel CP, Fischer B, et al. Assessment of lung volumes using helical CT at inspiration and expiration: comparison with pulmonary function tests. AJR Am J Roentgenol 1998;171:1091–5.
68. Mergo PJ, Williams WF, Gonzalez-Rothi R, et al. Three-dimensional volumetric assessment of abnormally low attenuation of the lung from routine helical CT: inspiratory and expiratory quantification. AJR Am J Roentgenol 1998;170: 1355–60.
69. Gillooly M, Lamb D. Airspace size in lungs of lifelong non-smokers: effect of age and sex. Thorax 1993;48:39–43.
70. Thurlbeck WM. Internal surface area and other measurements in emphysema. Thorax 1967;22:483–96.
71. Gevenois PA, Scillia P, de Maertelaer V, et al. The effects of age, sex, lung size, and hyperinflation on CT lung densitometry. AJR Am J Roentgenol 1996;167: 1169–73.
72. Soejima K, Yamaguchi K, Kohda E, et al. Longitudinal follow-up study of smoking-induced lung density changes by high-resolution computed tomography. Am J Respir Crit Care Med 2000;161:1264–73.
73. Foreman MG, Zhang L, Murphy J, et al. Early-onset chronic obstructive pulmonary disease is associated with female sex, maternal factors, and African American race in the COPDGene Study. Am J Respir Crit Care Med 2011;184: 414–20.
74. Hansel NN, Washko GR, Foreman MG, et al. Racial differences in CT phenotypes in COPD. COPD 2013;10:20–7.

75. Dunnill MS. The problem of lung growth. Thorax 1982;37:561–3.
76. Mishima M, Itoh H, Sakai H, et al. Optimized scanning conditions of high resolution CT in the follow-up of pulmonary emphysema. J Comput Assist Tomogr 1999;23:380–4.
77. Litmanovich D, Boiselle PM, Bankier AA. CT of pulmonary emphysema–current status, challenges, and future directions. Eur Radiol 2009;19:537–51.
78. Arakawa A, Yamashita Y, Nakayama Y, et al. Assessment of lung volumes in pulmonary emphysema using multidetector helical CT: comparison with pulmonary function tests. Comput Med Imaging Graph 2001;25:399–404.
79. Park KJ, Bergin CJ, Clausen JL. Quantitation of emphysema with three-dimensional CT densitometry: comparison with two-dimensional analysis, visual emphysema scores, and pulmonary function test results. Radiology 1999;211:541–7.
80. Nakano Y, Coxson HO, Bosan S, et al. Core to rind distribution of severe emphysema predicts outcome of lung volume reduction surgery. Am J Respir Crit Care Med 2001;164:2195–9.
81. Nakano Y, Sakai H, Muro S, et al. Comparison of low attenuation areas on computed tomographic scans between inner and outer segments of the lung in patients with chronic obstructive pulmonary disease: incidence and contribution to lung function. Thorax 1999;54:384–9.
82. Mishima M, Hirai T, Itoh H, et al. Complexity of terminal airspace geometry assessed by lung computed tomography in normal subjects and patients with chronic obstructive pulmonary disease. Proc Natl Acad Sci U S A 1999;96:8829–34.
83. Yamashiro T, Matsuoka S, Bartholmai BJ, et al. Collapsibility of lung volume by paired inspiratory and expiratory CT scans: correlations with lung function and mean lung density. Acad Radiol 2010;17:489–95.
84. Martinez FJ, Foster G, Curtis JL, et al. Predictors of mortality in patients with emphysema and severe airflow obstruction. Am J Respir Crit Care Med 2006;173:1326–34.
85. Johannessen A, Skorge TD, Bottai M, et al. Mortality by level of emphysema and airway wall thickness. Am J Respir Crit Care Med 2013;187:602–8.
86. Gurney JW, Jones KK, Robbins RA, et al. Regional distribution of emphysema: correlation of high-resolution CT with pulmonary function tests in unselected smokers. Radiology 1992;183:457–63.
87. Saitoh T, Koba H, Shijubo N, et al. Lobar distribution of emphysema in computed tomographic densitometric analysis. Invest Radiol 2000;35:235–43.
88. Aziz ZA, Wells AU, Desai SR, et al. Functional impairment in emphysema: contribution of airway abnormalities and distribution of parenchymal disease. AJR Am J Roentgenol 2005;185:1509–15.
89. McDonough JE, Yuan R, Suzuki M, et al. Small-airway obstruction and emphysema in chronic obstructive pulmonary disease. N Engl J Med 2011;365:1567–75.
90. Hogg JC, Macklem PT, Thurlbeck WM. Site and nature of airway obstruction in chronic obstructive lung disease. N Engl J Med 1968;278:1355–60.
91. Van Brabandt H, Cauberghs M, Verbeken E, et al. Partitioning of pulmonary impedance in excised human and canine lungs. J Appl Physiol 1983;55:1733–42.
92. Yanai M, Sekizawa K, Ohrui T, et al. Site of airway obstruction in pulmonary disease: direct measurement of intrabronchial pressure. J Appl Physiol 1992;72:1016–23.

93. Weibel E. The morphometry of human lung. New York: Academic Press; 1963. p. 110–35.
94. Knowles MR, Boucher RC. Mucus clearance as a primary innate defense mechanism for mammalian airways. J Clin Invest 2002;109:571–7.
95. Abbas AK, Lichtman AH, Pober JS. Cellular and molecular immunology. 4th edition. Philadelphia: W.B. Saunders Company; 2000.
96. Jones JG, Minty BD, Lawler P, et al. Increased alveolar epithelial permeability in cigarette smokers. Lancet 1980;1:66–8.
97. Simani AS, Inoue S, Hogg JC. Penetration of the respiratory epithelium of guinea pigs following exposure to cigarette smoke. Lab Invest 1974;31:75–81.
98. Orlandi I, Moroni C, Camiciottoli G, et al. Chronic obstructive pulmonary disease: thin-section CT measurement of airway wall thickness and lung attenuation. Radiology 2005;234:604–10.
99. Patel BD, Coxson HO, Pillai SG, et al. Airway wall thickening and emphysema show independent familial aggregation in chronic obstructive pulmonary disease. Am J Respir Crit Care Med 2008;178:500–5.
100. Bankier AA, Fleischmann D, Mallek R, et al. Bronchial wall thickness: appropriate window settings for thin-section CT and radiologic-anatomic correlation. Radiology 1996;199:831–6.
101. Bankier AA, Fleischmann D, De Maertelaer V, et al. Subjective differentiation of normal and pathological bronchi on thin-section CT: impact of observer training. Eur Respir J 1999;13:781–6.
102. Hogg JC, McDonough JE, Suzuki M. Small airway obstruction in COPD: new insights based on micro-CT imaging and MRI imaging. Chest 2013;143: 1436–43.
103. Nakano Y, Wong JC, de Jong PA, et al. The prediction of small airway dimensions using computed tomography. Am J Respir Crit Care Med 2005;171:142–6.
104. Achenbach T, Weinheimer O, Brochhausen C, et al. Accuracy of automatic airway morphometry in computed tomography–correlation of radiological-pathological findings. Eur J Radiol 2012;81:183–8.
105. Berger P, Perot V, Desbarats P, et al. Airway wall thickness in cigarette smokers: quantitative thin-section CT assessment. Radiology 2005;235:1055–64.
106. King GG, Muller NL, Pare PD. Evaluation of airways in obstructive pulmonary disease using high-resolution computed tomography. Am J Respir Crit Care Med 1999;159:992–1004.
107. King GG, Muller NL, Whittall KP, et al. An analysis algorithm for measuring airway lumen and wall areas from high-resolution computed tomographic data. Am J Respir Crit Care Med 2000;161:574–80.
108. McNamara AE, Müller NL, Okazawa M, et al. Airway narrowing in excised canine lungs measured by high-resolution computed tomography. J Appl Physiol 1992;73:307–16.
109. Montaudon M, Berger P, de Dietrich G, et al. Assessment of airways with three-dimensional quantitative thin-section CT: in vitro and in vivo validation. Radiology 2007;242:563–72.
110. Nakano Y, Muro S, Sakai H, et al. Computed tomographic measurements of airway dimensions and emphysema in smokers. Correlation with lung function. Am J Respir Crit Care Med 2000;162:1102–8.
111. Xie X, de Jong PA, Oudkerk M, et al. Morphological measurements in computed tomography correlate with airflow obstruction in chronic obstructive pulmonary disease: systematic review and meta-analysis. Eur Radiol 2012;22: 2085–93.

112. McNitt-Gray MF, Goldin JG, Johnson TD, et al. Development and testing of image-processing methods for the quantitative assessment of airway hyperresponsiveness from high-resolution CT images. J Comput Assist Tomogr 1997;21: 939–47.
113. Amirav I, Kramer SS, Grunstein MM, et al. Assessment of methacholine-induced airway constriction by ultrafast high-resolution computed tomography. J Appl Physiol 1993;75:2239–50.
114. Wood SA, Zerhouni EA, Hoford JD, et al. Measurement of three-dimensional lung tree structures by using computed tomography. J Appl Physiol 1995;79: 1687–97.
115. Nakano Y, Whittall K, Kalloger S, et al. Development and validation of human airway analysis algorithm using multidetector row CT. Proc SPIE 2002;4683: 460–9.
116. Saba OI, Hoffman EA, Reinhardt JM. Maximizing quantitative accuracy of lung airway lumen and wall measures obtained from X-ray CT imaging. J Appl Physiol 2003;95:1063–75.
117. Achenbach T, Weinheimer O, Biedermann A, et al. MDCT assessment of airway wall thickness in COPD patients using a new method: correlations with pulmonary function tests. Eur Radiol 2008;18:2731–8.
118. Achenbach T, Weinheimer O, Dueber C, et al. Influence of pixel size on quantification of airway wall thickness in computed tomography. J Comput Assist Tomogr 2009;33:725–30.
119. Matsuoka S, Yamashiro T, Washko GR, et al. Quantitative CT assessment of chronic obstructive pulmonary disease. Radiographics 2010;30:55–66.
120. Mets OM, de Jong PA, van Ginneken B, et al. Quantitative computed tomography in COPD: possibilities and limitations. Lung 2012;190:133–45.
121. Shuping RE, Judy PF. Resolution and contrast reduction. Med Phys 1978;5: 491–6.
122. Zerhouni EA, Spivey JF, Morgan RH, et al. Factors influencing quantitative CT measurements of solitary pulmonary nodules. J Comput Assist Tomogr 1982; 6:1075–87.
123. Washko GR, Dransfield MT, Estepar RS, et al. Airway wall attenuation: a biomarker of airway disease in subjects with COPD. J Appl Physiol 2009;107: 185–91.
124. Yamashiro T, Matsuoka S, Estepar RS, et al. Quantitative assessment of bronchial wall attenuation with thin-section CT: an indicator of airflow limitation in chronic obstructive pulmonary disease. AJR Am J Roentgenol 2010;195:363–9.
125. Boiselle PM, Litmanovich DE, Michaud G, et al. Dynamic expiratory tracheal collapse in morbidly obese COPD patients. COPD 2013. [Epub ahead of print].
126. Boiselle PM, Litmanovich DE, Michaud G, et al. Dynamic expiratory tracheal collapse in morbidly obese COPD patients. COPD 2013;10(5):604–10.
127. Lee HJ, Seo JB, Chae EJ, et al. Tracheal morphology and collapse in COPD: correlation with CT indices and pulmonary function test. Eur J Radiol 2011;80: e531–5.
128. Fujimoto K, Kitaguchi Y, Kubo K, et al. Clinical analysis of chronic obstructive pulmonary disease phenotypes classified using high-resolution computed tomography. Respirology 2006;11:731–40.
129. Kitaguchi Y, Fujimoto K, Kubo K, et al. Characteristics of COPD phenotypes classified according to the findings of HRCT. Respir Med 2006;100:1742–52.
130. Kim WD, Ling SH, Coxson HO, et al. The association between small airway obstruction and emphysema phenotypes in COPD. Chest 2007;131:1372–8.

131. Parraga G, Ouriadov A, Evans A, et al. Hyperpolarized 3He ventilation defects and apparent diffusion coefficients in chronic obstructive pulmonary disease: preliminary results at 3.0 Tesla. Invest Radiol 2007;42:384–91.

132. Patel B, Make B, Coxson HO, et al. Airway and parenchymal disease in chronic obstructive pulmonary disease are distinct phenotypes. Proc Am Thorac Soc 2006;3:533.

133. Han MK, Kazerooni EA, Lynch DA, et al. Chronic obstructive pulmonary disease exacerbations in the COPDGene study: associated radiologic phenotypes. Radiology 2011;261:274–82.

134. Albert P, Agusti A, Edwards L, et al. Bronchodilator responsiveness as a phenotypic characteristic of established chronic obstructive pulmonary disease. Thorax 2012;67:701–8.

135. Matsuoka S, Washko GR, Yamashiro T, et al. Pulmonary hypertension and computed tomography measurement of small pulmonary vessels in severe emphysema. Am J Respir Crit Care Med 2010;181:218–25.

136. Matsuoka S, Yamashiro T, Diaz A, et al. The relationship between small pulmonary vascular alteration and aortic atherosclerosis in chronic obstructive pulmonary disease: quantitative CT analysis. Acad Radiol 2011;18:40–6.

137. Rich JD, Archer SL, Rich S. Noninvasive cardiac output measurements in patients with pulmonary hypertension. Eur Respir J 2013;42:125–33.

138. Romme EA, Murchison JT, Edwards LD, et al. CT-measured bone attenuation in patients with chronic obstructive pulmonary disease: relation to clinical features and outcomes. J Bone Miner Res 2013;28:1369–77.

139. Clini EM, Beghe B, Fabbri LM. Chronic obstructive pulmonary disease is just one component of the complex multimorbidities in patients with COPD. Am J Respir Crit Care Med 2013;187:668–71.

140. Wells JM, Washko GR, Han MK, et al. Pulmonary arterial enlargement and acute exacerbations of COPD. N Engl J Med 2012;367:913–21.

141. Donaldson GC, Seemungal TA, Patel IS, et al. Airway and systemic inflammation and decline in lung function in patients with COPD. Chest 2005;128:1995–2004.

142. Palange P, Testa U, Huertas A, et al. Circulating haemopoietic and endothelial progenitor cells are decreased in COPD. Eur Respir J 2006;27:529–41.

143. Sin DD, Man SF. Why are patients with chronic obstructive pulmonary disease at increased risk of cardiovascular diseases? The potential role of systemic inflammation in chronic obstructive pulmonary disease. Circulation 2003;107:1514–9.

144. Budoff MJ, Nasir K, Kinney GL, et al. Coronary artery and thoracic calcium on noncontrast thoracic CT scans: comparison of ungated and gated examinations in patients from the COPD Gene cohort. J Cardiovasc Comput Tomogr 2011;5: 113–8.

Tobacco Smoking and Environmental Risk Factors for Chronic Obstructive Pulmonary Disease

Sundeep Salvi, MD, DNB, PhD

KEYWORDS

- Chronic obstructive pulmonary disease • Risk factors • Environmental
- Tobacco smoking • Biomass smoke

KEY POINTS

- A better understanding of the risk factors associated with chronic obstructive pulmonary disease (COPD) is important to help prevent the development and progression of COPD.
- Tobacco smoking is an established risk factor for COPD. Tobacco can be smoked in different forms apart from cigarettes, many of which are more harmful. Exposure to second-hand smoke is also a risk factor for COPD.
- However, many other risk factors associated with COPD remain underappreciated or neglected. More than 50% of cases of COPD can be attributed to nonsmoking risk factors.
- Exposure to indoor air pollution resulting from the burning of biomass fuels is a major risk factor for COPD, especially in developing countries.
- Other indoor air pollutants and outdoor air pollutants also contribute to the risk of COPD.
- Occupational causes contribute to up to 30% of COPD cases, but very little is known about this risk factor. Farming is a neglected risk factor for COPD.

INTRODUCTION

Chronic obstructive pulmonary disease (COPD) is a chronic progressive disease of the airways and lung parenchyma that is associated with exposure to tobacco smoke and other environmental insults in genetically susceptible individuals. The damaged lungs in COPD are difficult to revert back to normal. Current management is therefore aimed at reducing the symptoms and rapid decline in lung function, and preventing acute exacerbations. The economic burden associated with COPD is huge. Preventing the development of COPD, therefore, seems to be the only cost-effective public health

This article originally appeared in *Clinics in Chest Medicine*, Volume 35, Issue 1, March 2014.
Chest Research Foundation, Marigold Complex, Kalyaninagar, Pune 411014, India
E-mail address: ssalvi@crfindia.com

Clinics Collections 6 (2015) 225–240
http://dx.doi.org/10.1016/j.ccol.2015.05.041

intervention strategy that can reduce the global burden. Understanding the risk factors associated with the development of COPD is important so that primary, secondary, and even tertiary preventive strategies can be developed.

The development of COPD is multifactorial, and the risk factors include both genetic and environmental factors. The association between tobacco smoking and chronic bronchitis was first highlighted in 1955 by Oswald and Medvei.[1] However, the landmark study that established the association between tobacco smoking and COPD was the 8-year prospective study of 792 British men by Feltcher and Peto,[2] which observed that susceptible smokers showed a sharp and progressive decline in lung function that was the hallmark of this disease. The larger and longer Framingham study from the United States has confirmed these earlier reports.[3] For the last 5 decades, tobacco smoking has remained the most important risk factor associated with COPD across the world. In fact, the term COPD is used synonymously with smoking-induced lung disease.

As early as 1958, Fairbairn and Reid[4] reported that outdoor air pollution was an important risk factor for COPD, and in 1963 Phillips[5] reported that risk factors other than tobacco smoking were associated with COPD. However, the overwhelming interest in smoking as the main risk factor for COPD overshadowed these nonsmoking causes. In 2003, Lundbäck and colleagues[6] from Sweden and Mannino and colleagues[7] from the United States reported that the population-attributable risk of tobacco smoking for COPD was 45% and 44%, respectively, indicating that more than half of the cases of COPD were due to nonsmoking causes. In the same year, Ezatti and Lopez[8] published global mortality rates attributable to smoking from all causes in *The Lancet*, and reported that 47% of COPD deaths in men and 78% of COPD deaths in women were not attributable to tobacco smoking (**Fig. 1**). In 2009, Salvi and Barnes[9] reviewed the global literature on the prevalence of COPD among never-smokers, and reported that between 25% and 45% of patients with COPD across the globe had never smoked; highlighting the fact that COPD in never-smokers is much more common than was previously believed. A recent study on COPD prevalence from 14 countries, defined by postbronchodilator spirometry values, reported that 23.3% of the COPD subjects were never-smokers.[10]

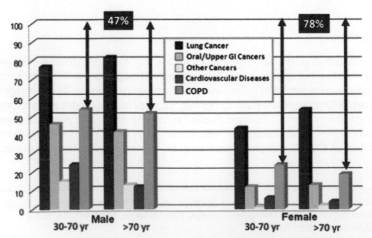

Fig. 1. Global mortality attributable to smoking: 47% of male COPD deaths and 78% of female COPD deaths are not attributable to tobacco smoking. (*Data from* Ezatti M, Lopez AD. Estimates of global mortality attributable to smoking in 2000. Lancet 2003;362(9387):847–52.)

This article describes the role of tobacco smoking and the various environmental risk factors associated with the development of COPD. Other risk factors for COPD such as poorly treated chronic severe asthma, status post pulmonary tuberculosis, poor socioeconomic status, and nutritional factors are not covered herein, and for a discussion of these factors the reader is referred to the review by Salvi and Barnes.[9]

TOBACCO SMOKING

The cigarette looks deceptively simple, but it is one of the most effectively engineered inhaler devices that delivers a steady dose of nicotine to the human body. Nicotine is present in the tobacco leaf, and its concentration varies depending on the variety of tobacco leaf. For example, the bright variety, which was originally grown in Virginia, United States, contains 2.5% to 3% nicotine, whereas the burley type of tobacco contains 3.5% to 4% nicotine and the oriental tobacco type contains less than 2% nicotine.

Nicotine is an alkaloid that is an extremely powerful drug. It stimulates the central nervous system and also increases the heart rate and blood pressure. Nicotine causes addiction similar to that of heroin and cocaine,[11] and is contained in the moisture of the tobacco leaf. When the cigarette is lit it evaporates, attaching itself to minute droplets in the tobacco smoke inhaled by the smoker. After being deposited in the lung, nicotine is absorbed very quickly and reaches the brain within 10 to 19 seconds. The damage that occurs in the lungs of tobacco smokers is mainly mediated by the tar present in the smoke, whereas the nicotine is relatively harmless.

Tar is the sticky brown substance that stains smokers' fingers and teeth yellow-brown. All cigarettes produce tar, but different brands produce different amounts. Earlier cigarettes (1950s) contained 30 mg tar per cigarette, but because of strict legislation modern cigarettes have tar levels lower than 11 mg per cigarette. According to the European Union directives, upper limits of tar, nicotine, and carbon monoxide have been set at 10 mg, 1 mg, and 10 mg, respectively. The type of paper used in the cigarette determines the amount of tar and nicotine that will be delivered into the lungs. Using more porous paper will let more air into the cigarette, diluting the smoke and reducing the amount of tar and nicotine entering into the lungs. Filters are made of cellulose acetate, and trap some of the tar and smoke particles from the inhaled smoke. Filters also cool the smoke slightly, making it easier to breathe.

Apart from the dried tobacco leaf, the cigarette also contains fillers made from the stems and other bits of tobacco, which are otherwise waste products. These fillers are mixed with water and various flavorings and additives. Additives are used to make the tobacco products more acceptable to the smoker, and include humectants (moisturizers) to prolong shelf life, and sugars to make the smoke milder and easier to inhale. A total of 600 such additives have been permitted by the Department of Health in the United States. Although many of these additives may seem quite harmless on their own, they may be toxic in their combination with other substances. Tobacco smoke contains 4000 chemicals, at least 20 of which are known to be carcinogenic.

Tobacco is inhaled in various other forms also. In India and other Asian countries, tobacco is rolled in dried tendu leaves (*Diospyros melanoxylon*), called bidi, and smoked (**Fig. 2**). Seventy percent of people in India smoke bidis mainly because they are cheap and easily available. Compared with cigarettes, bidis contain lesser amounts of nicotine (one-fourth of that in a cigarette) but produce 3 to 5 times the amount of tar, making it more harmful than cigarettes. Moreover, bidi smoking requires the person to smoke continuously and deeper to keep the bidi lit, which further increases the tar deposition in the lungs. Other forms of tobacco smoking include the

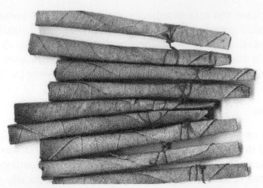

Fig. 2. Bidi: Tobacco wrapped in dried tendu leaf. (*From* Shutterstock, with permission. Available at: www.shutterstock.com.)

hookah or water-pipe and the chillum, which also contain other additives apart from tobacco leaf. These forms of smoking have been shown to be more harmful than cigarette smoke.[12] Water-pipe smoking, which is common in the Middle East and Asia (**Fig. 3**), is perceived to be safer than cigarettes because the smoke passes through water, but studies have shown that this smoke is as harmful as cigarette smoke.[13]

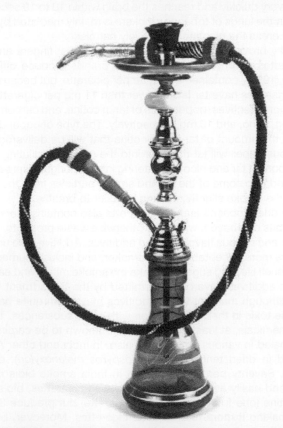

Fig. 3. Water-pipe smoker or hookah. (*From* Shutterstock, with permission. Available at: www.shutterstock.com.)

Associations between tobacco smoking and COPD have been shown in a large number of studies.[14] It was earlier reported that 15% of smokers develop COPD, indicating a strong genetic basis, because a significant proportion of smokers do not develop COPD. However, Lundbäck and colleagues[6] have reported that up to 50% of smokers can develop COPD, indicating that tobacco smoking poses a substantial risk for COPD in the general population.

SECOND-HAND SMOKE OR ENVIRONMENTAL TOBACCO SMOKE

The sidestream smoke from the burning of cigarettes is called second-hand smoke or environmental tobacco smoke, which mainly comes from the burning tip of the cigarette. Many toxins are present in higher concentrations in the sidestream smoke than in the mainstream smoke.[15] Typically, 85% of smoke in a room is due to sidestream smoke. Woodruff and colleagues[16] and, more recently, Goldklang and colleagues[17] studied the mechanisms by which second-hand smoke causes emphysema in animal experiments. Apart from cellular and mediator inflammation triggered by second-hand smoke, they report evidence of recruitment and activation of alveolar macrophages along with generation of reactive oxygen species, which together trigger the development of alveolar wall destruction. Exposure to second-hand smoke in human subjects has been shown to cause degradation of body elastin and possible injury to lung structure, thereby indicating a mechanism by which second-hand smoke can lead to the development of emphysema.[18]

Earlier observational studies reported an association between exposure to second-hand tobacco smoke and the risk of COPD.[19–21] A case-control study conducted by Kalandidi and colleagues[19] reported that women married to smokers and exposed to 1 pack per day or less were at a 2.5-times greater risk of having COPD than those married to nonsmokers. Sandler and colleagues[20] followed 14,783 healthy subjects exposed to second-hand smoke for 12 years and reported that the estimated relative risk of death from COPD was 5.65. Female spouses of smokers from Italy were reported to be at a 2.24-fold greater risk of developing obstructive lung disease than those married to nonsmokers.[21]

A cross-sectional study from China reported an association between self-reported exposure to passive smoking at home and work and the risk of COPD.[22] An average exposure of 40 hours per week for more than 5 years was associated with a 48% increased odds of contracting COPD. A similar cross-sectional study from the United States involving 2113 adults between the ages of 55 and 75 years reported that exposure to second-hand smoke was associated with a 36% greater odds of contracting COPD.[23] More recently, a study from Taiwan reported that women exposed to second-hand smoke had a 3.65-fold greater risk of being diagnosed with COPD, and that the duration of exposure to second-hand smoke correlated positively with the severity of COPD. The population-attributable risk for COPD from exposure to second-hand smoke was 47.3%.[24] Because the prevalence of cigarette smoking among Taiwanese men is high (55%–60%) and is low in women (3%–4%), a large number of Taiwanese nonsmoking women exposed to second-hand smoke seem to be at a greater risk of developing COPD. A recent prospective study conducted in 910 Chinese men and women for a period of 17 years reported that exposure to second-hand tobacco smoke was associated with a dose-dependent and 2.3-fold greater risk of COPD.[25]

However, not all studies have shown a positive association between second-hand tobacco smoke exposure and the risk of developing COPD.[26] More work needs to be done to study the true impact of second-hand smoke on COPD.

EXPOSURE TO INDOOR BIOMASS FUEL SMOKE

An estimated 50% of the world's population and 90% of the rural population of Africa and Asia use biomass fuels for cooking and heating purposes, accounting for more than 3 billion persons exposed to biomass smoke.[27] Biomass fuels include wood, animal dung, crop residues, dried twigs, dried grass, and fossil coal (**Fig. 4**). These fuels are cheap and easily available in rural settings, and are therefore widely used by poor people. Even modern homes in many developed countries are shifting their fuels from electricity and gas to biomass because of the increasing cost of cleaner fuels.[28]

Biomass fuels are inefficient because they not only produce less heat but also burn incompletely to release many noncombustible air pollutants. Crop residues are the least efficient, followed by animal dung and wood. Burning of biomass fuels produces more than 200 known chemical compounds, more than 90% of which can penetrate deep into the lungs.[29] These pollutants are classified into gaseous pollutants (carbon monoxide, sulfur dioxide, nitrogen dioxide) and particulate pollutants (PM10 and PM2.5, which are particles with a mass median aerodynamic diameter of 10 μm and 2.5 μm, respectively). These tiny particles are made up of black carbon, polyaromatic hydrocarbons, chlorinated dioxins, arsenic, lead, and transition metals such as nickel and vanadium. The indoor levels of PM10 in homes that use biomass fuel for cooking are often 5 to 50 times above the safety limits prescribed by the World Health Organization.[30] As many as 14 carcinogenic compounds, 6 cilia-toxic compounds and mucus-coagulating agents, and 4 cocarcinogenic or cancer-promoting agents have been identified in biomass fuel smoke.[31]

Women are typically exposed to high levels of biomass smoke pollutants for between 3 and 7 hours each day during cooking, often in poorly ventilated homes. On average, women spend 60,000 hours during their lifetime cooking near the biomass stove, during which period they inhale more than 25 million liters of highly polluted air.[32]

Two large meta-analyses investigated the association between exposure to biomass smoke and the risk of developing COPD. Hu and colleagues[33] analyzed 15 published studies and concluded that people exposed to biomass smoke had a 2.44-fold increased risk of COPD compared with those not exposed. Po and colleagues[34] analyzed 25 studies, and also reported a 2.4-fold increased odds of COPD among women exposed to biomass smoke. Of note, these odds are similar to those observed in chronic smokers who develop COPD. Compared with 1.1 billion smokers worldwide, 3 billion people are exposed to biomass smoke. It has therefore been argued that exposure to biomass smoke is probably a bigger risk factor for

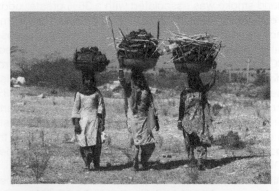

Fig. 4. Different types of biomass fuels (animal dung, wood, crop residues). (*From* Shutterstock, with permission. Available at: www.shutterstock.com.)

COPD than tobacco smoking from a global perspective.[32] The association between exposure to biomass smoke and COPD is seen in both developing and developed countries. Sood and colleagues[28] reported that exposure to wood smoke was associated with a 70% greater prevalence of COPD in New Mexico County in the United States. The reader is referred to the article by Sood and colleagues[28] for more information on the impact of biomass smoke on COPD.

Preliminary work from the author's laboratory indicates that subjects exposed to biomass smoke who develop COPD have a cellular and mediator inflammatory profile in the airways similar to that of tobacco smoke–induced COPD as evaluated by induced sputum.[35] Apart from greater small-airway obstruction in biomass smoke–induced COPD, the extent of physiologic impairment is similar to that of tobacco smoke–induced COPD.[36] More recently, the author compared the quality of life of patients with COPD caused by biomass smoke exposure and those with tobacco smoke–induced COPD using the St George questionnaire, and observed that subjects with COPD from biomass smoke had the same degree of impairment in quality of life (unpublished observations by the author, September 2013). Dutta and colleagues[37] have recently demonstrated that biomass users showed greater amounts of inflammatory cells, cytokines (eg, interleukin-6, interleukin-8, tumor necrosis factor α), and oxidative stress in the induced sputum in comparison with women who use cleaner fuels.

Exposure to biomass smoke is now recognized as an important risk factor for COPD. Several interventional studies examining the impact of improved cooking stoves (reducing biomass smoke) have reported improvements in lung function, symptoms, and the prevalence of COPD.[38–40] However, more work is needed to better understand the impact of different interventions that reduce indoor biomass smoke on the burden of COPD.

OTHER INDOOR AIR POLLUTANTS

The other indoor air pollutant that could pose a significant risk for COPD in tropical countries is smoke from mosquito coils (**Fig. 5**). It has been shown that burning one mosquito coil over a period of 8 hours emits as much particulate matter and formaldehyde as that equivalent to 100 cigarettes and 51 cigarettes, respectively.[41] Smoke from the burning of mosquito coils may therefore pose a significant risk for the development

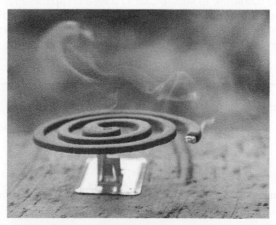

Fig. 5. A mosquito coil produces particulate matter equivalent to around 100 cigarettes. (*From* Shutterstock, with permission. Available at: www.shutterstock.com.)

of COPD, as these are widely used in many African and Asian countries to drive mosquitos away during sleeping hours. Moreover, mosquito-coil smoke has been shown to contain other harmful air pollutants, such as carbon monoxide, isoprene and benzene, and heavy metals such as lead, nickel, chromium, and tin. Smoke from mosquito coils has been shown to be a risk factor for lung cancer in Taiwan.[42] Animals exposed to mosquito-coil smoke have been shown to have significant histopathologic changes in the lung, such as loss of cilia, emphysema, metaplasia of epithelial cells, and morphologic alterations in alveolar macrophages.[43] Despite the concern over the risk of developing COPD from mosquito-coil smoke, very little research has been done on this aspect, even in countries where the use of these coils is common.

Other indoor air pollutants that are of potential risk in the development of COPD include cooking-oil smoke, kerosene smoke, incense smoke, pesticides, and volatile organic compounds from furnishings. However, there is very little information on these pollutants as potential risk factors for COPD.

OCCUPATIONAL COPD

Studies from developed countries indicate that the population-attributable fraction for COPD associated with occupational exposure varies between 9% and 31%.[44] A study from the United States estimated the population-attributable risk for COPD due to occupation to be 43%.[45] A prospective cohort study among Swiss workers reported that the population-attributable risk of COPD was 31% among smokers and 50% among nonsmokers in workers exposed to biological dusts.[46] The prevalence of occupational COPD is likely to be greater in developing countries because of the lack of stringent regulations at workplaces and the lack of adequate protective gear.

Several occupations are associated with an increased risk for COPD, and these are listed in **Box 1**.

Farming

Farming is one of the most common and neglected occupations associated with an increased risk of COPD. Studies in crop farmers from Canada[47,48] and the United States[49] have reported higher prevalence of chronic bronchitis and lower lung function compared with controls. Lamprecht and colleagues[50] reported that 30.2% of the farmers in rural Austria showed evidence of poorly reversible mild airway obstruction and that 7.7% had moderate to severe COPD based on spirometry. Similar observations have been reported from Spain,[51] and more recently from the Philippines[52] and China.[53] In the Philippines, farming for more than 40 years was found to be associated with a 2.5-fold greater risk of COPD and was similar to the risk associated with

---

Box 1
Occupations associated with COPD

- Dust exposures: coal mining, hard rock mining, concrete manufacturing, construction, tunneling, brick manufacturing, iron and steel founding, gold mining
- Animal farming: organic dust, ammonia, hydrogen sulfide, bacteria
- Crop farming: organic and inorganic dust
- Chemical exposure: plastic, textiles, rubber industry, leather manufacturing
- Diesel exhaust: trucking, transportation, automotive repair
- Road dust: sweeping

smoking tobacco for more than 20 pack-years.[52] In China, the prevalence of COPD was found to be 24.3%, 20.8%. 17.9%, and 12.6% among fungus greenhouse farmers, poultry greenhouse farmers, flower greenhouse farmers, and vegetable greenhouse farmers, respectively,[53] although it is not known whether smoking was a major confounder in this study.

Several cross-sectional studies have shown that animal farming is also associated with a greater risk of COPD. Poultry farming,[54] pig farming,[55] and dairy farming[56] have been shown to be strongly associated with COPD. Poultry-farm workers (**Fig. 6**) are often exposed to total inhalable dust levels exceeding 10 mg/m^3 during most activities.[57] The composition of dust in animal farms ranges from wood dust to a complex mixture of organic material derived from feed, litter, fecal material, dander, feather, and microorganisms. A Norwegian study reported that livestock farmers had a 40% greater risk of COPD than crop farmers, and this was strongly associated with ambient levels of ammonia, hydrogen sulfide, and organic dusts.[58] Farmers rearing more than one type of livestock, for example, sheep, goats, and poultry, had a significantly higher risk of COPD than those rearing only 1 type. Multiple etiologic factors are linked to the risk of developing COPD at farm locations, including organic dusts, endotoxins, peptidoglycans, and gases. Feeding operations in situations of large animal confinement also contain a wide diversity of microbes such as gram-positive bacteria and archaebacteria.[59] It has been suggested that chronic exposure to these inhalants has a

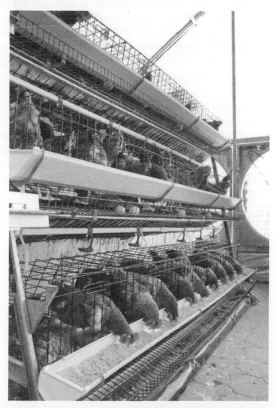

Fig. 6. Animal farming is an important occupation associated with COPD. (*From* Shutterstock, with permission. Available at: www.shutterstock.com.)

significant impact on local and systemic inflammatory responses that may underlie the development of chronic disease of the airways.[60]

Apart from organic dust, farmers are also exposed to significant amounts of inorganic soil dust (**Fig. 7**). The highest dust exposures occur during soil = preparation activities (eg, plowing, disking, and planting). Tractors pulling soil-preparation equipment generate large dust clouds, with particle concentrations reaching levels of up to 20 mg/m^3, and sometimes even 100 mg/m^3.[61] Total respirable dust concentrations in tractor cans reach levels between 1 and 5 mg/m^3. It has been shown that respirable quartz exposures in agriculture commonly exceed industrial standards. Silicates are the predominant inorganic fraction found in most soils, but in arid locations soil content is dominated by calcium carbonate and other soluble salts, whereas in warm humid climates soil dust is made up of oxides and hydroxides of iron and aluminum.[62]

Farming-induced COPD is poorly recognized across the world. Clinicians and policy makers need to be made aware of this association, so that early diagnosis and appropriate preventive strategies can be instituted. Farming-induced COPD can be prevented by controlling harmful exposures to organic dust, toxic gases, and chemicals on farms through improvements in animal-rearing techniques, ventilation of animal accommodation, careful drying and storage of animal feedstuffs, crops, and other products, and use of personal protective equipment.[63]

Other Occupations Associated with COPD

Mining and quarrying were the first occupations associated with significant reductions in lung function and the development of irreversible airflow obstruction. Coal mining has been shown to be associated with the risk of developing emphysema, 6 times more so than in nonminers.[64,65] Other mining activities that are generally characterized by silica exposure, such as gold, iron, and copper mining, and quarrying industries such as talc, potash, slate, and kaolin quarrying, have been reported to carry an increased risk of COPD.[66]

Petrochemical, mining, and steel industries are associated with chronic exposures to metals that are associated with an increased risk of COPD. A Danish study reported that cement and concrete workers have a higher risk of being hospitalized with COPD in comparison with gainfully employed men.[67] Occupations associated with exposure to diesel exhaust, such as transportation, trucking, construction, and vehicle mechanics, have been shown to be associated with an increased risk of COPD, but the evidence is weak.[68]

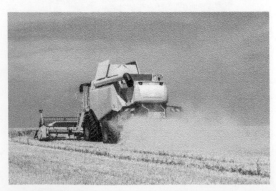

Fig. 7. Dust exposure during farming, both organic and inorganic, is a risk factor associated with COPD. (*From* Shutterstock, with permission. Available at: www.shutterstock.com.)

More recently, road sweepers from Pakistan have been shown to have a higher prevalence of COPD, which was proportional to the duration of exposure to road dust.[69]

In comparison with occupational asthma there is very little literature on the management and prevention of occupational COPD, and there are no published guidelines. The diagnosis of occupational COPD is infrequently made in clinical practice, and the clinician must therefore be attentive to all potential occupational causes in patients who have poorly reversible airway obstruction, especially among never-smokers.[70] Effective management should necessarily focus on medical treatment of already prevalent COPD and efforts to prevent and/or limit ongoing further damage via reduction of exposure.[70] The reader is referred to a review on this topic recently published in *Clinics in Chest Medicine*.[70]

OUTDOOR AIR POLLUTION

Outdoor air pollution, mainly from motor vehicular and industrial emissions, has been shown to be associated with various respiratory adverse effects, especially lung development in children aged 10 to 18 years.[71] The effects on adults are not clear, but women seem to be more affected than men.[72] In one of the largest published studies on the impact of traffic exposure on lung function in the United States, heavier traffic density was associated with greater decrements in lung function as evaluated by spirometry; when the distance from the main road was used as a parameter, the closer was the residence from the main road, the lower was the lung function.[72] Several biological mechanisms have been proposed to explain the harmful effects of ambient air pollutants, namely, increase in bronchial hyperresponsiveness, oxidative stress, airway inflammation, amplification of viral infections, and damage to ciliary activity of the airways.[73]

Few studies have investigated the effects of ambient air pollution on the risk of COPD prevalence. A German study of 4757 women living in the Rhine-Ruhr Basin reported that ambient PM10 levels were significantly associated with the risk of COPD. A 7-μg/m^3 increase in 5-year means of PM10 was associated with a 33% increased odds of contracting COPD. Moreover, women living within 100 m from the main road had 79% greater odds of presenting with COPD than those who lived more than 100 m away.[74] When the same cohort was followed up after 10 years, the prevalence of COPD had reduced as the levels of PM10 reduced.[75] A large cross-sectional study from Denmark showed a strong association between 35-year mean NO$_2$ levels and the risk of being hospitalized for COPD.[76]

A recent longitudinal cohort study from Vancouver, Canada, which examined the long-term exposure to elevated traffic-related air pollution with the risk of COPD hospitalization and mortality, reported that even a small increase in ambient black carbon air pollutants was associated with an increase in COPD hospitalizations and an increase in COPD mortality after adjustment for covariates.[77] A study from Rome, Italy reported that patients with COPD had 5 times greater mortality associated with ambient PM10 and NO$_2$ levels in comparison with normal subjects. Moreover, preexisting heart-conduction disorders and cerebrovascular diseases were found to have stronger effects in older men with COPD.[78]

Despite all the evidence, it remains unclear whether ambient air pollution may lead to a decline in lung function and subsequent development of COPD. Because few studies have confirmed COPD by spirometry and the published data are conflicting, a causal relationship between outdoor air pollution and COPD cannot be drawn at this stage.[73] A study from Nottingham, United Kingdom did not report any association between ambient levels of air pollutants and COPD.[79] A recent meta-analysis of 8 morbidity and 6 mortality studies reported that the evidence of chronic effects of air pollution on the prevalence and incidence of COPD among adults was suggestive but not conclusive, despite plausible biological mechanisms and good evidence that air pollution affects lung development in childhood and triggers exacerbations in COPD patients. The investigators recommend that larger studies with longer follow-up periods, specific definitions of COPD phenotypes, and more refined and source-specific exposure assessments are needed before any conclusive statement can be made.[80]

SUMMARY

Tobacco smoking is an important and preventable risk factor for the development and progression of COPD. Apart from the cigarette, several other devices are used to inhale tobacco smoke, many of which are in fact more harmful than cigarettes. However, tobacco smoking is not the only risk factor associated with COPD. Second-hand exposure to tobacco smoke has also been shown to be associated with the risk of COPD, although more robust evidence needs to be generated. Exposure to biomass smoke occurs in 50% of the world's population, especially in Africa and Asia, and is a major risk factor for COPD that is often neglected. Other indoor air pollutants are also important. Occupational causes contribute to up to 30% of COPD, and several occupations are associated with a greater risk of developing COPD. Farming is an important and neglected occupation associated with COPD. Cross-sectional studies have shown as association between outdoor air pollution and COPD, but more robust evidence is required.

A better understanding of the risk factors and their relative contribution to the development of COPD will help guide policy makers and health care providers to take appropriate interventional measures for primary as well as secondary prevention. Only then will the global burden of COPD be reduced.

REFERENCES

1. Oswald NC, Medvei VC. Chronic bronchitis: the effect of cigarette smoking. Lancet 1955;269:843–4.
2. Fletcher C, Peto R. The natural history of chronic airflow obstruction. BMJ 1977;1: 645–8.
3. Kohansal R, Martinez-Camblor P, Agusti A, et al. The natural history of chronic airflow obstruction revisited: an analysis of the Framingham offspring cohort. Am J Respir Crit Care Med 2009;180:3–10.
4. Fairbairn AS, Reid DD. Air pollution and other local factors in respiratory disease. Br J Prev Soc Med 1958;12:94–103.
5. Phillips AM. The influence of environmental factors in chronic bronchitis. J Occup Med 1963;5:468–75.
6. Lundbäck B, Lindberg A, Lindström M, et al. Not 15 but 50% of smokers develop COPD? Report from the Obstructive Lung Disease in Northern Sweden Studies. Respir Med 2003;97(2):115–22.
7. Mannino DM, Buist AS, Petty TL, et al. Lung function and mortality in the United States: data from the First National Health and Nutrition Examination Survey follow up study. Thorax 2003;58(5):388–93.
8. Ezatti M, Lopez AD. Estimates of global mortality attributable to smoking in 2000. Lancet 2003;362(9387):847–52.
9. Salvi SS, Barnes PJ. Chronic obstructive pulmonary disease in non-smokers. Lancet 2009;374:733–43.

10. Lamprecht B, McBurnie MA, Vollmer WM, et al. COPD in never smokers: results from the population-based burden of obstructive lung disease study. Chest 2011; 139(4):752–63.
11. Nicotine Addiction in Britain. A report of the Tobacco Advisory Group of the Royal College of Physicians. London: Royal College of Physicians; 2000.
12. Singh S, Soumya M, Saini A, et al. Breath carbon monoxide levels in different forms of smoking. Indian J Chest Dis Allied Sci 2011;53(1):25–8.
13. Raad D, Gaddam S, Schunemann HJ, et al. Effects of water-pipe smoking on lung function: a systemic review and meta-analysis. Chest 2011;139(4):764–74.
14. Bartal M. COPD and tobacco smoke. Monaldi Arch Chest Dis 2005;63(4):213–5.
15. California Environment Protection Agency. Health effects of exposure to environmental tobacco smoke. Tob Control 1997;6:346–53.
16. Woodruff PG, Ellwanger A, Solon M, et al. Alveolar macrophage recruitment and activation by chronic secondhand smoke exposure in mice. COPD 2009;6(2): 86–94.
17. Goldklang MP, Marks SM, D'Armiento JM. Second hand smoke and COPD. Lessons from animal studies. Front Physiol 2013;4(30):1–8.
18. Slowik N, Ma S, He J, et al. The effect of second hand smoke exposure on markers of elastic degradation. Chest 2011;140(4):946–53.
19. Kalandidi A, Trichopoulos D, Hatzakis A, et al. Passive smoking and chronic obstructive lung disease. Lancet 1987;2(8571):1325–6.
20. Sandler DP, Comstock GW, Helsing KJ, et al. Deaths from all causes in nonsmokers who lived with smokers. Am J Public Health 1989;79(2):163–7.
21. Simoni M, Baldacci S, Puntoni R, et al. Respiratory symptoms/diseases and environmental tobacco smoke (ETS) in never smoker Italian women. Respir Med 2007;101(3):531–8.
22. Yin P, Jiang CQ, Cheng KK, et al. Passive smoking exposure and risk of COPD among adults in China: The Guangzhou Biobank Cohort Study. Lancet 2007; 370:751–7.
23. Eisner MD, Balmes J, Katz PP, et al. Lifetime environmental tobacco smoke exposure and the risk of COPD. Environ Health 2005;4:7.
24. Wu CF, Feng NH, Chong IW, et al. Second hand smoke and chronic bronchitis in Taiwanese women: a health care based study. BMC Public Health 2010;10:44.
25. He Y, Jiang B, Li LS, et al. Second hand smoke exposure predicted COPD and other tobacco-related mortality in a 17-year cohort study in China. Chest 2012; 142(4):909–18.
26. Jaakkola MS, Jaakkola JJ. Effects of environmental tobacco smoke on respiratory health of adults. Scand J Work Environ Health 2002;28(Suppl 2):52–70.
27. World resources institute, UNEP, UNDP, World Bank. 1998-99 world resources: a guide to global environment. Oxford (United Kingdom): Oxford University Press; 1998.
28. Sood A, Petersen H, Blanchette CM, et al. Wood smoke exposure and gene promoter methylation are associated with increased risk for COPD in smokers. Am J Respir Crit Care Med 2010;182(9):1098–104.
29. Torres-Duque C, Maldonado D, Perez-Padilla R, et al. Biomass fuels and respiratory diseases: a review of the evidence. Proc Am Thorac Soc 2008;5(5): 577–90.
30. Kodgule R, Salvi S. Exposure to biomass smoke as a cause for airway disease in women and children. Curr Opin Allergy Clin Immunol 2012;12(1):82–90.
31. Balkrishnan K, Mehta S, Kumar P, et al. Indoor air pollution associated with household fuel use in India. India: ESMAP, World Bank; 2004.

32. Salvi S, Barnes PJ. Is exposure to biomass smoke the biggest risk factor for COPD globally? Chest 2010;138:3–6.
33. Hu G, Zhou Y, Tian J, et al. Risk of COPD from exposure to biomass smoke: a meta-analysis. Chest 2010;138(1):20–31.
34. Po JT, Fitzgerald JM, Carlsten C. Respiratory disease associated with solid biomass fuel exposure in rural women and children: systematic review and meta-analysis. Thorax 2011;66:232–9.
35. Brashier B, Vanjare N, Londhe J, et al. Comparison of airway cellular and mediator profiles between tobacco smoke-induced COPD and biomass fuel exposure-induced COPD in an Indian Population. Eur Respir J 2011;734.
36. Brashier B, Vanjare N, Vincent V, et al. Lung function differences in subjects with tobacco smoke-induced COPD (TS-COPD) and biomass smoke-induced COPD (BS-COPD) in an Indian population. Eur Respir J 2011;918.
37. Dutta A, Roychoudhury S, Chowdhury S, et al. Changes in sputum cytology, airway inflammation and oxidative stress due to chronic inhalation of biomass smoke during cooking in premenopausal rural Indian women. Int J Hyg Environ Health 2013;216(3):301–8.
38. Smith-Siversten T, Diaz E, Pope D, et al. Effect of reducing indoor air pollution on women's respiratory symptoms and lung function: the RESPIRE randomized trial, Guatemala. Am J Epidemiol 2009;170(2):211–20.
39. Romieu I, Riojas-Rodriguez H, Marron-Mares AT, et al. Improved biomass stove intervention in rural Mexico. Impact on the respiratory health of women. Am J Respir Crit Care Med 2009;180(7):649–56.
40. Chapman RS, He X, Blair AE, et al. Improvement in household cookstoves and risk of COPD in Xuanwei, China: Retrospective cohort study. BMJ 2005;331:1050.
41. Liu W, Zhang J, Hashim JH, et al. Mosquito coil emissions and health implications. Environ Health Perspect 2003;111(12):1454–60.
42. Chen SC, Wong RH, Shiu LJ, et al. Exposure to mosquito coil smoke may be a risk factor for lung cancer in Taiwan. J Epidemiol 2008;18(1):19–25.
43. Liu WK, Wong MH. Toxic effects of mosquito coil smoke on rats. II. Morphological changes of the respiratory system. Toxicol Lett 1987;39(2):231–9.
44. Trupin L, earnest G, San Pedro M, et al. The occupational burden of chronic obstructive pulmonary disease. Eur Respir J 2003;22:561–9.
45. Weinmann S, Vollmer WM, Breen V, et al. COPD and occupational exposures: a case control study. J Occup Environ Med 2008;50(5):561–9.
46. Mehta AJ, Miedinger D, Keidel D, et al. Occupational exposures to dusts, gases, and fumes and incidence of COPD in the Swiss cohort study on air pollution and lung and heart diseases in adults. Am J Respir Crit Care Med 2012;185:1292–300.
47. Dosman JA, Graham BL, Hall D, et al. Respiratory symptoms and pulmonary function in farmers. J Occup Med 1987;29(1):38–43.
48. Kennedy SM, Dimich-Ward H, Desjardins A, et al. Respiratory health among retired grain elevator workers. Am J Respir Crit Care Med 1994;150(1):59–65.
49. Gamsky TE, Schenker MB, McCurdy SA, et al. Smoking, respiratory symptoms and pulmonary function among a population of Hispanic farmworkers. Chest 1992;101(5):1361–8.
50. Lamprecht B, Schirnhofer L, Kaiser B, et al. Farming and the prevalence of non-reversible airways obstruction: results from a population based study. Am J Ind Med 2007;50(6):421–6.
51. Monso E. Bronchial colonization in chronic obstructive pulmonary disease: what's hiding under the rug. Arch Bronconeumol 2004;40(12):543–6.

52. Idolor LF, de Guia TS, Francisco NA, et al. Burden of obstructive lung disease in a rural setting in the Philippines. Respirology 2011;16(7):1111–8.
53. Liu S, Wen DL, Li LY, et al. Chronic pulmonary disease group of greenhouse farmers in Liaoning Province. Zhonghua Jie He He Hu Xi Za Zhi 2011;34(10): 753–6.
54. Viegas S, Faisca VM, Dias H, et al. Occupational exposure to poultry dust and effects on the respiratory system in workers. J Toxicol Environ Health 2013; 76(4–5):230–9.
55. Costa M, Teixeira PJ, Freitas PF. Respiratory manifestations and respiratory diseases: prevalence and risk factors among pig farmers in Braco de Norte, Brazil. J Bras Pneumol 2007;33(4):380–8.
56. Jouneau S, Boche A, Brinchault G, et al. On-site screening of farming-induced chronic obstructive pulmonary disease with the use of an electronic mini-spirometer: results of a pilot study in Britanny, France. Int Arch Occup Environ Health 2012;85(6):623–30.
57. Crook B, Easterbrook A, Stagg S. Exposure to dust and bioaerosols in poultry farming. Summary of observations and data. Health and Safety Laboratory. 2008. vii. Available at: http://www.hse.gov.uk/research/rrpdf/rr655.pdf. Accessed August 1, 2013.
58. Eduard W, Pearce N, Douwes J. Chronic bronchitis, COPD, and lung function in farmers: the role of biological agents. Chest 2009;136(3):716–25.
59. May S. Respiratory health effects of large animal farming environments. J Toxicol Environ Health 2012;15(8):524–41.
60. Sahlander K, Larsson K, Palmberg L. Altered innate immune response in farmers and smokers. Innate Immun 2010;16(1):27–38.
61. Nieuwenhuijsen MJ, Kruize H, Schenker MB. Exposure to dust, noise and pesticides, their determinants and the use of protective equipment among California farm operators. Appl Occup Environ Hyg 1996;11:1217–25.
62. Schenker M. Exposures and health effects from inorganic agricultural dusts. Environ Health Perspect 2000;108(4):661–4.
63. Linaker C, Smedley J. Respiratory illness in agriculture workers. Occup Med 2002;52(8):451–9.
64. Kuempel ED, Wheeler MW, Smith RJ, et al. Contributions of dust exposure and cigarette smoking to emphysema severity in coal miners in the United States. Am J Respir Crit Care Med 2009;180(3):257–64.
65. Santo-Tomas LH. Emphysema and COPD in coal miners. Curr Opin Pulm Med 2011;17(2):123–5.
66. Becklake MR. Chronic airflow limitation: its relationship to work in dusty occupations. Chest 1985;88(4):608–17.
67. Molgaard EF, Hannerz H, Tuchsen F, et al. Chronic lower respiratory diseases among demolition and cement workers: a population-based register study. BMJ Open 2013;3(1). http://dx.doi.org/10.1136/bmjopen-2012-001938.
68. Hart JE, Eisen EA, Laden F. Occupational diesel exhaust exposure as a risk factor for COPD. Curr Opin Pulm Med 2012;18(2):151–4.
69. Anwar SK, Mehmood N, Nasim N, et al. Sweeper's lung disease: a cross sectional study of an overlooked illness among sweepers of Pakistan. Int J Chron Obstruct Pulmon Dis 2013;8:193–7.
70. Diaz-Guzman E, Aryal S, Mannino DM. Occupational COPD. An update. Clin Chest Med 2012;33:625–36.
71. Gauderman WJ, Avol E, Gilliland F, et al. The effect of air pollution on lung development from 10-18 years of age. N Engl J Med 2004;351:1057–67.

72. Kan H, Heiss G, Rose KM, et al. Traffic exposure and lung function in adults: the atherosclerosis risk in communities study. Thorax 2007;62:873–9.
73. Ko FW, Hui DS. Air pollution and COPD. Respirology 2012;17:395–401.
74. Schikowski T, Sugiri D, Ranft U, et al. Long-term air pollution exposure and living close to busy roads are associated with COPD in women. Respir Res 2005;6:152.
75. Schikowski T, Ranft U, Sugiri D, et al. Decline in air pollution and change in prevalence in respiratory symptoms and COPD in elderly women. Respir Res 2010; 11:113.
76. Andersen ZH, Hvidberg M, Jensen SS, et al. COPD and long term exposure to traffic related air pollution: a cohort study. Am J Respir Crit Care Med 2011; 183(4):455–61.
77. Gan WQ, Fitzgerald JM, Carlsten C, et al. Associations of ambient air pollution with COPD hospitalisation and mortality. Am J Respir Crit Care Med 2013; 187(7):721–7.
78. Faustini A, Stafoggia M, Cappai G, et al. Short-term effects of air pollution in a cohort of patients with COPD. Epidemiology 2012;23(6):861–79.
79. Pujades-Rodriguez M, McKeever T, Lewis S, et al. Effect of traffic pollution on respiratory and allergic disease in adults: cross sectional and longitudinal analyses. BMC Pulm Med 2009;9:42.
80. Schikowski T, Mills IC, Andersen HR, et al. Ambient air pollution—a cause for COPD? Eur Respir J 2013. [Epub ahead of print].

How Phosphodiesterase 4 Inhibitors Work in Patients with Chronic Obstructive Pulmonary Disease of the Severe, Bronchitic, Frequent Exacerbator Phenotype

Mark A. Giembycz, BSc, PhD[a],*, Robert Newton, BSc, PhD[b]

KEYWORDS

- Phosphodiesterase 4 inhibitors • Roflumilast • COPD phenotypes
- Gene transactivation • Combination therapies • Acute exacerbations

KEY POINTS

- The novel, antiinflammatory drug, roflumilast, is efficacious in patients with severe chronic obstructive pulmonary disease (COPD) who have chronic bronchitis and a history of frequent exacerbations.
- This COPD phenotype is associated with mucus hypersecretion, an increased risk of bacterial colonization and infection, and a high level of inflammation. Such patients are most likely to derive clinical benefit from antiinflammatory drugs, such as the phosphodiesterase 4 inhibitor, roflumilast.
- The antiinflammatory benefit of roflumilast alone and in the presence of an inhaled corticosteroid/long-acting β_2-adrenoceptor agonist combination therapy may be caused, in part, by the de novo expression of a variety of antiinflammatory genes.

This article originally appeared in *Clinics in Chest Medicine*, Volume 35, Issue 1, March 2014. Financial disclosures and conflicts of interest: Grant support for M.A. Giembycz is from the Canadian Institutes for Health Research (CIHR; MOP 93742), the Lung Association, Alberta and North West Territories, Takeda, Gilead Sciences, GlaxoSmithKline, and AstraZeneca. Grant support for R. Newton is from the CIHR (MOP 68828), the Lung Association, Alberta and North West Territories, Takeda, Gilead Sciences, GlaxoSmithKline, and AstraZeneca. The authors state no conflict of interest.
[a] Department of Physiology & Pharmacology, Airways Inflammation Research Group, Snyder Institute for Chronic Diseases, University of Calgary, 3280 Hospital Drive Northwest, Calgary, Alberta T2N 4N1, Canada; [b] Department of Cell Biology & Anatomy, Airways Inflammation Research Group, Snyder Institute for Chronic Diseases, University of Calgary, 3280 Hospital Drive Northwest, Calgary, Alberta T2N 4N1, Canada
* Corresponding author.
E-mail address: giembycz@ucalgary.ca

INTRODUCTION

Chronic obstructive pulmonary disease (COPD) is an umbrella term that describes a heterogeneous collection of distinct, debilitating, pulmonary-related disorders that, in many individuals, coexist. COPD is defined clinically by a progressive and largely irreversible decrement in expiratory airflow[1] that is often associated with airway collapse, fibrosis, edema, mucus hypersecretion, airway and systemic inflammation, skeletal muscle wasting, pulmonary hypertension, right sided heart failure, and venous thromboembolism. The variable extent to which an individual presents with one or more of these clinical entities accounts for the wide spectrum of disease seen in clinical practice. COPD typically affects middle-aged and elderly people, and it is a general perception that chronic cigarette smoking is the primary cause.[2,3] However, long-term exposure of individuals to biomass fuel combustion products, used largely in the process of indoor cooking, also is now recognized as a significant cause especially in developing countries.[4]

COPD heterogeneity is probably caused by a complex interplay between genetic factors, which remain largely indeterminate, and the environment, in which tobacco smoke and pollutants are primary players.[5–8] It is intuitive that phenotypic diversity of COPD precludes effective treatment. Because current pharmacotherapies were not rationally designed to target distinct phenotypes, the current one-size fits all approach to management is inherently flawed and poorly effective. Therefore, although COPD heterogeneity is problematic, it nevertheless creates potential opportunities for the design of therapies tailored to the phenotype of interest.[9] In 2012, 4 broad COPD clinical phenotypes (denoted A–D) were proposed based on prognostic and therapeutic relevance (**Fig. 1A**).[10,11] According to this taxonomy, which is distinct from the groups defined in the Global Initiative for Chronic Obstructive Lung Disease (GOLD) guidelines (see **Fig. 1B**; www.goldcopd.org/uploads/users/files/GOLD_Report_2013_Feb20.pdf), patients are categorized as having infrequent exacerbations (A), an asthma/COPD overlap (B), exacerbations with emphysema (C), or exacerbations with chronic bronchitis (D). This article focuses on patients of the D phenotype. These patients have severe disease (GOLD stage 3–4), present with a history of productive cough or expectoration (>3 months per year and for more than 2 consecutive years) and respond to the novel, antiinflammatory drug, roflumilast (marketed variably as Daxas, Daliresp, and Libertek). Frequent exacerbations of COPD are associated, maybe causally, with mucus hypersecretion, an increased risk of bacterial colonization and infection, and a high level of inflammation.[12] Together, these characteristics suggest that patients of a severe, bronchitic phenotype are most likely to derive clinical benefit from antiinflammatory drugs, such as the phosphodiesterase (PDE) 4 inhibitor, roflumilast. A post hoc analysis of 2 phase III studies (AURA, M2-124; HERMES, M2-125[13]) found that roflumilast (500 μg daily for 1 year) transformed patients classified as frequent exacerbators at the outset of the trial into a more stable, infrequent exacerbator phenotype.[14]

PDE4 INHIBITORS AND COPD

PDEs represent a superfamily of enzymes that degrade the second messenger molecules cyclic adensosine-3′,5′-monophosphate (cAMP) and/or cyclic guanosine-3′,5′-monophophate to the catalytically inactive, corresponding 5′-nucleoside monophosphates. Following the first identification of a PDE activity more than 50 years ago,[15] 11 molecularly, biochemically, and immunologically distinct enzyme families have been clearly defined.[16] Since then, there has been considerable interest in the cAMP-specific PDE4 family as an intracellular target that could be exploited to

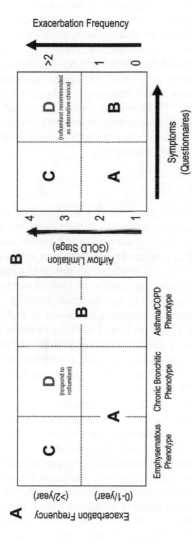

Fig. 1. Classification of COPD. (A) The subdivision of COPD into 4 broad phenotypes wherein patients are categorized as having infrequent exacerbations (A), an asthma/COPD overlap (B), exacerbations with emphysema (C), or exacerbations with chronic bronchitis (D). (B) The Global Initiative for Chronic Obstructive Lung Disease classification of COPD, which is based on airflow limitation, exacerbation history, and symptoms (determined by questionnaire). Patients are classified as low risk, fewer symptoms (A), low risk, more symptoms (B), high risk, fewer symptoms (C), or high risk, more symptoms (D). The phosphodiesterase (PDE) 4 inhibitor, roflumilast, is a recommended treatment option for group D patients in both classifications (shown in red). (*Adapted from* Miravitlles M, Jose Soler-Cataluna J, Calle M, et al. Treatment of COPD by clinical phenotypes. Putting old evidence into clinical practice. Eur Respir J 2013;41(6):1252–6.)

therapeutic advantage for a multitude of diseases associated with chronic inflammation, including COPD. Despite compelling preclinical evidence of efficacy,[17–19] the PDE4 inhibitors that have progressed to phase II and phase III clinical evaluation have had a regrettable rate of attrition, in part, because of unfavorable adverse-effect profiles.[20–22] However, after almost 30 years of research and development, the European Medicines Agency, in April 2010, recommended approval of the first PDE4 inhibitor, roflumilast, for the "maintenance treatment of patients with severe COPD associated with chronic bronchitis who have a history of frequent exacerbations" (www.ema.europa. eu/docs/en_GB/document_library/Summary_of_opinion_-_Initial_authorisation/human/ 001179/WC500089626.pdf). Roflumilast was subsequently approved by Health Canada (www.hc-sc.gc.ca/dhp-mps/prodpharma/applic-demande/regist/reg_innov_dr-eng.php), the United States Food and Drug Administration (www.fda.gov/NewsEvents/Newsroom/ PressAnnouncements/ucm244989.htm), and other regulatory agencies globally. The approval of roflumilast for COPD is significant because it is thought to provide clinical benefit by suppressing inflammation.[18,23,24] Moreover, the recommendation that roflumilast be used in a defined population of chronic bronchitic patients in whom exacerbation frequency is high and inflammation severe represents the first example of a drug that targets (albeit not by design) a specific COPD phenotype.

A TRIPLE COMBINATION THERAPY?

GOLD recently updated its recommendations for the treatment of stable COPD to include roflumilast as a second-choice medication in high-risk patients with severe (stages 3–4) symptomatic disease (www.goldcopd.org/uploads/users/files/GOLD_ Report_2013_Feb20.pdf). This clinical positioning dictates that roflumilast should be prescribed to patients with severe disease (defined as group D patients in both of the classifications shown in **Fig. 1**) taking, minimally, an inhaled corticosteroid (ICS)/ long-acting β_2-adrenoceptor agonist (LABA) combination therapy. Data accrued from the roflumilast clinical development program (reviewed in Refs.[23–27]) indicate that there may be a clinical rationale for combining a PDE4 inhibitor with an ICS or an ICS/LABA combination therapy. In a pooled post hoc analysis of 2 phase III studies (OPUS, M2-111; RATIO, M2-112), roflumilast reduced exacerbation frequency in a subgroup of patients with severe COPD who were taking an ICS concomitantly, whereas patients not taking an ICS derived no such benefit.[28] Lung function was also improved in patients diagnosed with COPD associated with chronic bronchitis, with or without coexisting emphysema, which was greater if they had received concomitant ICS relative to placebo.[28] However, 2 additional phase III trials (AURA, M2-124; HERMES, M2-125), also in patients with severe COPD, found that roflumilast reduced exacerbation rates in the absence of an ICS,[13] indicating that PDE4 inhibition alone is sufficient for clinical benefit to be realized. Although the reason(s) for this discrepancy is debatable, the possibility that the efficacy of roflumilast and an ICS together may be superior to either drug alone is attractive from a therapeutics standpoint. A meta-analysis of several trials involving almost 12,000 patients with COPD confirmed the superiority of an ICS/LABA combination therapy rather than a LABA alone in reducing the rate of acute exacerbations.[29] Given that LABAs and PDE4 inhibitors, which can both mediate their effects by increasing cAMP, are predicted to interact additively or, in theory, synergistically at the molecular level, the possibility that further improvement could be achieved with an ICS/LABA/PDE4 inhibitor triple combination therapy should be considered. Frequent exacerbations of COPD are associated with a high level of inflammation[12] and may be more responsive to these drug interventions if they are given in combination rather than individually as monotherapies. In 2011, the REACT (Roflumilast in the prevention of COPD Exacerbations while taking Appropriate Combination Treatment) study was initiated to test such a hypothesis. This 1-year investigation will compare the effects of roflumilast and placebo on exacerbation rates in patients with severe to very severe airflow limitation, symptoms of chronic bronchitis, and at least 2 exacerbations in the previous year, who are treated with ICS/LABA combination therapy, with or without a long-acting, muscarinic receptor antagonist.[30]

SCIENTIFIC RATIONALE FOR ADDING ON A PDE4 INHIBITOR TO AN ICS/LABA COMBINATION THERAPY: A CASE FOR GENE TRANSACTIVATION

Glucocorticoids as a monotherapy are poorly effective in COPD (cf asthma) and are contraindicated[31] because of doubts about efficacy and potential adverse effects including pneumonia and tuberculosis.[32,33] Nevertheless, the results of a recent meta-analysis suggest that the potential benefit of an ICS/LABA combination therapy is a reduction in acute exacerbations.[29] From a clinical perspective, this suggests that ICS/LABA combination therapies should only be used in patients classified as frequent exacerbators. Given that inflammation is assumed to be more prevalent and/or severe in these patients, adding on a PDE4 inhibitor might impart additional benefit through the ability of each component of the combination to act individually, additively, or cooperatively to repress inflammation. Notwithstanding multiple nongenomic mechanisms, which have been reviewed extensively elsewhere (see Ref.[18] for review), the remainder of this article focuses on the concept that the clinical efficacy of roflumilast in COPD is derived, in part, from its ability either alone or in combination with an ICS and LABA to induce and/or enhance the expression of a variety of genes that collectively suppress inflammation and improve lung function.

In considering the potential for drug interactions, a mechanistic basis is required. It is thought that the primary mode of action of glucocorticoids, more commonly known as corticosteroids or simply steroids, is to repress the expression of proinflammatory genes, including those that encode cytokines, chemokines, and growth factors.[34] Two general mechanisms have been described in which the glucocorticoid receptor (GR) may act either to directly repress gene transcription (transrepression) or to activate gene transcription (transactivation). In terms of antiinflammatory actions, the most widely accepted of these mechanisms is transrepression, in which the agonist-bound GR, through ill-defined tethering interactions, prevents transcription factors such as nuclear factor kappa B (NF-κB) and activator protein 1 (AP-1) from inducing the expression of target proinflammatory genes. Transrepression may also occur via a direct interaction of the agonist-bound GR to negative glucocorticoid response elements (GREs) located in the promoter regions of target genes.[35] However, glucocorticoids are often only partial inhibitors of proinflammatory gene transcription, implying that processes in addition to transcriptional repression must contribute to their in vivo antiinflammatory activity.[34,36] In this respect, considerable evidence is available that transactivation of genes encoding proteins with antiinflammatory properties also constitutes a major mechanism of glucocorticoid action.[37] For example, glucocorticoids are able to transcriptionally induce the expression of the NF-κB inhibitor protein, IκBα, and this represents a mechanism of repression that involves transactivation by GR.[38,39] The expression of the antiinflammatory gene, *GILZ* (glucocorticoid-induced leucine zipper; HUGO gene name, transforming growth factor β-stimulated clone 22; domain family member 3 [*TSC22D3*]), similarly is significantly upregulated in bronchial biopsies harvested from human asthmatic subjects given a high dose of budesonide by a mechanism thought to involve GR-mediated transactivation.[40]

The empirical demonstration that a glucocorticoid can promote gene transactivation in vivo in human subjects is of particular therapeutic relevance because cAMP can augment glucocorticoid-induced gene expression,[41] possibly by enhancing the binding of ligand-bound GRs to GREs on target genes.[42] This effect was initially reported in the early 1990s following overexpression of cAMP-dependent protein kinase (PKA) in cAMP response element binding protein (CREB)–deficient F9 embryonal carcinoma cells.[43] LABAs and other cAMP-increasing agents, including PDE4 inhibitors, produce the same effect by a mechanism that involves the activation of PKA.[41,44–47] Although this interaction was initially identified from experiments using artificial reporter constructs, it became clear that many bona fides glucocorticoid-inducible genes are regulated similarly.[41,44–47] In many cases, the cAMP-increasing agent alone is without effect, but interacts with glucocorticoid in a positive cooperative fashion. For example, LABAs and PDE4 inhibitors do not promote transcription of a simple GRE reporter. However, they markedly enhance the maximum response produced by the glucocorticoid without changing its potency,[41,46] which indicates that cAMP can boost the intrinsic efficacy (vide infra) of the GR agonist (**Fig. 2**A). In the presence of a LABA, or a PDE4 inhibitor, a glucocorticoid is therefore able to produce a given level of response but at a significantly lower concentration (see **Fig. 2**A). As an example, selective PDE4 inhibition with roflumilast potentiates the ability of formoterol to enhance the expression of luciferase from a GRE reporter stably transfected into the human BEAS-2B airway epithelial cell line (see **Fig. 2**A) as well as the expression of several putative, glucocorticoid-inducible antiinflammatory genes.[46] This effect is described pharmacologically by a sinistral displacement of the LABA concentration-response curve (see **Fig. 2**A), indicating that the cells are now more sensitive to the LABA. In the absence of evidence that cAMP can enhance GR-mediated transrepression, these

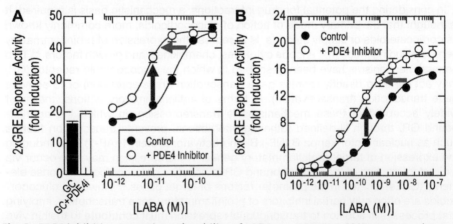

Fig. 2. PDE4 inhibition potentiates the ability of LABAs to promote cAMP response element (CRE)–dependent transcription and enhance GRE-dependent transcription. (*A*) The BEAS-2B human airway epithelial cell line was stably transfected with 2 copies of a GRE upstream of the luciferase gene and stimulated concurrently with the glucocorticoid (GC), fluticasone propionate (100 nM) and the LABA, formoterol, in the absence and presence of the PDE4 inhibitor (PDE4i), roflumilast. (*B*) The results of a similar study in which BEAS-2B cells were stably transfected with 6 copies of a CRE upstream of the same luciferase gene and exposed to the LABA, indacaterol, in the absence and presence of the PDE4 inhibitor, GSK 256066. In both cases, PDE4 inhibition produced a sinistral displacement of the LABA concentration-response curve (*red arrow*) and thereby augmented transcription, especially at low LABA concentrations (*blue arrow*).

results collectively add weight to the importance of transactivation as a mechanism of glucocorticoid action.[34] Moreover, the data also have potential clinical relevance because they provide a plausible explanation for the superior efficacy of ICS/LABA combination therapies in several respiratory diseases relative to an ICS alone as a monotherapy. Such positive interactions are clear for patients with moderate to severe asthma[48–51] and similar, albeit less impressive, data are available in COPD.[29] The treatment of acute bronchiolitis with a combination of dexamethasone and adrenaline (an endogenous agonist that activates the β_2-adrenoceptor) or salbutamol was recently reported to significantly reduce the frequency of acute hospitalizations relative to either treatment alone.[52,53] Although β_2-adrenoceptor agonists are not antiinflammatory as monotherapies, these data strongly suggest that they can interact with glucocorticoids to deliver enhanced clinical benefit that is superior to the effect of a glucocorticoid alone. On a molecular level, we suggest that these beneficial effects might derive, in part, from the ability of cAMP to enhance glucocorticoid-induced gene expression, which requires the activation of the canonical cAMP signaling cascade. Adding on a PDE4 inhibitor could therefore potentiate β_2-adrenoceptor–mediated cAMP formation and thereby further enhance antiinflammatory gene expression. This effect might be particularly relevant in cells in which β_2-adrenoceptor signaling is weak because of low receptor number and/or poor coupling efficiency. A PDE4 inhibitor might transform a proinflammatory or immune cell that is normally insensitive to a LABA into one that generates a cAMP signal of sufficient magnitude to enhance glucocorticoid-induced gene expression (vide infra).

PDE4 inhibitors and LABAs alone and in combination could also impart clinical benefit in COPD by promoting the transactivation of antiinflammatory genes that is independent of their ability to enhance the genomic effects of glucocorticoids. A prior microarray study in the BEAS-2B human bronchial epithelial cell line identified more than 200 genes that were upregulated more than 2-fold by the LABA, indacaterol, and the PDE4 inhibitor, GSK 256066 (authors' unpublished data). Many of these genes are glucocorticoid insensitive but, nevertheless, have documented antiinflammatory activity. Moreover, on some genes, the PDE4 inhibitor and LABA in combination could interact synergistically (see **Fig. 2**B). Thus, superior efficacy of a triple combination therapy can be envisaged by considering that each component can work in several distinct, and mutually cooperative, ways, Stated differently, the rationale for combining these drugs is based on the assumption that distinct subpopulations of genes exist that are induced by glucocorticoid alone, cAMP alone, and by both glucocorticoid and cAMP with potential for additivity and/or synergy. In this last group, it is conceivable that genes could respond to both glucocorticoid and cAMP in combination, but not necessarily to each individually. The possibility that LABAs and PDE4 inhibitors can also upregulate distinct subpopulations of cAMP-inducible genes is also worthy of consideration in view of the mounting evidence that distinct subcellular compartments of cyclic nucleotides can be generated in an agonists-dependent manner.

WHY ICS/LABA COMBINATION THERAPIES ARE NOT ENOUGH

Logic dictates that, for a glucocorticoid and a LABA to interact additively or synergistically, target tissues must express functional GR and β_2-adrenceptors in sufficient numbers. Although GR is expressed ubiquitously, consistent with the pleiotropic effects produced by cortisol in humans, its density varies considerably across tissues.[54] In immune and proinflammatory cells, the rank order of GR expression (high to low) is estimated to be airway smooth muscle $\geq$ bronchial epithelium > alveolar macrophages > eosinophils $\geq$ peripheral blood mononuclear cells (lymphocytes and monocytes) > neutrophils.[55–58] Based on this ranking, it can be speculated that low GR number in neutrophils may explain, in part, why inflammation in COPD is insensitive to glucocorticoids as a monotherapy.[59] In these same cell types, β_2-adrenoceptor density is also low and/or coupling to downstream effectors inefficient. Compared with airway myocytes and epithelial cells, which express approximately 30,000 to 40,000 and 8000 to 9000 sites/cell respectively,[60–62] alveolar macrophages,[63] eosinophils,[64] neutrophils,[65] and T lymphocytes[66] express few β_2-adrenoceptors ($\sim$6000, $\sim$4000, $\sim$900, and $\sim$750 sites/cell respectively). The ability of a LABA to enhance the expression of glucocorticoid-inducible antiinflammatory genes could therefore be minimal or not happen at all in cell types in which functional β_2-adrenoceptor number is limiting. This effect is compounded if functional GR number is also low. It is in these β_2-adrenoceptor–poor cells that the potential therapeutic benefit of adding on a PDE4 inhibitor could be most realized. This concept is illustrated in **Fig. 3**, which shows responses in 2 hypothetical cells, A and B, that express the β_2-adrenoceptor in high and low copy number respectively. In each panel, the term system maximum (E_m) is indicated. E_m is the maximum achievable tissue (but not necessarily agonist) response and is both an agonist-dependent and tissue-dependent parameter. In a cell with high β_2-adrenoceptor density (eg, an airway myocyte; A), a LABA might produce a response that equates to E_m. As a result, the amplitude of that response is unaffected by a PDE4 inhibitor but, because of second messenger amplification, the concentration-response curve is displaced to the left (ie, the system is now more sensitive to the LABA). In contrast, the same LABA in a cell with low β_2-adrenoceptor density or poor coupling efficiency (eg, a neutrophil; B), might produce a response considerably less than the E_m. In this

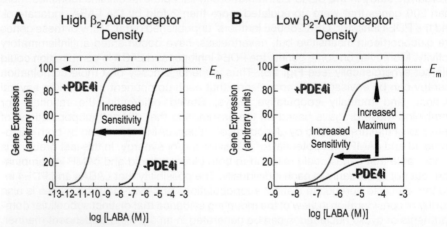

Fig. 3. Theoretical effects of PDE4 inhibition on LABA concentration-response curves constructed in cells expressing high and low β_2-adrenoceptor density. In each panel, the term system maximum (E_m) is indicated, which is the maximum achievable tissue response. In a cell with high β_2-adrenoceptor density (*A*) a LABA produces a response that equates to E_m (*red curve*). In the presence of a PDE4i, the amplitude of the LABA response is unaffected but the concentration-response curve is displaced to the left (*blue curve*). (*B*) A cell with low β_2-adrenoceptor density on which a LABA produces a response that is considerably less than the E_m. In this situation, PDE4 inhibition enhances the maximal effect of the LABA toward E_m, without changing its half maximal effective concentration [EC_{50}]. However, the cell is sensitized because a given level of response in the presence of a PDE4 inhibitor can now be produced by a lower concentration of the LABA.

situation, PDE4 inhibition could enhance the maximal effect toward E_m. Although there may be little change in agonist potency (quantified as the half maximal effective concentration [EC_{50}]), the system has, nevertheless, been sensitized such that a given level of response in the presence of a PDE4 inhibitor can now be produced by a lower concentration of the LABA (see **Fig. 3**). For a PDE4 inhibitor to work optimally in cells in which β_2-adrenoceptor number is limiting, the intrinsic efficacy of the LABA is an important parameter and highly relevant for the design of new ICS/LABA combination therapies. The term intrinsic efficacy, as given by Furchgott,[67] is defined as a quantal unit of stimulus given to a receptor and is solely an agonist-dependent parameter. Therefore, the ability of an agonist to produce response in a given tissue (ie, its efficacy) is the product of intrinsic efficacy (agonist dependent) and receptor number (tissue dependent). This pharmacodynamic concept is seen in eosinophils (low β_2-adrenoceptor density) in which salmeterol behaves as a β_2-adrenoceptor antagonist under conditions in which formoterol, which has a higher intrinsic efficacy, is an effective agonist.[68,69]

An additional theoretical advantage of a PDE4 inhibitor is its ability to potentiate the antiinflammatory activity of endogenous agonists that act through G-protein–coupled receptors (GPCRs) coupled to cAMP formation such as catecholamines, certain prostaglandins, and adenosine.

CANDIDATE ANTIINFLAMMATORY GENES

Several glucocorticoid and/or cAMP-inducible genes have recently been identified that, when expressed together, could collectively impart a clinically beneficial impact on those mechanisms that promote inflammation and predispose susceptible patients to acute exacerbations (vide infra). Moreover, their expression could contribute to the therapeutic benefit of roflumilast seen in patients with severe, bronchitic disease who have frequent, acute exacerbations. As transactivation becomes more accepted as a mechanism that contributes to the beneficial actions of glucocorticoids (rather than an entrenched and inaccurate view that it mediates only side effects)[70] it is likely that many more genes will be discovered that, when upregulated, would be advantageous in chronic inflammatory diseases such as COPD.

Mitogen-activated Protein Kinase Phosphatase 1

Mitogen-activated protein (MAP) kinases are central regulators of virtually all aspects of the inflammatory process, including proinflammatory gene expression.[71] The activity of these enzyme cascades is tightly controlled by reversible phosphorylation. Termination of MAP kinase signaling is mediated by a several phosphatases that dephosphorylate 2 critical amino acids that are targeted by upstream activating kinases. One of these phosphatases is MAP kinase phosphatase (MKP) 1 (HUGO gene name, dual-specificity phosphatase 1 [*DUSP1*]), for which extracellular-signal-regulated kinase, p38 MAP kinase and *c-jun*-N-terminal kinase (JNK), are substrates.[72] In humans and other species, *MKP-1* is profoundly induced by glucocorticoids through the activation of a glucocorticoid-responsive region (located between −1380 and −1266bp of the *MKP-1* promoter)[73] and is implicated in the repression of several proinflammatory genes.[74–76] MKP-1 can prevent the activation of key proinflammatory transcription factors (eg, NF-κB, AP-1)[77,78] and also promote the destabilization of proinflammatory gene mRNAs.[74,79] In vivo, the ability of glucocorticoids to repress proinflammatory gene expression is impaired in *mkp-1*–deficient mice.[80] Acetylcholine-induced airways hyper-responsiveness in mice exposed to ozone is normalized by dexamethasone through the upregulation of *mkp-1*.[81]

In human bronchial epithelial cells and airway myocytes, *MKP-1* is also induced by cAMP-increasing agents, including LABAs and PDE4 inhibitors, by activating the canonical cAMP/PKA signaling cascade.[41,73,82] The human *MKP-1* promoter contains 2 *cis*-acting cAMP response elements[83] that can be activated by the transcription factor, CREB.[84] Moreover, a LABA and a glucocorticoid in combination have been shown to activate a human *MKP-1* promoter construct in an additive manner, indicating that these are transcriptionally regulated events.[73,82]

The mucus hypersecretion that can often occur in COPD is thought to be caused by overexpression of *MUC5AC,* which encodes a major gel-forming mucin.[85,86] Acute, bacteria-induced exacerbations of COPD are associated, maybe causally, with enhanced mucus production.[87] It has been shown recently that PDE4 inhibitors, by selectively targeting the PDE4B subtype, can attenuate *Streptococcus pneumoniae*–induced *MUC5AC* gene expression in human airway epithelial cells in vitro and in an in vivo murine model of otitis media by enhancing the expression of MKP-1.[75] This effect is thought to be transcriptional, because similar data were obtained with a MUC5AC luciferase reporter.[75] It is possible that some form of additional upregulation of MKP-1 could be produced when a PDE4 inhibitor is added on to a glucocorticoid alone or in combination with a LABA.

Glucocorticoid-induced Leucine Zipper

Glucocorticoid-induced leucine zipper (GILZ) is typically described as a very highly glucocorticoid-inducible gene.[88] Expression levels can increase dramatically in a range of cell types relevant to airways inflammatory disorders including bronchial epithelial cells, mast cells, airway myocytes, and T lymphocytes.[40,41,89,90] GILZ blocks the activity of certain key proinflammatory transcription factors including NF-κB and AP-1.[89] There are 2 principal ways that inhibition may occur. One process involves the physical interaction of GILZ with NF-κB and AP-1 in the nucleus to inhibit their ability to promote transcription,[89,91,92] whereas other studies show that GILZ is localized to the cytoplasm[40] where it may suppress MAP kinase signaling.[93] Whichever mechanism applies, it is clear that GILZ can inhibit the expression of proinflammatory genes such as interleukin (IL)-8.[94]

Neither LABAs nor PDE4 inhibitors induce *GILZ* and their ability to enhance glucocorticoid-induced GILZ expression is modest compared with many of the other genes described here. However, in certain cells, such as human primary airway epithelia, synergy has been reported with formoterol and a high concentration of roflumilast.[46]

Regulator of G-protein Signaling 2

Regulators of G-protein signaling (RGS) represent a large group of GTPase-activating proteins that act as critical, negative modulators of GPCRs. By enhancing the intrinsic GTPase activity of active G proteins, RGSs promote guanosine 5′-monophosphate (GTP) hydrolysis and return the GPCR-G-protein complex to the resting state. RGS2 is selective for Gq[95] and inactivates receptors that typically mediate airway smooth muscle contraction. In mice lacking *rgs2,* the muscarinic M_3-receptor agonist, methacholine, produces exaggerated contractile responses of tracheal smooth muscle, whereas in vivo such animals display airways hyper-reactivity.[96] In human ASM cells, LABAs, including formoterol and salmeterol, induce *RGS2.* The magnitude of this effect is enhanced and the kinetics significantly protracted in the presence of a glucocorticoid, affording a long-lasting protection of the muscle against constrictor stimuli.[96] Similar data have been found in human airway epithelial cells in which RGS2 upregulation could suppress proinflammatory responses mediated through

Gq-linked GPCRs. RGS2 is reported to attenuate *MUC5AC* expression in human airway epithelial cells following activation of GPR68, a proton-sensing Gq-linked receptor that is more commonly known as ovarian cancer G-protein–coupled receptor-1.[97] Of particular interest is the finding that the PDE4 inhibitor, roflumilast, further enhanced the expression of RGS2 in these cells to a level greater than that produced by a combination of fluticasone propionate and formoterol.[46] If this also occurs in airways smooth muscle, the degree and/or duration of bronchoprotection afforded by ICS/LABA combination therapy could be extended further.

Cluster of Differentiation 200

Cluster of differentiation (CD) 200 is a transmembrane glycoprotein expressed on a variety of cells of both hematopoietic and nonhematopoietic origin (eg, neutrophils, airway epithelia, alveolar macrophages, mast cells, dendritic cells, lymphocytes). The receptor for CD200, CD200R, has a more restricted expression profile, being found primarily on myeloid and lymphoid cells. Together, CD200 and CD200R form an inhibitory ligand-receptor pair that results in a unidirectional, downregulation of proinflammatory responses in CD200R-bearing cells. In mice infected with influenza virus, the CD200/CD200R interaction blunts the activation of alveolar macrophages (which have high constitutive expression of CD200R compared with their systemic counterparts) as measured by proinflammatory cytokine generation.[98] Because acute exacerbations of COPD are triggered, primarily, by acute bouts of excessive inflammation in response to bacterial and viral infections, upregulation of *CD200* on epithelial and other airway cells could, by this mechanism, help reduce exacerbation frequency.[98] In this context, *CD200* is modestly induced on human airway epithelial cells by the glucocorticoid, fluticasone propionate. However, this effect is significantly enhanced by formoterol alone and, even more dramatically, in combination with roflumilast.[46]

Cysteine-rich Secretory Protein Limulus Clotting Factor C, Cochlin, Lgl1 Domain-containing 2

A similar function to CD200 may be attributed to CRISPLD2 (cysteine-rich secretory protein limulus clotting factor C, cochlin, Lgl1 domain-containing 2), which can function as a secreted lipopolysaccharide-binding protein in mice and humans.[99] The expression of this gene could also help reduce COPD exacerbations in response to infections with gram-negative bacteria by downregulating Toll-like receptor-4 (TLR4)–mediated proinflammatory responses. *CRISPLD2* was originally identified as a glucocorticoid-induced gene in rat lung[100] and, subsequently, shown to be upregulated in human airway epithelial cells by both fluticasone propionate and formoterol, which interact in a synergistic manner.[46] Moreover, although roflumilast at clinically relevant concentrations failed to increase *CRISPLD2* mRNA levels, it potentiated the induction produced by fluticasone propionate and formoterol in combination. CRISPLD2 also plays a critical role in branching morphogenesis in fetal lung and in the development of alveolae.[100] Whether these functions are pertinent in adults with emphysema is unclear.

p57^{kip2}

An inhibitor of certain G1 cyclin/cyclin-dependent kinase complexes, p57^{kip2} (kinase inhibitor protein 2 of 57 kDa; HUGO gene name, cyclin-dependent kinase inhibitor 1C [*CDKN1C*]), was originally reported to be involved in the antiproliferative actions of glucocorticoids in HeLa cells.[101] The findings that glucocorticoids induce *p57^{kip2}* in airways smooth muscle and human bronchial epithelial cells[41] suggests that it may subserve a similar function in other tissues. In the context of COPD, the expression of p57[kip2] in airway structural cells could arrest mitogenesis and suppress airways remodeling, which is a characteristic feature of COPD.[102] In bovine airway myocytes, the combination of low concentrations of fluticasone propionate and formoterol inhibits the induction of a proliferative, hypocontractile phenotype produced by platelet-derived growth factor.[102] The findings that glucocorticoid-induced p57[kip2] expression is enhanced by formoterol alone, and more impressively by formoterol and roflumilast in combination, raises the possibility that an even greater effect could be produced with an ICS/LABA/PDE4 inhibitor triple combination therapy.[46,102] In addition, p57[kip2] may also block proinflammatory responses through its ability to inhibit JNK, one of the core MAP kinases.[103]

Suppressor of Cytokine Signaling 3

Suppressors of cytokine signaling (SOCS) are a family of 8 related proteins that terminate signals emanating from the interaction of proinflammatory mediators with IL-6Rα, IL-12Rβ2, and receptors for interferon-γ, granulocyte colony–stimulating factor, and leptin.[104] In vascular endothelial cells, SOCS3 is a cAMP-inducible gene that is regulated independently of PKA by mechanisms that involve, minimally, cAMP-guanine nucleotide exchange factor-1 and downstream small GTPases, Rap1 and Ras.[105] The expression of SOCS3 is also upregulated by cAMP-increasing agents in human airway epithelial cells[47,106] and synergy has been reported with a LABA (salmeterol) and a glucocorticoid (fluticasone propionate) in combination.[106] Moreover, in airway epithelial cells exposed to tobacco smoke, basal SOCS3 expression was significantly downregulated and this was rescued by fluticasone propionate and salmeterol in combination.[106] Additivity or further synergy might be predicted in the presence of a PDE4 inhibitor. Given that IL-6 and leptin are increased in COPD and may correlate with disease severity,[107,108] the expression of SOCS3 by an ICS/LABA/PDE4 inhibitor triple combination therapy could help attenuate proinflammatory signals mediated by their cognate receptors.

Cylindromatosis

Polyubiquitination is an enzymatic process whereby ubiquitin molecules are added sequentially to susceptible protein substrates through the formation of covalent, intermolecular glycine-lysine (K) bonds.[109] Ubiquitin chains linked via K48 typically mark a given protein for proteosomal degradation. However, linkage via other lysines (eg, K63) facilitates several nondegradative processes[109] including the activation of the proinflammatory transcription factor, NF-κB,[110] and of JNK signaling cascades.[111] There is evidence that several upstream, K63-linked ubiquitinated proteins including tumor necrosis factor receptor-associated factor (TRAF) 6 and NF-κB essential modulator (NEMO) are required for an active NF-κB signaling complex to form.[112,113] Ubiquitination is a reversible process and the opposite reaction is catalyzed by a large group deubiquitinases that deconjugate protein-bound ubiquitin chains. A novel deubiquitinase, cylindromatosis (CYLD), was recently identified as an inducible, negative regulator of NF-κB through its ability to cleave ubiquitin molecules from several substrates including TRAF6 and NEMO and so prevent the formation of an active NF-κB signaling complex.[112,113] In the context of COPD exacerbations, several reports have documented that CYLD is upregulated by both gram-positive (eg, S pneumoniae) and gram-negative (eg, nontypeable Haemophilus influenzae [NTHi], Escherichia coli) bacteria to repress inflammation,[114] which may represent an autoinhibitory (protective) mechanism to oppose the deleterious effects of TLR4 activation.[115,116] Moreover, Komatsu and colleagues[117] reported in 2013 that inhibition of PDE4, specifically the

PDE4B isoform, augments the induction of *CYLD* in human airway epithelial cells in response to NTHi and in the lungs of NTHi-infected mice. By using siRNA technology and *cyld*$^{-/-}$ mice, the same investigators showed that the PDE4 inhibitors, rolipram and roflumilast, suppressed proinflammatory cytokine generation in vitro and indices of pulmonary inflammation in vivo by a CYLD-dependent mechanism.[117] The sensitivity of *CYLD* to LABAs has not been investigated, but similar results in β_2-adrenoceptor-expressing cells might be expected and for there to be some form of positive interaction with a PDE4 inhibitor. It is not known whether *CYLD* is a glucocorticoid-inducible gene.

Tristetraprolin

Posttranscriptional mechanisms are central to regulating gene expression. In this respect, the mRNA destabilizing protein, tristetraprolin (TTP; HUGO gene name, zinc finger protein 36 homologue [*ZFP36*]), by binding to regulatory sequences in the 3′-untranslated regions of target mRNAs, provides feedback control of many inflammatory genes, including *TNF, IL1B, IL8,* and *CSF2*.[118] Thus, although *TTP* is primarily induced by inflammatory stimuli,[119] it is also upregulated by glucocorticoids to exert repression.[47,120,121] In addition, *TTP* is induced by β_2-adrenceptor agonists, PDE inhibitors (including inhibitors of PDE4), and other cAMP-increasing agents.[47,122] Such data support the beneficial effects of the cAMP and glucocorticoid pathways on TTP expression, but no obvious combinatorial effect was noted in BEAS-2B human bronchial epithelial cells treated with LABAs and glucocorticoid,[41] although additivity was reported when the same cells were exposed to glucocorticoid and the adenosine A_{2B}-receptor agonist, Bay 60–6583.[47]

GENE TRANSACTIVATION AND GLUCOCORTICOID RESISTANCE

The concept of gene transactivation as a mechanism of action of glucocorticoids also has relevance to the clinical phenomenon of reduced glucocorticoid responsiveness (variably reported as resistance, tolerance, insensitivity, or subsensitivity) such as that seen in COPD. Compelling evidence is available that the ability of glucocorticoids to induce transcriptional responses is impaired by a variety of proinflammatory stimuli including tobacco smoke extract, cytokines, growth factors, and viruses (both respiratory syncytial virus and human rhinovirus).[123–126] The expression of *GILZ*, *p57*[kip2], and *RGS2*, which may exert antiinflammatory, antiproliferative, and bronchoprotective effects respectively (vide supra), is inhibited by one or more of these proinflammatory insults.[123–127] The finding that LABAs can functionally rescue cells and tissues from this form of glucocorticoid subsensitivity[96,123] provides an attractive mechanism to explain the superior clinical benefit of ICS/LABA combination therapies. A PDE4 inhibitor, as part of a triple combination therapy, could further boost the transactivation potential of a glucocorticoid alone and in combination with a LABA in addition to any effect it might produce by itself.

A NOTE ON CAMP-INDUCED, ADVERSE-EFFECT GENES

A clinical concern of β_2-adrenoceptor agonists as monotherapies is their ability to upregulate the expression of a variety of proinflammatory signaling molecules including IL-6, IL-6R, IL-8, IL-11, IL-15, and IL-20Rβ (authors' unpublished observations).[128] In asthmatic patients, this is an important issue because regular administration of β_2-adrenoceptor agonists is reported to promote pulmonary eosinophilia.[129,130] Whether this proinflammatory liability is also realized in patients with COPD is, currently, vague but should not be ignored. It is intuitive that the upregulation of adverse-effect genes could be replicated by a PDE4 inhibitor and be more pronounced if the PDE4 inhibitor is combined with a LABA because of their potential to synergize. Although this possibility needs to be carefully evaluated, it may not be problematic in the context of a triple combination therapy because a large number of these cAMP-inducible genes are repressed by glucocorticoids.[37,128] Unwanted actions of LABAs may also be mediated by $Gs\beta\gamma$ heterodimers or through promiscuous coupling of the β_2-adrenoceptor to Gi.[131] At present, there is little evidence for such signal transduction in native systems (but see Refs.[132,133]) and, regardless, PDE4 inhibitors are not expected to potentiate responses mediated by these alternative signaling cascades.

SUMMARY AND FUTURE DIRECTIONS

Current international guidelines recommend that roflumilast be added on to an ICS/LABA combination therapy in high-risk patients with severe, bronchitic COPD who have frequent acute exacerbations. Evidence is presented here that a glucocorticoid, LABA, and PDE4 inhibitor in combination can interact in a complex manner to induce a panel of genes that could act collectively to suppress inflammation and improve lung function. Central to this concept is that this drug combination produces a unique gene induction fingerprint that is not reproduced by any components of the triple therapy alone. The clinical efficacy of roflumilast, when combined with an ICS and a LABA, is therefore attributable, in part, to the individual, additive, and often cooperative actions of these drugs on gene transcription.[134] In this respect, the results of the ongoing REACT study[30] are awaited with anticipation.

At present, side effects remain a continuing problem with PDE4 inhibitors, including roflumilast.[20,22] However, several strategies may result in the discovery of compounds with improved therapeutic ratios. These strategies include the selective targeting of certain PDE4 subtypes and the development of allosteric PDE4 inhibitors.[135,136] The possibility that multivalent (multifunctional) ligands, which feature 2 or more pharmacophores, may deliver superior efficacy is also an approach that is being explored. Single molecules that inhibit PDE4 and activate β_2-adrenoceptors at similar concentrations have been described.[137,138] These drugs would not have the potential disadvantage of an inhaled combination therapy in which unequal deposition of each component is always possible.

ACKNOWLEDGMENTS

We thank our colleague, Dr Richard Leigh, Department of Medicine, University of Calgary, for constructive comments on this article.

REFERENCES

1. Pauwels RA, Buist AS, Calverley PM, et al. Global strategy for the diagnosis, management, and prevention of chronic obstructive pulmonary disease. NHLBI/WHO Global Initiative for Chronic Obstructive Lung Disease (GOLD) workshop summary. Am J Respir Crit Care Med 2001;163:1256–76.
2. Hogg JC. Pathophysiology of airflow limitation in chronic obstructive pulmonary disease. Lancet 2004;364:709–21.
3. Hogg JC, Chu F, Utokaparch S, et al. The nature of small-airway obstruction in chronic obstructive pulmonary disease. N Engl J Med 2004;350:2645–53.
4. Laumbach RJ, Kipen HM. Respiratory health effects of air pollution: update on biomass smoke and traffic pollution. J Allergy Clin Immunol 2012;129:3–11.

5. Walter R, Gottlieb DJ, O'Connor GT. Environmental and genetic risk factors and gene-environment interactions in the pathogenesis of chronic obstructive lung disease. Environ Health Perspect 2000;108(Suppl 4):733–42.
6. Kleeberger SR, Cho HY. Gene-environment interactions in environmental lung diseases. Novartis Found Symp 2008;293:168–78.
7. Caramori G, Adcock I. Gene-environment interactions in the development of chronic obstructive pulmonary disease. Curr Opin Allergy Clin Immunol 2006; 6:323–8.
8. Kleeberger SR, Peden D. Gene-environment interactions in asthma and other respiratory diseases. Annu Rev Med 2005;56:383–400.
9. Rennard SI, Vestbo J. The many "small COPDs": COPD should be an orphan disease. Chest 2008;134:623–7.
10. Miravitlles M, Soler-Cataluna JJ, Calle M, et al. A new approach to grading and treating COPD based on clinical phenotypes: summary of the Spanish COPD guidelines (GesEPOC). Prim Care Respir J 2013;22:117–21.
11. Miravitlles M, Jose Soler-Cataluna J, Calle M, et al. Treatment of COPD by clinical phenotypes. Putting old evidence into clinical practice. Eur Respir J 2013; 41(6):1252–6.
12. Perera WR, Hurst JR, Wilkinson TM, et al. Inflammatory changes, recovery and recurrence at COPD exacerbation. Eur Respir J 2007;29:527–34.
13. Calverley PM, Rabe KF, Goehring UM, et al. Roflumilast in symptomatic chronic obstructive pulmonary disease: two randomised clinical trials. Lancet 2009;374: 685–94.
14. Wedzicha1 JA, Rabe KF, Martinez FJ, et al. Efficacy of roflumilast in the chronic obstructive pulmonary disease frequent exacerbator phenotype. Chest 2012; 143(5):1302–11.
15. Butcher RW, Sutherland EW. Adenosine 3',5'-phosphate in biological materials. I. Purification and properties of cyclic 3',5'-nucleotide phosphodiesterase and use of this enzyme to characterize adenosine 3',5'-phosphate in human urine. J Biol Chem 1962;237:1244–50.
16. Bender AT, Beavo JA. Cyclic nucleotide phosphodiesterases: molecular regulation to clinical use. Pharmacol Rev 2006;58:488–520.
17. Dastidar SG, Rajagopal D, Ray A. Therapeutic benefit of PDE4 inhibitors in inflammatory diseases. Curr Opin Investig Drugs 2007;8:364–72.
18. Hatzelmann A, Morcillo EJ, Lungarella G, et al. The preclinical pharmacology of roflumilast - a selective, oral phosphodiesterase 4 inhibitor in development for chronic obstructive pulmonary disease. Pulm Pharmacol Ther 2010;23: 235–56.
19. Torphy TJ. Phosphodiesterase isozymes: molecular targets for novel antiasthma agents. Am J Respir Crit Care Med 1998;157:351–70.
20. Oba Y, Lone NA. Efficacy and safety of roflumilast in patients with chronic obstructive pulmonary disease: a systematic review and meta-analysis. Ther Adv Respir Dis 2013;7:13–24.
21. Giembycz MA. Life after PDE4: overcoming adverse events with dual-specificity phosphodiesterase inhibitors. Curr Opin Pharmacol 2005;5: 238–44.
22. Giembycz MA. An update and appraisal of the cilomilast phase III clinical development programme for chronic obstructive pulmonary disease. Br J Clin Pharmacol 2006;62:138–52.
23. Giembycz MA, Field SK. Roflumilast: first phosphodiesterase 4 inhibitor approved for treatment of COPD. Drug Des Devel Ther 2010;4:147–58.

24. Gross NJ, Giembycz MA, Rennard SI. Treatment of chronic obstructive pulmonary disease with roflumilast - a new phosphodiesterase 4 inhibitor. COPD 2010; 7:141–53.
25. Field SK. Roflumilast, a novel phosphodiesterase 4 inhibitor, for COPD patients with a history of exacerbations. Clin Med Insights Circ Respir Pulm Med 2011;5: 57–70.
26. Cazzola M, Picciolo S, Matera MG. Roflumilast in chronic obstructive pulmonary disease: evidence from large trials. Expert Opin Pharmacother 2010;11:441–9.
27. Antoniu SA. New therapeutic options in the management of COPD - focus on roflumilast. Int J Chron Obstruct Pulmon Dis 2011;6:147–55.
28. Rennard SI, Calverley PM, Goehring UM, et al. Reduction of exacerbations by the PDE4 inhibitor roflumilast–the importance of defining different subsets of patients with COPD. Respir Res 2011;12:18.
29. Nannini LJ, Lasserson TJ, Poole P. Combined corticosteroid and long-acting β_2-agonist in one inhaler versus long-acting β_2-agonists for chronic obstructive pulmonary disease. Cochrane Database Syst Rev 2012;(9):CD006829.
30. Calverley PM, Martinez FJ, Fabbri LM, et al. Does roflumilast decrease exacerbations in severe COPD patients not controlled by inhaled combination therapy? The REACT study protocol. Int J Chron Obstruct Pulmon Dis 2012;7:375–82.
31. O'Donnell DE, Aaron S, Bourbeau J, et al. Canadian Thoracic Society recommendations for management of chronic obstructive pulmonary disease - 2007 update. Can Respir J 2007;14(Suppl B):5B–32B.
32. Brassard P, Suissa S, Kezouh A, et al. Inhaled corticosteroids and risk of tuberculosis in patients with respiratory diseases. Am J Respir Crit Care Med 2011; 183:675–8.
33. Ernst P, Gonzalez AV, Brassard P, et al. Inhaled corticosteroid use in chronic obstructive pulmonary disease and the risk of hospitalization for pneumonia. Am J Respir Crit Care Med 2007;176:162–6.
34. Newton R, Leigh R, Giembycz MA. Pharmacological strategies for improving the efficacy and therapeutic ratio of glucocorticoids in inflammatory lung diseases. Pharmacol Ther 2010;125:286–327.
35. Surjit M, Ganti KP, Mukherji A, et al. Widespread negative response elements mediate direct repression by agonist-liganded glucocorticoid receptor. Cell 2011;145:224–41.
36. Clark AR. Anti-inflammatory functions of glucocorticoid-induced genes. Mol Cell Endocrinol 2007;275:79–97.
37. King EM, Chivers JE, Rider CF, et al. Glucocorticoid repression of inflammatory gene expression shows differential responsiveness by transactivation- and transrepression-dependent mechanisms. PLoS One 2013;8:e53936.
38. Scheinman RI, Cogswell PC, Lofquist AK, et al. Role of transcriptional activation of IκBα in mediation of immunosuppression by glucocorticoids. Science 1995; 270:283–6.
39. Auphan N, DiDonato JA, Rosette C, et al. Immunosuppression by glucocorticoids: inhibition of NF-κB activity through induction of IκB synthesis. Science 1995;270:286–90.
40. Kelly MM, King EM, Rider CF, et al. Corticosteroid-induced gene expression in allergen-challenged asthmatic subjects taking inhaled budesonide. Br J Pharmacol 2012;165:1737–47.
41. Kaur M, Chivers JE, Giembycz MA, et al. Long-acting β_2-adrenoceptor agonists synergistically enhance glucocorticoid-dependent transcription in human airway epithelial and smooth muscle cells. Mol Pharmacol 2008;73:201–14.

42. Roth M, Johnson PR, Rudiger JJ, et al. Interaction between glucocorticoids and β₂ agonists on bronchial airway smooth muscle cells through synchronised cellular signalling. Lancet 2002;360:1293–9.
43. Rangarajan PN, Umesono K, Evans RM. Modulation of glucocorticoid receptor function by protein kinase A. Mol Endocrinol 1992;6:1451–7.
44. Miller AH, Vogt GJ, Pearce BD. The phosphodiesterase type 4 inhibitor, rolipram, enhances glucocorticoid receptor function. Neuropsychopharmacology 2002;27:939–48.
45. Wilson SM, Shen P, Rider CF, et al. Selective prostacyclin receptor agonism augments glucocorticoid-induced gene expression in human bronchial epithelial cells. J Immunol 2009;183:6788–99.
46. Moodley T, Wilson SM, Joshi T, et al. Phosphodiesterase 4 inhibitors augment the ability of formoterol to enhance glucocorticoid-dependent gene transcription in human airway epithelial cells: a novel mechanism for the clinical efficacy of roflumilast in severe COPD. Mol Pharmacol 2013;83:894–906.
47. Greer S, Page CW, Joshi T, et al. Concurrent agonism of adenosine A₂ʙ- and glucocorticoid receptors in human airway epithelial cells cooperatively induces genes with anti-inflammatory potential: a novel approach to treat COPD. J Pharmacol Exp Ther 2013;346(3):473–85.
48. Ducharme FM, Ni CM, Greenstone I, et al. Addition of long-acting β₂-agonists to inhaled corticosteroids versus same dose inhaled corticosteroids for chronic asthma in adults and children. Cochrane Database Syst Rev 2010;(5):CD005535.
49. Frois C, Wu EQ, Ray S, et al. Inhaled corticosteroids or long-acting β-agonists alone or in fixed-dose combinations in asthma treatment: a systematic review of fluticasone/budesonide and formoterol/salmeterol. Clin Ther 2009;31:2779–803.
50. Pauwels RA, Lofdahl CG, Postma DS, et al. Effect of inhaled formoterol and budesonide on exacerbations of asthma. Formoterol and Corticosteroids Establishing Therapy (FACET) International Study Group. N Engl J Med 1997;337:1405–11.
51. Shrewsbury S, Pyke S, Britton M. Meta-analysis of increased dose of inhaled steroid or addition of salmeterol in symptomatic asthma (MIASMA). BMJ 2000;320:1368–73.
52. Plint AC, Johnson DW, Patel H, et al. Epinephrine and dexamethasone in children with bronchiolitis. N Engl J Med 2009;360:2079–89.
53. Kuyucu S, Unal S, Kuyucu N, et al. Additive effects of dexamethasone in nebulized salbutamol or L-epinephrine treated infants with acute bronchiolitis. Pediatr Int 2004;46:539–44.
54. Su AI, Wiltshire T, Batalov S, et al. A gene atlas of the mouse and human protein-encoding transcriptomes. Proc Natl Acad Sci U S A 2004;101:6062–7.
55. Pujols L, Mullol J, Roca-Ferrer J, et al. Expression of glucocorticoid receptor α- and β-isoforms in human cells and tissues. Am J Physiol Cell Physiol 2002;283:C1324–31.
56. Plumb J, Gaffey K, Kane B, et al. Reduced glucocorticoid receptor expression and function in airway neutrophils. Int Immunopharmacol 2012;12:26–33.
57. Miller AH, Spencer RL, Pearce BD, et al. Glucocorticoid receptors are differentially expressed in the cells and tissues of the immune system. Cell Immunol 1998;186:45–54.
58. Adcock IM, Gilbey T, Gelder CM, et al. Glucocorticoid receptor localization in normal and asthmatic lung. Am J Respir Crit Care Med 1996;154:771–82.
59. Schleimer RP. Effects of glucocorticosteroids on inflammatory cells relevant to their therapeutic applications in asthma. Am Rev Respir Dis 1990;141:S59–69.

60. Johnson M. Effects of β_2-agonists on resident and infiltrating inflammatory cells. J Allergy Clin Immunol 2002;110:S282–90.
61. Penn RB, Kelsen SG, Benovic JL. Regulation of β-agonist- and prostaglandin E_2-mediated adenylyl cyclase activity in human airway epithelial cells. Am J Respir Cell Mol Biol 1994;11:496–505.
62. Kelsen SG, Higgins NC, Zhou S, et al. Expression and function of the β-adrenergic receptor coupled-adenylyl cyclase system on human airway epithelial cells. Am J Respir Crit Care Med 1995;152:1774–83.
63. Liggett SB. Identification and characterization of a homogeneous population of β_2-adrenergic receptors on human alveolar macrophages. Am Rev Respir Dis 1989;139:552–5.
64. Yukawa T, Ukena D, Kroegel C, et al. β_2-Adrenergic receptors on eosinophils. Binding and functional studies. Am Rev Respir Dis 1990;141: 1446–52.
65. Galant SP, Underwood S, Duriseti L, et al. Characterization of high-affinity β_2-adrenergic receptor binding of (-)-[^{3}H]-dihydroalprenolol to human polymorphonuclear cell particulates. J Lab Clin Med 1978;92:613–8.
66. Martinsson A, Larsson K, Hjemdahl P. Studies *in vivo* and *in vitro* of terbutaline-induced β-adrenoceptor desensitization in healthy subjects. Clin Sci (Lond) 1987;72:47–54.
67. Furchgott RF. The use of β-haloalkylamines in the differentiation of receptors and in the determination of dissociation constants of receptor-agonist complexes. Adv Drug Res 1966;3:21–55.
68. Rabe KF, Giembycz MA, Dent G, et al. Salmeterol is a competitive antagonist at β-adrenoceptors mediating inhibition of respiratory burst in guinea-pig eosinophils. Eur J Pharmacol 1993;231:305–8.
69. Munoz NM, Rabe KF, Vita AJ, et al. Paradoxical blockade of β-adrenergically-mediated inhibition of stimulated eosinophil secretion by salmeterol. J Pharmacol Exp Ther 1995;273:850–4.
70. Newton R. Molecular mechanisms of glucocorticoid action: what is important? Thorax 2000;55:603–13.
71. Kyriakis JM, Avruch J. Mammalian mitogen-activated protein kinase signal transduction pathways activated by stress and inflammation. Physiol Rev 2001;81:807–69.
72. Clark AR, Martins JR, Tchen CR. Role of dual specificity phosphatases in biological responses to glucocorticoids. J Biol Chem 2008;283:25765–9.
73. Manetsch M, Ramsay EE, King EM, et al. Corticosteroids and β_2-agonists upregulate mitogen-activated protein kinase phosphatase 1: in vitro mechanisms. Br J Pharmacol 2012;166:2049–59.
74. Quante T, Ng YC, Ramsay EE, et al. Corticosteroids reduce IL-6 in ASM cells via up-regulation of MKP-1. Am J Respir Cell Mol Biol 2008;39:208–17.
75. Lee J, Komatsu K, Lee BC, et al. Phosphodiesterase 4B mediates extracellular signal-regulated kinase-dependent up-regulation of mucin MUC5AC protein by *Streptococcus pneumoniae* by inhibiting cAMP-protein kinase A-dependent MKP-1 phosphatase pathway. J Biol Chem 2012;287:22799–811.
76. Issa R, Xie S, Khorasani N, et al. Corticosteroid inhibition of growth-related oncogene protein-alpha via mitogen-activated kinase phosphatase-1 in airway smooth muscle cells. J Immunol 2007;178:7366–75.
77. King EM, Holden NS, Gong W, et al. Inhibition of NF-κB-dependent transcription by MKP-1: transcriptional repression by glucocorticoids occurring via p38 MAPK. J Biol Chem 2009;284:26803–15.

78. Diefenbacher M, Sekula S, Heilbock C, et al. Restriction to Fos family members of Trip6-dependent coactivation and glucocorticoid receptor-dependent transrepression of activator protein-1. Mol Endocrinol 2008;22:1767–80.

79. Lasa M, Abraham SM, Boucheron C, et al. Dexamethasone causes sustained expression of mitogen-activated protein kinase (MAPK) phosphatase 1 and phosphatase-mediated inhibition of MAPK p38. Mol Cell Biol 2002;22: 7802–11.

80. Abraham SM, Lawrence T, Kleiman A, et al. Antiinflammatory effects of dexamethasone are partly dependent on induction of dual specificity phosphatase 1. J Exp Med 2006;203:1883–9.

81. Li F, Zhang M, Hussain F, et al. Inhibition of p38 MAPK-dependent bronchial contraction after ozone by corticosteroids. Eur Respir J 2011;37:933–42.

82. Manetsch M, Rahman MM, Patel BS, et al. Long-acting β_2-agonists increase fluticasone propionate-induced mitogen-activated protein kinase phosphatase 1 (MKP-1) in airway smooth muscle cells. PLoS One 2013;8:e59635.

83. Kwak SP, Hakes DJ, Martell KJ, et al. Isolation and characterization of a human dual specificity protein-tyrosine phosphatase gene. J Biol Chem 1994;269: 3596–604.

84. Cho IJ, Woo NR, Shin IC, et al. H89, an inhibitor of PKA and MSK, inhibits cyclic-AMP response element binding protein-mediated MAPK phosphatase-1 induction by lipopolysaccharide. Inflamm Res 2009;58:863–72.

85. Innes AL, Woodruff PG, Ferrando RE, et al. Epithelial mucin stores are increased in the large airways of smokers with airflow obstruction. Chest 2006;130:1102–8.

86. Caramori G, Casolari P, Di Gregorio C, et al. MUC5AC expression is increased in bronchial submucosal glands of stable COPD patients. Histopathology 2009;55: 321–31.

87. Dohrman A, Miyata S, Gallup M, et al. Mucin gene (MUC2 and MUC5AC) upregulation by Gram-positive and Gram-negative bacteria. Biochim Biophys Acta 1998;1406:251–9.

88. Ayroldi E, Riccardi C. Glucocorticoid-induced leucine zipper (GILZ): a new important mediator of glucocorticoid action. FASEB J 2009;23:3649–58.

89. Mittelstadt PR, Ashwell JD. Inhibition of AP-1 by the glucocorticoid-inducible protein GILZ. J Biol Chem 2001;276:29603–10.

90. Godot V, Garcia G, Capel F, et al. Dexamethasone and IL-10 stimulate glucocorticoid-induced leucine zipper synthesis by human mast cells. Allergy 2006;61:886–90.

91. Ayroldi E, Migliorati G, Bruscoli S, et al. Modulation of T-cell activation by the glucocorticoid-induced leucine zipper factor via inhibition of nuclear factor kappaB. Blood 2001;98:743–53.

92. Di Marco B, Massetti M, Bruscoli S, et al. Glucocorticoid-induced leucine zipper (GILZ)/NF-κB interaction: role of GILZ homo-dimerization and C-terminal domain. Nucleic Acids Res 2007;35:517–28.

93. Ayroldi E, Zollo O, Macchiarulo A, et al. Glucocorticoid-induced leucine zipper inhibits the Raf-extracellular signal-regulated kinase pathway by binding to Raf-1. Mol Cell Biol 2002;22:7929–41.

94. Eddleston J, Herschbach J, Wagelie-Steffen AL, et al. The anti-inflammatory effect of glucocorticoids is mediated by glucocorticoid-induced leucine zipper in epithelial cells. J Allergy Clin Immunol 2007;119:115–22.

95. Heximer SP, Watson N, Linder ME, et al. RGS2/G0S8 is a selective inhibitor of Gqα function. Proc Natl Acad Sci U S A 1997;94:14389–93.

96. Holden NS, Bell MJ, Rider CF, et al. β_2-Adrenoceptor agonist-induced RGS2 expression is a genomic mechanism of bronchoprotection that is enhanced by glucocorticoids. Proc Natl Acad Sci U S A 2011;108:19713–8.

97. Liu C, Li Q, Zhou X, et al. Regulator of G-protein signaling 2 inhibits acid-induced mucin5AC hypersecretion in human airway epithelial cells. Respir Physiol Neurobiol 2013;185:265–71.

98. Snelgrove RJ, Goulding J, Didierlaurent AM, et al. A critical function for CD200 in lung immune homeostasis and the severity of influenza infection. Nat Immunol 2008;9:1074–83.

99. Wang ZQ, Xing WM, Fan HH, et al. The novel lipopolysaccharide-binding protein CRISPLD2 is a critical serum protein to regulate endotoxin function. J Immunol 2009;183:6646–56.

100. Kaplan F, Ledoux P, Kassamali FQ, et al. A novel developmentally regulated gene in lung mesenchyme: homology to a tumor-derived trypsin inhibitor. Am J Physiol 1999;276:L1027–36.

101. Samuelsson MK, Pazirandeh A, Davani B, et al. p57^{kip2}, a glucocorticoid-induced inhibitor of cell cycle progression in HeLa cells. Mol Endocrinol 1999;13:1811–22.

102. Dekkers BG, Pehlic A, Mariani R, et al. Glucocorticosteroids and β_2-adrenoceptor agonists synergize to inhibit airway smooth muscle remodeling. J Pharmacol Exp Ther 2012;342:780–7.

103. Chang TS, Kim MJ, Ryoo K, et al. p57^{KIP2} modulates stress-activated signaling by inhibiting c-*Jun* NH$_2$-terminal kinase/stress-activated protein kinase. J Biol Chem 2003;278:48092–8.

104. Yoshimura A, Naka T, Kubo M. SOCS proteins, cytokine signalling and immune regulation. Nat Rev Immunol 2007;7:454–65.

105. Milne GR, Palmer TM, Yarwood SJ. Novel control of cAMP-regulated transcription in vascular endothelial cells. Biochem Soc Trans 2012;40:1–5.

106. Nasreen N, Khodayari N, Sukka-Ganesh B, et al. Fluticasone propionate and salmeterol combination induces SOCS-3 expression in airway epithelial cells. Int Immunopharmacol 2012;12:217–25.

107. Liang R, Zhang W, Song YM. Levels of leptin and IL-6 in lungs and blood are associated with the severity of chronic obstructive pulmonary disease in patients and rat models. Mol Med Rep 2013;7:1470–6.

108. Barnes PJ. The cytokine network in COPD. Am J Respir Cell Mol Biol 2009;41:631–8.

109. Hershko A, Ciechanover A. The ubiquitin system. Annu Rev Biochem 1998;67:425–79.

110. Jono H, Lim JH, Chen LF, et al. NF-kappaB is essential for induction of CYLD, the negative regulator of NF-κB: evidence for a novel inducible autoregulatory feedback pathway. J Biol Chem 2004;279:36171–4.

111. Reiley W, Zhang M, Sun SC. Negative regulation of JNK signaling by the tumor suppressor CYLD. J Biol Chem 2004;279:55161–7.

112. Lim JH, Jono H, Komatsu K, et al. CYLD negatively regulates transforming growth factor-β-signalling via deubiquitinating Akt. Nat Commun 2012;3:771.

113. Sun SC. CYLD: a tumor suppressor deubiquitinase regulating NF-κB activation and diverse biological processes. Cell Death Differ 2010;17:25–34.

114. Lim JH, Ha UH, Woo CH, et al. CYLD is a crucial negative regulator of innate immune response in *Escherichia coli* pneumonia. Cell Microbiol 2008;10:2247–56.

115. Lim JH, Jono H, Koga T, et al. Tumor suppressor CYLD acts as a negative regulator for non-typeable *Haemophilus influenza*-induced inflammation in the middle ear and lung of mice. PLoS One 2007;2:e1032.

116. Lim JH, Stirling B, Derry J, et al. Tumor suppressor CYLD regulates acute lung injury in lethal *Streptococcus pneumoniae* infections. Immunity 2007;27:349–60.
117. Komatsu K, Lee JY, Miyata M, et al. Inhibition of PDE4B suppresses inflammation by increasing expression of the deubiquitinase CYLD. Nat Commun 2013;4: 1684.
118. Anderson P. Post-transcriptional control of cytokine production. Nat Immunol 2008;9:353–9.
119. King EM, Kaur M, Gong W, et al. Regulation of tristetraprolin expression by interleukin-1β and dexamethasone in human pulmonary epithelial cells: roles for nuclear factor-κB and p38 mitogen-activated protein kinase. J Pharmacol Exp Ther 2009;330:575–85.
120. Smoak K, Cidlowski JA. Glucocorticoids regulate tristetraprolin synthesis and post-transcriptionally regulate tumor necrosis factor α inflammatory signaling. Mol Cell Biol 2006;26:9126–35.
121. Ishmael FT, Fang X, Galdiero MR, et al. Role of the RNA-binding protein tristetraprolin in glucocorticoid-mediated gene regulation. J Immunol 2008;180: 8342–53.
122. Jalonen U, Leppanen T, Kankaanranta H, et al. Salbutamol increases tristetraprolin expression in macrophages. Life Sci 2007;81:1651–8.
123. Rider CF, King EM, Holden NS, et al. Inflammatory stimuli inhibit glucocorticoid-dependent transactivation in human pulmonary epithelial cells: rescue by long-acting β2-adrenoceptor agonists. J Pharmacol Exp Ther 2011;338:860–9.
124. Salem S, Harris T, Mok JS, et al. Transforming growth factor-β impairs glucocorticoid activity in the A549 lung adenocarcinoma cell line. Br J Pharmacol 2012; 166:2036–48.
125. Hinzey A, Alexander J, Corry J, et al. Respiratory syncytial virus represses glucocorticoid receptor-mediated gene activation. Endocrinology 2011;152: 483–94.
126. Rider CF, Miller-Larsson A, Proud D, et al. Modulation of transcriptional responses by poly(I:C) and human rhinovirus: effect of long-acting β2-adrenoceptor agonists. Eur J Pharmacol 2013;708:60–7.
127. Xie Y, Jiang H, Nguyen H, et al. Regulator of G protein signaling 2 is a key modulator of airway hyperresponsiveness. J Allergy Clin Immunol 2012;130:968–76.
128. Holden NS, Rider CF, Bell MJ, et al. Enhancement of inflammatory mediator release by β2-adrenoceptor agonists in airway epithelial cells is reversed by glucocorticoid action. Br J Pharmacol 2010;160:410–20.
129. Manolitsas ND, Wang J, Devalia JL, et al. Regular albuterol, nedocromil sodium, and bronchial inflammation in asthma. Am J Respir Crit Care Med 1995;151: 1925–30.
130. Gauvreau GM, Jordana M, Watson RM, et al. Effect of regular inhaled albuterol on allergen-induced late responses and sputum eosinophils in asthmatic subjects. Am J Respir Crit Care Med 1997;156:1738–45.
131. Giembycz MA, Newton R. Beyond the dogma: novel β2-adrenoceptor signalling in the airways. Eur Respir J 2006;27:1286–306.
132. Lecuona E, Ridge K, Pesce L, et al. The GTP-binding protein RhoA mediates Na, K-ATPase exocytosis in alveolar epithelial cells. Mol Biol Cell 2003;14: 3888–97.
133. Wang WC, Schillinger RM, Malone MM, et al. Paradoxical attenuation of β2-AR function in airway smooth muscle by Gi-mediated counterregulation in transgenic mice over-expressing type 5 adenylyl cyclase. Am J Physiol Lung Cell Mol Physiol 2011;300:L472–8.

134. Giembycz MA, Newton R. Harnessing the clinical efficacy of phosphodiesterase 4 inhibitors in inflammatory lung diseases: dual-selective phosphodiesterase inhibitors and novel combination therapies. Handb Exp Pharmacol 2011;204: 415–46.
135. Giembycz MA. Can the anti-inflammatory potential of PDE4 inhibitors be realized: guarded optimism or wishful thinking? Br J Pharmacol 2008;155:288–90.
136. Burgin AB, Magnusson OT, Singh J, et al. Design of phosphodiesterase 4D (PDE4D) allosteric modulators for enhancing cognition with improved safety. Nat Biotechnol 2010;28:63–70.
137. Shan WJ, Huang L, Zhou Q, et al. Dual β_2-adrenoceptor agonists-PDE4 inhibitors for the treatment of asthma and COPD. Bioorg Med Chem Lett 2012;22: 1523–6.
138. Liu A, Huang L, Wang Z, et al. Hybrids consisting of the pharmacophores of salmeterol and roflumilast or phthalazinone: dual β_2-adrenoceptor agonists-PDE4 inhibitors for the treatment of COPD. Bioorg Med Chem Lett 2013;23:1548–52.

New Drug Therapies for COPD

Clare L. Ross, MRCP, Trevor T. Hansel, FRCPath, PhD*

KEYWORDS

- COPD • Pharmacology • Bronchodilators • Antiinflammatory drugs • Antioxidants
- Protease inhibitors • Fibrosis • Lung regeneration

KEY POINTS

- It is proving a major challenge to produce new effective drugs for chronic obstructive pulmonary disease (COPD).
- Improved understanding of COPD pathophysiology, novel clinical trial designs, endpoints, imaging and biomarkers, noninvasive sampling, patient stratification, challenge models, and clinical trial designs is necessary to facilitate development of new drugs for COPD.
- Smoking cessation is fundamental and new approaches include antinicotine vaccines, cannabinoid receptor antagonists, and dopamine D3 receptor antagonists.
- Novel combinations of inhaled bronchodilators and corticosteroids are being introduced.
- Antiinfective drugs are important, with a recent focus on the viruses that commonly cause exacerbations.
- Antiinflammatory drugs are in development, including kinase inhibitors, chemokine receptor antagonists, inhibitors of innate immune mechanisms, and statins.
- Biologics used in rheumatoid diseases may also have a role; anti-IL-6 (tocilizumab) is promising.
- Antioxidants, mucolytics, antiproteases, and antifibrotics are all under active development.
- Aids to lung regeneration have potential to alter the natural history of COPD, including retinoids and mesenchymal stem cell therapy.

INTRODUCTION

New drugs for chronic obstructive pulmonary disease (COPD) have been largely based on existing classes of current therapies, involving new inhaled combinations of long-acting muscarinic antagonists (LAMAs), long-acting beta2-agonists (LABAs), and inhaled corticosteroids (ICS) **(Table 1)**.[1] A useful reference source for new

This article originally appeared in *Clinics in Chest Medicine*, Volume 35, Issue 1, March 2014.
Imperial Clinical Respiratory Research Unit (ICRRU), Biomedical Research Centre (BMRC), Centre for Respiratory Infection (CRI), National Heart and Lung Institute (NHLI), St Mary's Hospital, Imperial College, Praed Street, Paddington, London W2 INY, UK
* Corresponding author.
E-mail address: t.hansel@imperial.ac.uk

Clinics Collections 6 (2015) 263–291
http://dx.doi.org/10.1016/j.ccol.2015.05.043

2352-7986/15/$ – see front matter © 2015 Elsevier Inc. All rights reserved.

Table 1 Drugs to aid smoking cessation	
Current treatments	First-line: • Nicotine replacement therapy • Bupropion • Varenicline (partial agonist for $\alpha4\beta2$ nicotinic acetylcholine receptors) Second-line: • Nortriptyline • Clonidine
New approaches	• Antinicotine vaccines: NicVAX, SEL-068 • Electronic cigarettes • Novel nicotine formulations: eg, inhaled aerosolized nicotine (ARD-1600) • Nicotine partial agonist: cytisine • Cannabinoid receptor 1 antagonists: taranabant • Dopamine D3 receptor antagonists: GSK598809 • Monoamine oxidase inhibitors: selegiline

COPD medicines in development is the Pharmaceutical Research and Manufacturers of America (www.phrma.org). There is also an excellent series of topical articles on "The COPD Pipeline" provided by Nicholas J. Gross in the journal COPD (22 articles as of mid-2012). Although recent increases in knowledge of the inflammatory components contributing to COPD have led to many new targets for COPD treatment,[2] very few new classes of drugs are being licensed, making this a controversial area for new drug development.[3]

Clinical studies with new drugs for COPD have been difficult for several reasons[4]:

- The immunopathology of COPD is complex and variable (**Fig. 1**). Cigarette smoke has widespread effects beyond the respiratory system, involving the large airways (bronchitis), small airways (bronchiolitis), lung interstitium (emphysema and interstitial lung disease), pulmonary vasculature (pulmonary artery hypertension), and systemic complications.[5–7] Pathologic features such as mucus hypersecretion, small airway fibrosis, and lung destruction (emphysema) are notoriously difficult to reverse with drugs.
- COPD may be caused by the innate immune response to oxidants and microbes, with accelerated aging and autoimmune features. Bacteria and viruses may become more important in more severe COPD.[8]
- Preclinical models need to be improved for in vitro and in vivo (animal) studies.[9]
- COPD patients are often elderly, frail, and have multiple diseases associated with smoking. Cardiovascular diseases, metabolic syndrome, and malignancies may be present. Hence, these patients may be on a variety of medications. These factors may mean that it is difficult to recruit patients when there are strict entry criteria.
- A new therapy is more likely to be effective when used early in the natural history of COPD, before irreversible disease has occurred. However, delays in diagnosis are common and the disease is notoriously underdiagnosed.
- Small proof-of-concept studies in humans are poorly predictive of efficacy in clinical practice. Some clinical development plans for COPD have been discontinued after large-scale clinical trials, including Viozan, recombinant DNase (Pulmozyme), and cilomilast (Ariflo).
- Challenge models looking at the effects of cigarette smoke,[10] ozone, or lipopolysaccharide have been developed. On the other hand, smoking cessation is part

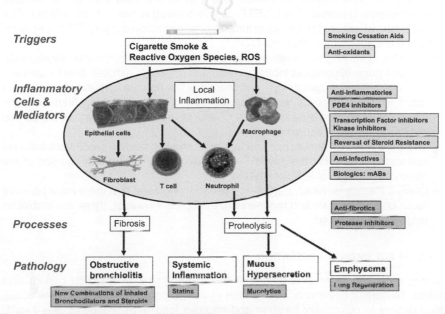

Fig. 1. Pathology, targets, and new drugs for COPD. An overview of some of the pathophysiologic processes involved in COPD, highlighting potential therapeutic targets for novel therapies. Cigarette smoke contains reactive oxygen species, particulates, and chemicals, which lead to a range of inflammatory effects: macrophage, epithelial cell, and CD8+ T cell activation. These cells in turn release neutrophil chemotactic factors. Numerous local inflammatory mediators are then released, along with proteases, which break down connective tissue in the lung, causing emphysema. Proteases are also important in stimulating mucus hypersecretion, which may manifest as chronic bronchitis. Profibrotic mediators are also released by epithelial cells, contributing to fibroblast proliferation and small airway fibrosis. Novel therapies include those aimed at local as well as systemic inflammation. The most ambitious target is to regenerate lung tissue in response to emphysema. mABs, monoclonal antibodies; PDE4, phosphodiesterase 4.

of COPD patient care, providing an interesting situation of withdrawal of the stimulus.[10–12] As a model of COPD exacerbations, live experimental challenge can be performed with human rhinovirus (HRV) in patients with COPD.[13] Novel large scale clinical trial designs for COPD are also needed.[14]

- There is a need to identify and validate endpoints that can capture the considerable heterogeneity of pulmonary and systemic features. Forced expiratory volume in 1 second (FEV_1) is a commonly used endpoint in most clinical COPD trials. However, recently, the Evaluation of COPD Longitudinally to Identify Predictive Surrogate Endpoints (ECLIPSE) study has demonstrated that the annual rate of change in FEV_1 in COPD is highly variable in different subjects.[15] In addition, given that the FEV_1 declines very slowly during the natural history of COPD, an estimated 1000 subjects per sample group must be followed for a minimum of 3 years to have sufficient power to detect a 50% improvement in disease progression.[16]
- Phenotypes of COPD need to be defined and validated in order to tailor drugs to individual patients; it is becoming increasing clear that "one size does not fit all"

in COPD.[17] This was demonstrated clearly by recent trials such as the National Emphysema Treatment Trial (NETT), which showed a mortality benefit in only a subgroup of patients undergoing lung volume reduction surgery.[18] Of special interest are approaches that use CT.[7,19]

- Samples of varying invasiveness and from different compartments are required. Sputum gene expression looks promising,[20] although exhaled breath condensate has been disappointing,[21] and there are few studies with exhaled nitric oxide.[22] However, assessment by proteomics of epithelial lining fluid from the airway of COPD patients is feasible,[23] and bronchial brushings can be carried out to assess gene expression.[24]
- There is a need to identify and validate biomarkers that may predict potential responders for specific therapy.[25–27] Gene expression or transcriptomics of the airway in COPD is of special interest.[20,24]
- Current therapy is merely palliative; it is becoming clear that there must be more focus on preventative and regenerative therapies. However, these are ambitious targets for new drugs.

DRUGS TO AID SMOKING CESSATION

Smoking cessation is the first priority in the management of a COPD patient who smokes. To date, it is the only intervention shown to convincingly reduce the accelerated decline in pulmonary function and improve long-term prognosis (see **Fig. 1**, **Table 1**).[28,29] Success in quitting is increased by behavioral support in addition to a range of pharmacotherapies.[30] However, a recent systematic review has concluded that, in contrast to non-COPD smokers, neither the intensity of counseling nor the type of antismoking drug make a significant difference in smoking cessation results.[31]

The most widely used agents include nicotine replacement (in a variety of preparations), antidepressants such as bupropion and nortriptyline, and nicotine partial receptor agonists such as varenicline (which remains the most efficacious monotherapy for smoking cessation[32]). Cytisine, a partial agonist that binds with high affinity to the $\alpha4\beta2$ subtype of the nicotine acetylcholine receptor is effective in sustaining abstinence at 12 months.[33] Other approaches currently under investigation include nicotine vaccines (with the associated benefits of infrequent dosing and prolonged effect); however, large trials of the current front-runners (NicVAx and NIC002) have been disappointing.[34,35] Both agents stimulate the production of antibodies that bind to nicotine and prevent it from crossing the blood-brain barrier. Novel nicotine products that can be given via the inhaled, topical (in the form of a spray) or orally dissolving film route are also under development, and detailed in a recent review.[36] Compounds are also being explored to target other neurotransmitters implicated in nicotine dependence such as dopamine, γ- aminobutyric acid (GABA), and glutamate.[37] These include trials of monoamine oxidase inhibitors such as selegiline.[36] The cannabinoid receptor system is thought to inhibit indirectly the dopamine-mediated rewarding properties of food and tobacco, and cannabinoid receptor 1 antagonists are undergoing evaluation, although trials have so far been disappointing.[36] There is increasing popularity of electronic cigarettes, which deliver nicotine via an electronic battery-powered device resembling a cigarette, despite no formal demonstration of the efficacy and safety of such devices. These devices have the potential advantage of tackling the psychological and physical components of nicotine addiction; therefore, several large prospective studies are now underway.[38]

INHALED BRONCHODILATORS AND CORTICOSTEROIDS
Inhaled Bronchodilators

The development of improved bronchodilators has focused on finding better inhaled LABAs and LAMAs (**Table 2**).[39–41] Novel classes of bronchodilator have been difficult to develop because they often have additional unwanted effects on vascular smooth muscle, producing postural hypotension and headaches. Until recently, all LABAs required twice-daily dosing, but newer once-daily agents, ultra-LABAs (ULABAs), such as indacaterol, olodaterol, vilanterol, and carmoterol are proving to be effective.[39,42–44] Aclidinium bromide is a new LAMA that has an acute onset of action (compared with tiotropium's slower onset of action) but has disappointed in trials to date.[45,46] Other LAMAs with a more rapid onset of action are in development. Glycopyrronium bromide/NVA237 has been shown to provide comparable effects to tiotropium.[47–49] Another company is soon to start phase III trials with nebulized LAMA, EP-101, a glycopyrrolate solution. Two single-molecule, dual-action bronchodilators, muscarinic antagonist and beta2-agonists (MABAs), are in phase I and II trials, including GSK961081.

Studies looking at the benefits of dual LABA or LAMA (salmeterol or formoterol with tiotropium) therapy have demonstrated greater bronchodilation and fewer symptoms when the drugs are combined, than with either agent alone.[50–52] New ULABAs allow for once-daily administration of LABA-LAMA combination inhaler, and a recent study

Table 2 Inhaled bronchodilators and corticosteroids and corticosteroid-related approaches	
Ultralong-acting β2-agonists	Abadeterol AZD3199 Olodaterol (BI1744CL) Carmoterol Vilanterol (GSK642444) Indacaterol (QAB149)
LAMA	Aclidinium (LAS-34273) AZD8683 Umeclidinium (GSK573719) Glycopyrronium (NVA237)
Muscarinic antagonist and β2-agonist	AZD2115 GSK961081
LABA + LAMA	Formoterol + aclidinium Olodaterol + tiotropium Vilanterol + umeclidinium Indacaterol + glycopyrronium (QVA149)
ICS + Ultralong-acting β2-agonists	Beclomethasone + formoterol (Fostair) Fluticasone + vilanterol (Relovair) Mometasone + formoterol (Dulera) Fluticasone + formoterol (Flutiform) Mometasone + indacaterol (QMF149) Ciclesonide + formoterol
New corticosteroid-related approaches	Nonglucocorticoid steroids Selective glucocorticoid receptor agonists
Reversal of steroid resistance	Theophylline (histone deacetylase 2 activators) Phosphoinositide-3-kinase inhibitors LABAs and phosphodiesterase 4/LABAs (via phosphoinositide-3-kinase inhibition)

has demonstrated significant benefits in FEV_1 using QVA149 (a combination of glyco-pyrronium bromide and indacaterol) versus indacaterol alone or placebo.[53] Aclidinium has been combined with formoterol as a LAMA and LABA combination.[46]

Attempts to combine existing classes of drugs with additional agents have proved less successful, as demonstrated by the arrested development of the novel D2 dopamine receptor–β2 adrenoreceptor agonist sibenadet (Viozan). The rationale for this agent was based on observations that sensory afferent nerves were key mediators of COPD symptoms such as breathlessness, cough, and excess sputum production, and advocates of Viozan hypothesized that that activation of D2-receptors on such nerves would modulate their activity.[54] Although initial short-term studies were promising, the duration of the bronchodilator effect diminished as studies progressed and no sustained benefit was reported in a 1-year large-scale trial.[55]

ICS

Current United Kingdom and international guidance, despite little supporting evidence, recommend ICS for symptomatic patients with an FEV_1 lower than 50% and/or frequent exacerbations. These are usually prescribed in the form of a combination inhaler containing LABA. In reality ICS-LABA inhalers may be used inappropriately in an excessive number of COPD patients who do not meet the criteria outlined by the Global Initiative for Chronic Obstructive Lung Disease (GOLD) guidelines.[56] A Spanish study found a rate of inappropriate ICS use of 18.2%.[57]

A Cochrane review of the role of ICS included studies published up until July 2011.[58] This review concluded that long-term (>6 months) ICS use did not consistently reduce the rate of decline in FEV_1 in COPD patients. There was no statistically significant effect on mortality in COPD subjects, but long-term use of ICS did reduce the mean rate of exacerbations in those studies in which pooling of data was possible. In addition, there was slowing of the rate of decline in quality of life (measured by the St. George's Respiratory Questionnaire). There was an increased risk of oropharyngeal candidiasis and hoarseness with ICS use and, in the long-term studies, the rate of pneumonia was increased in the ICS group compared with the placebo group. Although ICS does seem to have some beneficial effects in COPD, when compared with long-acting bronchodilators, the latter agents seem to provide similar benefits to ICS or ICS-LABA combinations in exacerbation reduction without the side effects associated with ICS use.[59]

One alternative may be the use of nonglucocorticoid steroids. EPI-12323 is a once-daily, small molecule, inhaled nonglucocorticoid steroid and may not exhibit any of the classic side effects of glucocorticoid steroids. It may also be possible to avoid the unwanted side effects of glucocorticoids by selectively inducing transrepression genomic mechanisms (which are responsible for many desirable antiinflammatory and immunomodulating effects), whereas transactivation processes (associated with frequently occurring side effects) are simultaneously less affected.[60,61] An inhaled selective glucocorticoid receptor agonist is currently undergoing clinical trials.

For patients who remain symptomatic despite LABA-ICS combination, GOLD recommends triple therapy with LAMA, LABA, and ICS. The rationale behind this seems logical because all three agents work via different mechanisms on different targets, potentially allowing for lower doses of the individual agents to be used, accompanied by improved side-effect profiles. However, there has been a lack of sufficiently powered studies primarily addressing the benefits of triple therapy versus LABA-ICS therapy, or, indeed, versus dual LABA-LAMA therapy.[62,63] A single inhaler combining all three agents is currently in formational development, although the ICS to be used has not been confirmed. Once-daily ICS are now in development to allow future trials with once-daily triple-therapy combined inhalers. These inhalers may well improve compliance, but titration of individual component drug doses may prove difficult, and disease severity seems to affect the drug dose-response curve.[64]

Steroid Resistance

Interestingly, ICS do not seem to suppress inflammation in COPD. One hypothesis attributes this to the marked reduction in histone deacetylase 2 (HDAC2), the nuclear enzyme that corticosteroids require to switch off activated inflammatory genes,[65] rendering these patients resistant to the effects of ICS. The reduction in HDAC2 is thought to be secondary to oxidative stress, both independent of and by way of activation of phosphoinositide-3-kinase-δ (PI3Kδ).[66] Inhibition of PI3Kδ has recently shown to restore corticosteroid sensitivity in mice[66] and may hold therapeutic promise.[67,68] One group has shown that formoterol reverses oxidative stress-induced corticosteroid insensitivity via PI3Kδ.[68] Low-dose theophylline has shown to enhance the antiinflammatory effects of steroids during exacerbations of COPD[69] and seems to have the capacity to restore the reduced HDAC2 activity in COPD macrophages.[70] More recently, roflumilast has shown to augment the ability of formoterol to enhance glucocorticoid-dependent gene transcription in human airway epithelial cells.[71]

ANTIINFECTIVE AND ANTIINFLAMMATORY AGENTS
Antibiotics

The Lung Health Study of North America revealed that lower respiratory tract illnesses promote FEV_1 decline in current smokers (**Table 3**).[72] There is growing evidence that exacerbations accelerate the progressive decline in lung function in COPD patients.[73] Several lines of evidence now implicate bacteria as an important cause of exacerbations[74] and bacterial colonization is frequently found in patients with COPD.[75] It is associated with the frequency of exacerbations.[76] There seems to be a correlation between bacterial colonization of lower airways and elevated levels of inflammatory mediators.[77] Finally, patients with severe COPD who receive inappropriate antibiotic treatment are vulnerable to multidrug-resistant infections.[78]

It has become increasingly difficult to develop new antibiotics, so that there is a need for novel types of therapy. Bacteriophages are bacterial viruses that are approximately 10 times more numerous than bacteria in nature. Although they have been used in Russia for many decades as antibacterial agents, they have been used less in Western medicine.[79] Lytic phages are highly specific to particular bacteria and are well tolerated, with no risk of overgrowth of intestinal flora. They may be administered by inhalation, so may be effective in the treatment of respiratory bacterial infections.

Antimicrobial peptides, including α-defensins, β-defensins, and cathelicidins, are produced from epithelial and other cells in the respiratory tract and play a key role in innate immunity and stimulating adaptive immune responses.[80] These peptides may also be considered potential future therapies.

Although the molecular mechanisms for these effects are not fully clear, 14- and 15-membered ring macrolide antibiotics have several antiinflammatory effects in addition to their antibacterial actions.[81] It has been shown that these drugs decrease the production of cytokines in the lungs.[82] A recent large clinical trial, with more than 1142 volunteers, randomized subjects to daily administration of 250 mg of azithromycin or placebo for 1 year.[83] The median time to the first acute exacerbation in the azithromycin group was increased by 92 days, and the frequency of exacerbations in the azithromycin group was significantly reduced. However, deafness was observed in the

Table 3
Antiinfective and antiinflammatory agents

Antibacterials	Antibiotics, antimicrobial peptides, bacteriophages, vaccines
Antivirals	Antivirals (eg, neuraminidase inhibitors for influenza) Vaccines for influenza, HRV, and respiratory syncytial virus
Agents acting on pattern recognition by the innate immune system	Toll-like receptor inhibitors 2, 4, and 9 NLR agonists or antagonists RLR agonists or antagonists
Antagonists of cell surface receptors	CXCR2 antagonists (AZD5069); GSK1325756 CCR2 antagonists (CCR2b antagonist: AZD2423) Chemoattractant receptor-homologous molecule expressed on Th2 cells antagonists LTB_4 receptor antagonists Selectin antagonists
Phosphodiesterase (PDE)-4 inhibitors	PDE4i: roflumilast, tetomilast Inhaled selective PDE4B inhibitor: GSK25066 Dual selective PDE inhibitors Novel combinations: PDE4 +7A inhibition PDE3 + PDE4 inhibition (RPL554)
Kinase inhibition	p38 mitogen-activated protein kinase inhibitors (inhaled GSK610677) JNK inhibitors Syk inhibitors JAK/STAT inhibitors: tofacitinib
Transcription inhibition	NF-κB inhibitors: IKK2 inhibitors PI3K-γ/δ inhibitors Peroxisome proliferator-activated receptor-γ antagonists (rosiglitazone) Cyclosporine-A (inhaled)
Combating systemic inflammation	Statins

treatment group as an adverse event. Another long-term, placebo-controlled clinical trial examining macrolides in the prevention of acute exacerbations used erythromycin at a dose of 250 mg twice daily for 1 year.[84] A nonantibiotic macrolide such as EM704, derived from the structure of erythromycin, has been shown to inhibit neutrophilic inflammation, the release of TGF-β, and fibrosis in a bleomycin model of pulmonary fibrosis.[85] Such nonantibiotic macrolides may be delivered by inhalation during an exacerbation and will not affect antibiotic resistance patterns.

Recently, pulsed antibiotic prophylaxis has been trialed. Moxifloxacin has shown to reduce the odds of exacerbation in stable COPD subjects when given once a day for 5 days every 8 weeks for 48 weeks.[86] New pneumococcal vaccines are also in development that may prove more effective than are their current counterparts.

Antivirals

With advances in diagnostic techniques for viruses, such as polymerase chain reaction, there is evidence that the most COPD exacerbations are associated with viral infections and that, of these, HRV is the most common cause[87] and can directly infect the lower respiratory tract.[88] Up-regulation of the HRV receptor, intercellular adhesion molecule 1, on epithelial cells occurs in COPD patients and this may cause predisposition to infection.[89] When infected, COPD primary bronchial epithelial cells elicit exaggerated antiviral therapies, especially in relation to HIV, development of resistance to proinflammatory response.[90] Although there have been remarkable strides in the development of antiviral therapies, especially in relation to HIV, development of resistance to viral therapy is a recurrent problem[91] and there are no effective antirhinoviral treatments to date. Recently, an important model of human RV16 challenge has been introduced as a model of exacerbations in patients with COPD.[13]

Respiratory syncytial virus (RSV) is increasingly recognized in adults with COPD[92] and it can persist in stable disease.[93] Treatment of RSV infection remains largely supportive, although a monoclonal antibody (MoAB) therapy against RSV F protein (palivizumab) is licensed for specialist use in restricted circumstances.[94]

Seasonal influenza is another important cause of exacerbations of COPD and there is the fear that an influenza pandemic could cause high mortality in patients with COPD.[95] It is important that all patients with COPD have adequate influenza immunization and that they be considered for early treatment in the event of an influenza-induced exacerbation of COPD. Apart from vaccines, there are two licensed antiviral agents against influenza: zanamivir and oseltamivir (Tamiflu).[96] Nevertheless, development of resistance is a major problem and new anti-influenza agents are being actively sought.[97]

Agents Acting on Innate Immunity

Cigarette smoke has long been known to increase the permeability of the respiratory epithelium, thus compromising the barrier function. Respiratory viruses have a particular predilection for respiratory epithelial cells and these can then initiate nonspecific inflammation. Once the respiratory physical barrier is penetrated, danger signals meet the next part of the immune system defense: the pattern recognition receptors (PRRs). Recently, there has been recent dramatic progress in the understanding of the molecular and cellular details of how the innate nonspecific immune system is activated.[98] PRRs are thought to be central to the activation of the innate immune system and they have the capacity to drive chronic lung inflammation,[99] repair processes, fibrosis, and proteolysis. A unified theory can be made of how the development of mild-to-moderate COPD, as well as exacerbations of COPD, is mediated through interaction of reactive oxidant species (ROS), viruses, and bacteria with the innate immune system.[100] Molecular signatures on ROS, viruses, and bacteria, as well as from dead and damaged cells, cause rapid activation of the family of PRRs. Pathogen-associated molecular patterns (PAMPs) are found especially in the nucleic acid of the viruses that infect the respiratory epithelium and in various cell wall and cytoplasmic components of bacteria.[101] A variety of damage-associated molecular patterns (DAMPs) has been proposed, including high-mobility group box 1, S100 proteins, heat shock proteins (HSP), and extracellular matrix hyaluronans.

ROS activate Toll-like receptor (TLR) 2[102] and TLR4 using MyD88 signaling,[103,104] but they can also cause damage to membrane lipids and to DNA and thus activate DAMPs.[105,106] The cell wall of gram-negative bacteria contains lipopolysaccharide that activates cell surface TLR4, whereas various other bacterial components activate different cell surface TLRs. In contrast, viral nucleic acid motifs activate TLR3, 7, and 9, which are found on the inner surface of the endosomal membrane.

PRRs undergo extensive cross-talk with TLRs,[101] scavenger receptors,[107] and receptor for advanced glycation end-products (RAGE).[91,108] In addition, there are TLRs on endosomes that recognize viral nucleic acids and cytoplasmic PRRs that consist of retinoic acid-inducible gene-1 (RIG-1)-like receptors (RLRs), and NOD-like receptors (NLRs). Activation of PRRs takes place in COPD on epithelial cells, neutrophils, macrophages, smooth muscle[109] fibroblasts, and other cells of the airways. Acute cigarette smoke activates MyD88, a common adapter protein that is involved in the signaling of several TLRs (including TLR2, 4, 7, 8, and 9).[104]

Therefore, blocking PRRs, including TLRs that recognize and are activated by PAMPs on oxidants and infectious agents, may be a potential way of modulating disease activity in COPD. There are now intensive efforts to develop TLR-agonists and antagonists for treatment of diseases like COPD that involve inflammation and infection.[110] Eritoran, a synthetic TLR4 antagonist, has been shown to block influenza-induced lethality in mice, and may well provide a novel therapeutic approach for other infections.[111] PRRs activate a variety of signal transduction pathways, including NF-κB and mitogen-activated protein (MAP) kinase pathways, as well as type I interferon pathways in the case of viruses.[112] MyD88 offers another target for therapy.[104,113]

Chemokine Receptor Antagonists

CXC and CC chemokine receptors are thought to be involved in COPD inflammation due to their role in neutrophil recruitment. The concentrations of CXC chemokines, including CXCL5 and CXCL8, are increased during exacerbations and, because they all signal through a common receptor, CXCR2, specific antagonists of this receptor may be useful in treating exacerbations. A small molecule CXCR1/2 antagonist (AZD8309) shows promise in inhibiting sputum neutrophils, after inhaled endotoxin, by approximately 80%,[114] suggesting that this could be useful in exacerbations and has the advantage of oral administration. A proof-of-principle study revealed that SCH527123, a novel, selective CXCR2 antagonist, causes significant attenuation of ozone-induced airway neutrophilia in healthy subjects.[115] However, experimental inflammation by ozone challenge is chiefly CXCL8-dependent, transient, and fully reversible in contrast to the pathologic inflammation occurring in the airways of subjects with COPD, which depends on multiple mediators and is chronic and largely irreversible. This highlights the difficulty with current models. Interestingly, SCH527123 has now undergone phase 2 studies in subjects with moderate-to-severe COPD, during which there were beneficial effects on sputum neutrophil counts and FEV_1 (reported at the ERS in 2010).

Several other oral CXCR2 antagonists such as AZD5069 are currently in phase II trials and include secondary outcome measures of circulating blood neutrophil levels.

CX3CL1 binds exclusively to CX3C chemokine receptor 1 (CX3CR1), and is unregulated in the lung tissue of smokers with COPD, making this an attractive target.[38]

An inhaled CCR1 antagonist (AZD4818) failed to show benefit in COPD,[116] although a CCR2b antagonist (AZD2423) is currently in trials.

Chemoattractant Receptor-homologous Receptor Antagonism

Chemoattractant receptor-homologous molecule expressed on Th2 cells (CRTH2) is a G-protein coupled receptor expressed by Th2 lymphocytes, eosinophils, and basophils. The receptor mediates the activation and chemotaxis of these cell types in response to prostaglandin D2 (PGD_2), the major prostanoid produced by mast cell degranulation typically in the initial phase of IgE-mediated reactions but also thought to occur at sites of inflammation, such as the bronchial mucosa. As such, selective PGD_2 receptor antagonists (CRTh2 antagonists) are mainly in development for asthma.[117]

LTB_4 Receptor Antagonists

Serum concentrations of LTB_4, a potent neutrophil chemoattractant, are increased in patients with COPD.[118] LTB_4 activates BLT_1-receptors, which are expressed on neutrophils and T lymphocytes. Although BLT_1-antagonists have a relatively small effect on neutrophil chemotaxis in response to COPD sputum[119] and they have not proved to be effective in treating stable COPD, it is possible that they would have greater efficacy if used acutely, due to observations that LTB_4 is especially elevated during COPD exacerbations.[7]

LTA4H has been proposed as another potential therapeutic target because it is the enzyme responsible for generation of LTB_4 from leukotriene A2. However, another role for LTA4H has been observed, whereby it degrades another neutrophil chemoattractant, namely proline-glycine-proline (PGP),[120] thus therapeutic strategies inhibiting LTA4H to prevent LTB_4 generation may not reduce neutrophil recruitment due to simultaneous elevation in PGP levels, once again demonstrating the complexity of manipulating inflammatory processes in COPD.

Selectin Antagonism

The selectin family is a group of adhesion molecules involved in the initial activation and adhesion of leukocytes on the vascular endothelium, which facilitates their migration into the surrounding tissue. In a phase II trial in 77 COPD subjects, 28 days of bimosiamose (an inhaled pan-selectin antagonist) led to a significant decrease in the sputum macrophage count, and decreased CXCL8 and matrix metalloprotease (MMP)-9, whereas most lung function parameters also showed a small numeric increase with no difference in adverse events.[121] Trials with longer treatment durations are now required and an antiselectin MoAB (EL246) is currently under predevelopment.[122]

Phosphodiesterase Inhibitors

Theophylline has some PDE inhibitor activities and it as been used in the treatment of COPD for more than 75 years. However, its use is limited by its narrow therapeutic range, side-effect profile, and drug interactions. Newer selective PDE inhibitors are anticipated to exhibit the beneficial effects of theophylline with an improved side-effect profile. PDE4 inhibitors have a broad spectrum of antiinflammatory effects and are effective in animal models of COPD. However, in human studies their effectiveness has been limited by side effects, such as nausea, diarrhea, and headaches.[123,124]

Development of selective orally active PDE4 inhibitors has predominantly involved cilomilast (Ariflo), roflumilast, and tetomilast in inflammatory bowel disease.[125] Cilomilast has been studied in five phase III studies: involving 2088 subjects on cilomilast and 1408 on placebo for 24 weeks.[126] Although an initial study was very encouraging in 424 patients with COPD assessed for 6 weeks,[127] benefits were not as great in a larger study for 6 months,[128] and cilomilast failed to convince in other phase III studies. As a result, the entire cilomilast program was terminated, providing a cautionary example of the difficulties in developing new drugs for COPD.

In contrast, roflumilast has proved more effective in long-term studies,[129–132] especially in decreasing exacerbations, and is now the first in this new class of agents licensed for treatment of severe COPD with bronchitis.[133,134] Roflumilast is given once daily (500 μg), but gastrointestinal adverse effects and weight loss are common on starting therapy. The Roflumilast in the Prevention of COPD Exacerbations While Taking Appropriate Combination Treatment (REACT) study aims to assess whether or not roflumilast will provide additional benefit when added to dual or triple therapy.[135] This will also go some way to confirming the safety of the drug and it's future use, although it may be that newer inhaled PDE4 inhibitors will prove preferable in terms of reduced side effects. To date, inhaled PDE4 inhibitors have been found to be ineffective.

Avoidance of targeting certain isoforms should help limit side effects because mouse studies have suggested that emesis is the result of PDE4D inhibition,[136] whereas PDE4B is the predominant subtype present in monocytes and neutrophils and is implicated in the inflammatory process. This insight has led to the design of PDE4 inhibitor modulators, which have one to two orders of magnitude less affinity for the PDE4D isoform, while maintaining other PDE4 inhibitory activities. However, more work is needed to confirm whether targeting specific subtypes really is more beneficial. In addition, mixed PDE4/7 inhibitors are under development that may have synergistic benefits. TPI 1100, which comprises two antisense oligonucleotides targeting the mRNA for the PDE4B/4D and PDE7A isoforms, has been shown to reduce neutrophil influx and key cytokines in an established smoking mouse model.[137] A final approach may be use of a PDE4 inhibitor in combination with other antiinflammatory drugs such as glucocorticoids[138] based on recent findings that these drugs together may impart clinical benefit beyond that achievable by an ICS or a PDE4 alone.[71]

Kinase Inhibitors

After decades of research on oral kinase inhibitors, a JAK inhibitor has been licensed in 2012 for the treatment of rheumatoid arthritis.[139] There is also progress with orally active Syk inhibitors in autoimmune disease. p38 (p38 MAP kinase) is activated by bacteria and viruses, as well as other inflammatory signals and, therefore, is another target for inhibition.[140,141] These phosphorylases are involved in cell-signaling cascades, which often result in the activation of proinflammatory nuclear transcription factors such as NF-κB. Several p38 MAP kinase inhibitors are now in clinical development, and the results of a phase II trial with losmapimod (an oral p38 MAP kinase inhibitor) were published last year. Although losmapimod did not have an effect on sputum neutrophils or lung function, there was a significant reduction in plasma fibrinogen levels after 12 weeks, and improvements in lung hyperinflation were noted.[142]

Other broad-spectrum antiinflammatory drugs in development include inhibitors of NF-κB and PI3K. However, there is much interaction between signaling pathways and it may be that a multipronged approach is required.[125,143] NF-κB inhibition can be attempted through a variety of approaches; namely by inhibiting the degradation of the inhibitor of NF-κB family of proteins (IκB), gene transfer of IκB or IκB kinase (IKK) inhibition. Several IKK inhibitors are in development.[38] PI3K inhibitors also have therapeutic potential,[144,145] and selective inhibition may restore glucocorticoid sensitivity.[146] There are drugs directed against both the δ- and γ-isoforms of PI3K,[147,148] as well as an inhaled dual γ/δ inhibitor.[149] In addition, peroxisome proliferator-activated receptor gamma (PPAR-γ) antagonists such as rosiglitazone may treat airway mucus hypersecretion.[150] Finally, new formulations of cyclosporine A (inhaled) are being developed for asthma and COPD.[151]

Statins

COPD is associated with a complex list of systemic manifestations, including systemic inflammation associated with cachexia and skeletal muscle weakness.[152,153] COPD also has an extensive association with comorbidities, such as cardiovascular diseases,[154] and it is recognized that new drugs are required for COPD and these comorbidities.[155] This subset of patients with persistent systemic inflammation has been associated with poor clinical outcomes, irrespective of their lung impairment.[156] It is recognized that skeletal muscle weakness and wasting may also be amenable to therapy.[157,158]

This has encouraged the use of statins in COPD because they have a range of systemic antiinflammatory effects.[159] Statins increase survival in patients with peripheral arterial disease and COPD,[160] and may reduce COPD exacerbations.[161] Furthermore, retrospective studies have shown that statins reduce the risk of death in patients with COPD.[162–164] The benefit on all-cause mortality depends on the level of underlying systemic inflammation, as assessed using high-sensitivity C-reactive protein (hsCRP) measurements.[165] Various academic institutions are currently conducting studies looking at the effect of statins on the frequency of COPD exacerbations in patients with moderate-to-severe COPD who are prone to exacerbations, but may not have other indications for statin treatment. In addition, statins have been associated with a reduced risk of extrapulmonary cancers in patients with COPD.[166]

MISCELLANEOUS ADDITIONAL CLASSES OF NEW DRUGS
Antioxidants

Each inhalation of cigarette smoke contains a large burden of ROS,[167] as well as many different chemical components that cause lung toxicity (**Table 4**).[168] In addition, oxidants are generated endogenously from activated inflammatory cells. Manipulation

Table 4
Miscellaneous additional classes of new drugs

Antioxidants	• Dietary antioxidants • N-acetyl-cysteine, N-acystelyn, N-isobutyryl-cysteine, erdosteine, procysteine, carbocysteine • Thiols, spin traps • Enzyme mimetics: superoxide dismutase, catalase and glutathione peroxidase • Polyphenols
Mucolytics	• N-acetyl-cysteine and carbocysteine • Epidermal growth factor receptor tyrosine kinase inhibitors
Protease inhibitors	• Neutrophil elastase inhibitors: sivelestat (ONO-5046), silanediol isosteres, AZD 9688 • MMP-9 & MMP-12 inhibitors • Broad-spectrum MMP inhibitors: ilomastat, marimastat
Antifibrotics	Agents used in idiopathic pulmonary fibrosis • Pirfenidone • Endothelin antagonists • PDE5 inhibitor: sildenafil • MoABs: anti-TGF-β, anti-FGF, anti-IL-13, anti-αvβ6 integrin (STX-100), anti-CCL2 (CNTO 888)
Drugs to combat cachexia and muscle wasting	Growth hormone releasing factor analogue (tesamorelin)
MoABs	• Anti-TNFα • Anti-IL-1β • Anti-IL-6 (tocilizumab) • Anti-CXCL8 (IL-8) • Anti-IL-17, anti-IL-13, anti-IgE • Anti-TGF-β
Drugs to slow aging	Sirtuin 1 activator (GSK2245840)
Lung regeneration	• Retinoids (γ-selective retinoid agonist, palovarotene) • Mesenchymal stem cell therapy • Gly-his-lys (GHK) tripeptide

of the oxidant–antioxidant balance, therefore, seems to be a logical therapeutic strategy and there is a range of novel targets.[169,170] Resveratrol is a cardioprotective antioxidant in red wine, whereas stilbenes are dietary antioxidants from tomatoes, but may not achieve sufficient levels in established COPD. Interestingly, resveratrol is also a sirtuin (SIRT) activator and this property has been proposed to account for anti-aging effects.[171] There are theories that COPD represents an accelerated form of lung aging,[172,173] and this concept suggests that antiaging molecules may have potential in COPD.[174] Other dietary components such as sulforaphanes and chalcones are potential therapeutic antioxidants in COPD.[175]

N-acetyl-cysteine (NAC) is a potent reducing agent capable of increasing intracellular glutathione levels. In addition, its mucolytic properties can improve sputum clearance in COPD. In preclinical studies, NAC attenuated elastase-induced emphysema in rats,[176] but later clinical studies have yielded mixed results. A Cochrane review reported the beneficial effects on exacerbation frequency of NAC in chronic bronchitis,[177] but this was later followed by a large multicenter trial in which NAC had no effect on exacerbation frequency or FEV_1 decline.[178] Carbocysteine may be more promising. The PEACE study revealed a significant decline in COPD exacerbations using 500 mg carbocysteine three times a day daily in Chinese patients with COPD.[179] Both of these agents are undergoing further studies in COPD.

Stable glutathione compounds, superoxide dismutase (SOD) analogues, and radical scavengers are in development. Enzyme mimetics are being developed that enhance the activity or expression of antioxidant enzymes such as SOD and glutathione peroxidase, which can neutralize cellular ROS. Nitrone spin-traps are potent antioxidants, which inhibit the formation of intracellular ROS by forming stable compounds, whereas thioredoxin is a redox sensor inhibitor. Hydrogen sulfide (H_2S) is a potent antioxidant and GYY4137 is a novel H_2S-releasing molecule that protects against endotoxic shock in the rat[180]; however, all these agents are still being assessed in animal models.

Mucoactive Drugs

Secretions can accumulate in airway lumens, exacerbating airflow obstruction and increasing susceptibility to infections in COPD. A variety of drugs has been developed to treat airway mucus hypersecretion, as well as mucoactive drugs,[181] in addition to NAC and carbocysteine mentioned above. These agents combat targets such as epidermal growth factor receptor, tyrosine kinase inhibitors, and human calcium-activated chloride channel (hCACL2). PPAR-γ is an exciting target for drugs to treat airway mucus hypersecretion.[150] Surfactant protein B has recently been found to be associated with COPD exacerbations.[182] It is important to stress that mucus can be both protective and harmful in different situations in COPD. In a study using inhaled recombinant DNAse to treat acute exacerbations of COPD, the study was terminated due to a trend toward increased mortality in the treatment arm.[183]

Proteases

α1-Antitrypsin deficiency is a genetic disease that illustrates the importance of proteases in causing a subtype of COPD.[134,135] There have been recent advances in provision of augmentation therapy for α1-antitrypsin deficiency.[184] Neutrophil elastase (NE),[136] MMP-9,[137] and MMP-12[185] have been implicated in the pathogenesis of COPD, and provide targets for novel therapies.[186]

A novel oral inhibitor of NE, AZD9668, underwent a 12-week dose-finding study in subjects with COPD treated with tiotropium, but failed to show benefit.[187,188] An inhibitory effect of heparin has been shown on neutrophil elastase release, which is independent of the anticoagulant activity of this molecule.[189] However, a phase II trial of O-desulfated heparin in subjects with exacerbations of COPD was terminated at the end of last year due to a lack of efficacy. Interestingly, heparin is also a known inhibitor of selectin-mediated interactions, but a phase II trial in COPD exacerbation patients with PGX-100 (2-O, 3-O desulfated heparin) also failed to demonstrate efficacy and was terminated early.[122]

Attempts to readdress the protease-antiprotease imbalance with synthetic MMP inhibitors have been attempted,[190] but the development of musculoskeletal syndrome with marimastat is a prominent adverse effect.[191] AZD1236, a novel more selective inhibitor of MMP-9 and MMP-12, has failed to demonstrate convincing clinical efficacy in two studies over 6 weeks.[192,193] The role of other proteases in COPD remains unclear, but inhibitors of cysteine proteases are under development.

Fibrosis and Remodeling

There have been dramatic advances in the understanding of lung injury and idiopathic pulmonary fibrosis (IPF).[194–196] This has resulted in a flurry of drug development, for which excellent reviews are available.[197,198] Inflammation and fibrosis are related processes, and COPD and IPF have some common features.[199,200] Airway inflammation, resulting in tissue injury can result in peribronchial fibrosis when lung injury exceeds the lung's ability to repair. The resulting airways become narrowed, leading to airway obstruction. However, although these processes, inflammation, and fibrosis, may be closely related, it has also been postulated that fibrosis may occur alone in COPD. For example, in IPF there can be very little inflammation.[201] The process of fibrosis is prominent in the small airways as obstructive bronchiolitis, but excessive fibrosis may also contribute to emphysema. It has been recently recognized that fibroblasts and myofibroblasts may be resident cells, derived from bone marrow stem cells and blood-borne fibrocytes, or may be derived by epithelial to mesenchymal transition (EMT).[202,203] Therefore, strategies used to treat IPF (eg, pirfenidone) may be of benefit in COPD, but more research is needed in this area.[194,204]

A recent study has demonstrated that cigarette smoke induces EMT in differentiated bronchial epithelial cells via release and autocrine action of transforming growth factor-$\beta1$ (TGF-$\beta1$) as well as by enhancing oxidative stress, thus suggesting that EMT could participate in the COPD remodeling process of small bronchi such as peribronchiolar fibrosis.[205] Small-molecule inhibitors of TGF-$\beta1$ receptor tyrosine kinase have been developed: SD-208, however, has been shown to inhibit airway fibrosis in a model of asthma.[206]

Biologics: MoABs

Tumor necrosis factor α (TNF-α) has been implicated in the pathogenesis of COPD and seems to be a good therapeutic target. Indeed, an observational study in rheumatoid arthritis patients demonstrated that etanercept (a TNF-receptor antagonist) led to a reduction of 50% in the rate of hospitalization due to COPD exacerbations.[207] Although blocking TNF-α was not effective in stable COPD patients,[208–210] it is possible that administration during an acute exacerbation might be effective in view of the acutely increased TNF-α concentrations. However, there are major concerns that the TNF antibody infliximab increased the incidence of respiratory cancers in a COPD study (although this was not statistically significant),[208] and increased other types of cancer as well as infections in a study in severe asthma.[211] Future efforts may consider a more tailored approach using these agents in a subset of patients defined by an increased TNF-α axis. In addition, cachectic patients were found to have a small improvement in exercise capacity in post hoc analysis.[208] Inhibition of

TNF-α production by inhibition of TNF-α converting enzyme is an alternative strategy.[38] A prominent effect of NF-κB and p38 MAP kinase inhibitor is the downstream inhibition of TNF-α synthesis.

An anti-CXCL8 (IL-8) MoAB was tested in COPD, but no improvement in health status or lung function was seen, possibly because the active bound form of CXCL8 was not recognized by the MoAB.[38] There is now special interest in assessing MoABs directed against IL-6, IL-1β, IL-17, IL-18, IL-1R, TGF-β, and granulocyte-macrophage colony-stimulating factor for effects in COPD. A humanized antibody against IL-6 receptors (tocilizumab) is effective in several other inflammatory diseases,[212] but there are no studies in COPD. Canakinumab, a MoAB to IL-1β, is already used in rare autoimmune diseases and is now in trials in COPD.[213] Th17 cells have recently been identified as a separate cell population that produce IL-17, which causes neutrophilia[214,215] and induce loss of HDAC2 and steroid insensitivity,[216] thus implicating another potential target, and phase II trials in psoriasis have been encouraging.[217,218] Finally, omalizumab, the anti-IgE MoAB approved for severe allergic asthma, has also now entered a study in a subgroup of COPD patients with elevated IgE levels.

Aging and Autoimmunity

COPD may be considered a disease of accelerated aging and geroprotectors are a novel therapeutic strategy.[219] SIRT1 and SIRT6 are attractive targets[220,221] because they can possess HDAC2 activity, protect against oxidative stress, and permit stabilization and repair of DNA. Another insight is that autoimmunity may have a role in COPD[222] and the immune system may be targeted against elastin[223] or epithelial cells.[224]

Lung Regeneration

Approaches to aid lung regeneration aim to correct the defect of emphysema and to replace destroyed lung interstitium. Human lungs have regenerative capacity, as demonstrated in Nepalese children given maternal vitamin A supplements.[225] This is not exclusive to children as demonstrated in an adult patient after pneumonectomy.[226] Attempts have been made to exploit this potential with new drugs to cause lung regeneration in COPD.[227–229]

Retinoids are known to promote alveolar septation in the developing lung and to stimulate alveolar repair in some animal models of emphysema. However, despite abrogation of elastase-induced emphysema in rats using all-trans retinoic acid,[230] subsequent attempts with retinoids and γ-retinoic acid receptor agonists in humans have been less promising.[231,232] The REPAIR study evaluated the effects of palovarotene (an oral γ-selective retinoid agonist) on lung density in emphysema secondary to α1-antitrypsin deficiency. Although effects on the primary endpoint were not significant, there was a trend toward an improvement in most functional parameters in subjects taking palovarotene for a year. Another group conducted a 2-year trial with this agent and reported their findings at the ATS in 2011. There was no overall improvement in FEV_1 in COPD subjects on the drug; however, subgroup analysis revealed a significant reduction in the rate of decline in FEV_1 and TLCO in subjects with lower lobe emphysema.

Mesenchymal stem cells (MSCs) also offer exciting regenerative potential.[228,233] MSCs exhibit potent antiinflammatory and immunomodulatory activities both in vitro and in vivo. This finding has led to a trial assessing the safety and efficacy of an IV preparation of allogenic MSCs (Prochymal).[234] The therapy was well tolerated and, although there were no significant differences in lung function tests or quality of life indicators, an early significant decrease in levels of circulating C-reactive protein was observed in some subjects. Another approach taken with MSCs was to populate a biologic connective tissue scaffold (which has been stripped of HLA-antigen expressing cells), which can then be used to grow autologous tissue before surgical implantation.[235]

SUMMARY

For the future treatment of COPD, it should be possible to have improved current drugs, antiinfective and antioxidant therapy, coupled with novel approaches directed against the innate immune system. In terms of the processes involved in COPD, there is rapid advancement of knowledge of viral responses and fibrosis, steroid-insensitive inflammation, autoimmunity, aberrant repair, accelerated aging, and appreciation of systemic disease and comorbidities. There is the need to develop validated noninvasive biomarkers for COPD and to have novel challenge models in animals and humans.[71] More interest has recently focused on cigarette-challenge models in an attempt to understand the exact immunologic responses to an acute smoke exposure event, to understand better the chronic changes that result from smoking.[68] In terms of clinical trial designs, these are adapted for bronchodilation, the natural history, and the prevention and treatment of COPD exacerbations and comorbidities. As is the case with many diseases, combinations of therapies may be the key to effective COPD treatment and prevention, and they may need to be given early in the disease. To develop novel drugs for COPD, it is clear that long-term studies in specific phenotypic groups, giving targeted therapy based on companion biomarkers, are needed. This would ideally use inhaled agents delivered directly to the intended site of action, with minimal unwanted side effects.[35] Overall, there is need for extensive collaboration between scientists, clinicians, the pharmaceutical industry, and drug regulators to identify and provide better therapy for patients with COPD.

REFERENCES

1. Ngkelo A, Adcock IM. New treatments for COPD. Curr Opin Pharmacol 2013; 13(3):362–9.
2. Gross NJ. Novel antiinflammatory therapies for COPD. Chest 2012;142(5): 1300–7.
3. Rabe KF, Wedzicha JA. Controversies in treatment of chronic obstructive pulmonary disease. Lancet 2011;378(9795):1038–47.
4. Martinez FJ, Donohue JF, Rennard SI. The future of chronic obstructive pulmonary disease treatment–difficulties of and barriers to drug development. Lancet 2011;378(9795):1027–37.
5. Hogg JC, Chu F, Utokaparch S, et al. The nature of small-airway obstruction in chronic obstructive pulmonary disease. N Engl J Med 2004;350(26):2645–53.
6. Hansel TT, Barnes PJ. New drugs for exacerbations of chronic obstructive pulmonary disease. Lancet 2009;374(9691):744–55.
7. McDonough JE, Yuan R, Suzuki M, et al. Small-airway obstruction and emphysema in chronic obstructive pulmonary disease. N Engl J Med 2011;365(17): 1567–75.
8. Brusselle GG, Joos GF, Bracke KR. New insights into the immunology of chronic obstructive pulmonary disease. Lancet 2011;378(9795):1015–26.
9. Churg A, Wright JL. Testing drugs in animal models of cigarette smoke-induced chronic obstructive pulmonary disease. Proc Am Thorac Soc 2009;6(6):550–2.

10. van der Vaart H, Postma DS, Timens W, et al. Acute effects of cigarette smoke on inflammation and oxidative stress: a review. Thorax 2004;59(8):713–21.

11. Willemse BW, Postma DS, Timens W, et al. The impact of smoking cessation on respiratory symptoms, lung function, airway hyperresponsiveness and inflammation. Eur Respir J 2004;23(3):464–76.

12. Willemse BW, ten Hacken NH, Rutgers B, et al. Effect of 1-year smoking cessation on airway inflammation in COPD and asymptomatic smokers. Eur Respir J 2005;26(5):835–45.

13. Papi A, Contoli M, Caramori G, et al. Models of infection and exacerbations in COPD. Curr Opin Pharmacol 2007;7(3):259–65.

14. Calverley PM, Rennard SI. What have we learned from large drug treatment trials in COPD? Lancet 2007;370(9589):774–85.

15. Vestbo J, Edwards LD, Scanlon PD, et al. Changes in forced expiratory volume in 1 second over time in COPD. N Engl J Med 2011;365(13):1184–92.

16. Anthonisen N, Connett J, Friedman B, et al. Design of a clinical trial to test a treatment of the underlying cause of emphysema. Ann N Y Acad Sci 1991; 624(Suppl):31–4.

17. Han MK, Agusti A, Calverley PM, et al. Chronic obstructive pulmonary disease phenotypes: the future of COPD. Am J Respir Crit Care Med 2010;182(5): 598–604.

18. National Emphysema Treatment Trial Research Group. Patients at high risk of death after lung-volume-reduction surgery. N Engl J Med 2001;345(15):1075–83.

19. Agusti A, Calverley PM, Celli B, et al. Characterisation of COPD heterogeneity in the ECLIPSE cohort. Respir Res 2010;11:122.

20. Qiu W, Cho MH, Riley JH, et al. Genetics of sputum gene expression in chronic obstructive pulmonary disease. PLoS One 2011;6(9):e24395.

21. MacNee W, Rennard SI, Hunt JF, et al. Evaluation of exhaled breath condensate pH as a biomarker for COPD. Respir Med 2011;105(7):1037–45.

22. Gelb AF, Barnes PJ, George SC, et al. Review of exhaled nitric oxide in chronic obstructive pulmonary disease. J Breath Res 2012;6(4):047101.

23. Franciosi L, Govorukhina N, Fusetti F, et al. Proteomic analysis of human epithelial lining fluid by microfluidics-based nanoLC-MS/MS: a feasibility study. Electrophoresis 2013. [Epub ahead of print].

24. Steiling K, van den Berge M, Hijazi K, et al. A dynamic bronchial airway gene expression signature of chronic obstructive pulmonary disease and lung function impairment. Am J Respir Crit Care Med 2013;187(9):933–42.

25. Woodruff PG. Novel outcomes and end points: biomarkers in chronic obstructive pulmonary disease clinical trials. Proc Am Thorac Soc 2011;8(4):350–5.

26. Verrills NM, Irwin JA, He XY, et al. Identification of novel diagnostic biomarkers for asthma and chronic obstructive pulmonary disease. Am J Respir Crit Care Med 2011;183(12):1633–43.

27. Rosenberg SR, Kalhan R. Biomarkers in chronic obstructive pulmonary disease. Transl Res 2012;159(4):228–37.

28. Scanlon PD, Connett JE, Waller LA, et al. Smoking cessation and lung function in mild-to-moderate chronic obstructive pulmonary disease. The lung health study. Am J Respir Crit Care Med 2000;161(2 Pt 1):381–90.

29. Tonnesen P, Carrozzi L, Fagerstrom KO, et al. Smoking cessation in patients with respiratory diseases: a high priority, integral component of therapy. Eur Respir J 2007;29(2):390–417.

30. Stead LF, Lancaster T. Combined pharmacotherapy and behavioural interventions for smoking cessation. Cochrane Database Syst Rev 2012;(10):CD008286.

31. Kanazawa H, Tochino Y, Asai K, et al. Validity of HMGB1 measurement in epithelial lining fluid in patients with COPD. Eur J Clin Invest 2012;42(4):419–26.
32. Williams JM, Steinberg MB, Steinberg ML, et al. Varenicline for tobacco dependence: panacea or plight? Expert Opin Pharmacother 2011;12(11): 1799–812.
33. West R, Zatonski W, Cedzynska M, et al. Placebo-controlled trial of cytisine for smoking cessation. N Engl J Med 2011;365(13):1193–200.
34. Hartmann-Boyce J, Cahill K, Hatsukami D, et al. Nicotine vaccines for smoking cessation. Cochrane Database Syst Rev 2012;(8):CD007072.
35. Hickey AJ. Back to the future: inhaled drug products. J Pharm Sci 2013;102(4): 1165–72.
36. Yasuda H, Soejima K, Nakayama S, et al. Bronchoscopic microsampling is a useful complementary diagnostic tool for detecting lung cancer. Lung Cancer 2011;72(1):32–8.
37. D'Souza MS, Markou A. Neuronal mechanisms underlying development of nicotine dependence: implications for novel smoking-cessation treatments. Addict Sci Clin Pract 2011;6(1):4–16.
38. Cazzola M, Page CP, Calzetta L, et al. Emerging anti-inflammatory strategies for COPD. Eur Respir J 2012;40(3):724–41.
39. Cazzola M, Page CP, Calzetta L, et al. Pharmacology and therapeutics of bronchodilators. Pharmacol Rev 2012;64(3):450–504.
40. Cazzola M, Page CP, Rogliani P, et al. Beta2-agonist therapy in lung disease. Am J Respir Crit Care Med 2013;187(7):690–6.
41. Cazzola M, Page C, Matera MG. Long-acting muscarinic receptor antagonists for the treatment of respiratory disease. Pulm Pharmacol Ther 2013;26(3): 307–17.
42. Vogelmeier C, Ramos-Barbon D, Jack D, et al. Indacaterol provides 24-hour bronchodilation in COPD: a placebo-controlled blinded comparison with tiotropium. Respir Res 2010;11:135.
43. Barnes PJ, Pocock SJ, Magnussen H, et al. Integrating indacaterol dose selection in a clinical study in COPD using an adaptive seamless design. Pulm Pharmacol Ther 2010;23(3):165–71.
44. Korn S, Kerwin E, Atis S, et al. Indacaterol once-daily provides superior efficacy to salmeterol twice-daily in COPD: a 12-week study. Respir Med 2011;105(5): 719–26.
45. Cazzola M. Aclidinium bromide, a novel long-acting muscarinic M3 antagonist for the treatment of COPD. Curr Opin Investig Drugs 2009;10(5):482–90.
46. Cazzola M, Rogliani P, Matera MG. Aclidinium bromide/formoterol fumarate fixed-dose combination for the treatment of chronic obstructive pulmonary disease. Expert Opin Pharmacother 2013;14(6):775–81.
47. Buhl R, Banerji D. Profile of glycopyrronium for once-daily treatment of moderate-to-severe COPD. Int J Chron Obstruct Pulmon Dis 2012;7:729–41.
48. Kerwin E, Hebert J, Gallagher N, et al. Efficacy and safety of NVA237 versus placebo and tiotropium in patients with COPD: the GLOW2 study. Eur Respir J 2012;40(5):1106–14.
49. Beeh KM, Singh D, Di SL, et al. Once-daily NVA237 improves exercise tolerance from the first dose in patients with COPD: the GLOW3 trial. Int J Chron Obstruct Pulmon Dis 2012;7:503–13.
50. van Noord JA, Aumann JL, Janssens E, et al. Combining tiotropium and salmeterol in COPD: effects on airflow obstruction and symptoms. Respir Med 2010; 104(7):995–1004.

51. van Noord JA, Aumann JL, Janssens E, et al. Effects of tiotropium with and without formoterol on airflow obstruction and resting hyperinflation in patients with COPD. Chest 2006;129(3):509–17.
52. Tashkin DP, Pearle J, Iezzoni D, et al. Formoterol and tiotropium compared with tiotropium alone for treatment of COPD. COPD 2009;6(1):17–25.
53. van Noord JA, Buhl R, LaForce C, et al. QVA149 demonstrates superior bronchodilation compared with indacaterol or placebo in patients with chronic obstructive pulmonary disease. Thorax 2010;65(12):1086–91.
54. Dougall IG, Young A, Ince F, et al. Dual dopamine D2 receptor and beta2-adrenoceptor agonists for the treatment of chronic obstructive pulmonary disease: the pre-clinical rationale. Respir Med 2003;97(Suppl A):S3–7.
55. Hiller FC, Alderfer V, Goldman M. Long-term use of Viozan (sibenadet HCl) in patients with chronic obstructive pulmonary disease: results of a 1-year study. Respir Med 2003;97(Suppl A):S45–52.
56. Vestbo J, Hurd SS, Agusti AG, et al. Global strategy for the diagnosis, management, and prevention of chronic obstructive pulmonary disease: GOLD executive summary. Am J Respir Crit Care Med 2013;187(4):347–65.
57. de Miguel-Diez J, Carrasco-Garrido P, Rejas-Gutierrez J, et al. Inappropriate overuse of inhaled corticosteroids for COPD patients: impact on health costs and health status. Lung 2011;189(3):199–206.
58. Yang IA, Clarke MS, Sim EH, et al. Inhaled corticosteroids for stable chronic obstructive pulmonary disease. Cochrane Database Syst Rev 2012;(7):CD002991.
59. Wedzicha JA, Calverley PM, Seemungal TA, et al. The prevention of COPD exacerbations by salmeterol/fluticasone propionate or tiotropium bromide. Am J Respir Crit Care Med 2007;177:19–26.
60. Ehrchen J, Steinmuller L, Barczyk K, et al. Glucocorticoids induce differentiation of a specifically activated, anti-inflammatory subtype of human monocytes. Blood 2007;109(3):1265–74.
61. Barnes PJ. Glucocorticosteroids: current and future directions. Br J Pharmacol 2011;163(1):29–43.
62. Cazzola M, Ando F, Santus P, et al. A pilot study to assess the effects of combining fluticasone propionate/salmeterol and tiotropium on the airflow obstruction of patients with severe-to-very severe COPD. Pulm Pharmacol Ther 2007;20(5):556–61.
63. Singh D, Brooks J, Hagan G, et al. Superiority of "triple" therapy with salmeterol/fluticasone propionate and tiotropium bromide versus individual components in moderate to severe COPD. Thorax 2008;63:592–8.
64. Renard D, Looby M, Kramer B, et al. Characterization of the bronchodilatory dose response to indacaterol in patients with chronic obstructive pulmonary disease using model-based approaches. Respir Res 2011;12:54.
65. Ito K, Ito M, Elliott WM, et al. Decreased histone deacetylase activity in chronic obstructive pulmonary disease. N Engl J Med 2005;352(19):1967–76.
66. Marwick JA, Caramori G, Stevenson CS, et al. Inhibition of PI3Kdelta restores glucocorticoid function in smoking-induced airway inflammation in mice. Am J Respir Crit Care Med 2009;179(7):542–8.
67. Ito K, Caramori G, Adcock IM. Therapeutic potential of phosphatidylinositol 3-kinase inhibitors in inflammatory respiratory disease. J Pharmacol Exp Ther 2007; 321(1):1–8.
68. Lo Tam Loi AT, Hoonhorst SJ, Franciosi L, et al. Acute and chronic inflammatory responses induced by smoking in individuals susceptible and non-susceptible

to development of COPD: from specific disease phenotyping towards novel therapy. Protocol of a cross-sectional study. BMJ Open 2013;3(2).

69. Cosio BG, Iglesias A, Rios A, et al. Low-dose theophylline enhances the anti-inflammatory effects of steroids during exacerbations of COPD. Thorax 2009; 64(5):424–9.

70. Cosio BG, Tsaprouni L, Ito K, et al. Theophylline restores histone deacetylase activity and steroid responses in COPD macrophages. J Exp Med 2004; 200(5):689–95.

71. Warnier MJ, van Riet EE, Rutten FH, et al. Smoking cessation strategies in patients with COPD. Eur Respir J 2013;41(3):727–34.

72. Kanner RE, Anthonisen NR, Connett JE. Lower respiratory illnesses promote FEV_1 decline in current smokers but not ex-smokers with chronic obstructive pulmonary disease: results from Lung Health Study. Am J Respir Crit Care Med 2001;164:358–64.

73. Donaldson GC, Seemungal TA, Bhowmik A, et al. Relationship between exacerbation frequency and lung function decline in chronic obstructive pulmonary disease. Thorax 2002;57(10):847–52.

74. Murphy TF. The role of bacteria in airway inflammation in exacerbations of chronic obstructive pulmonary disease. Curr Opin Infect Dis 2006;19(3):225–30.

75. Sethi S, Maloney J, Grove L, et al. Airway inflammation and bronchial bacterial colonization in chronic obstructive pulmonary disease. Am J Respir Crit Care Med 2006;173(9):991–8.

76. Patel IS, Seemungal TA, Wilks M, et al. Relationship between bacterial colonisation and the frequency, character, and severity of COPD exacerbations. Thorax 2002;57(9):759–64.

77. Barnes PJ. The cytokine network in asthma and chronic obstructive pulmonary disease. J Clin Invest 2008;118(11):3546–56.

78. Nseir S, Ader F. Prevalence and outcome of severe chronic obstructive pulmonary disease exacerbations caused by multidrug-resistant bacteria. Curr Opin Pulm Med 2008;14(2):95–100.

79. Hanlon GW. Bacteriophages: an appraisal of their role in the treatment of bacterial infections. Int J Antimicrob Agents 2007;30(2):118–28.

80. Serhan CN, Chiang N, Van Dyke TE. Resolving inflammation: dual anti-inflammatory and pro-resolution lipid mediators. Nat Rev Immunol 2008;8(5):349–61.

81. Tamaoki J, Kadota J, Takizawa H. Clinical implications of the immunomodulatory effects of macrolides. Am J Med 2004;117(Suppl 9A):5S–11S.

82. Kanoh S, Rubin BK. Mechanisms of action and clinical application of macrolides as immunomodulatory medications. Clin Microbiol Rev 2010;23(3):590–615.

83. Albert RK, Connett J, Bailey WC, et al. Azithromycin for prevention of exacerbations of COPD. N Engl J Med 2011;365(8):689–98.

84. Seemungal TA, Wilkinson TM, Hurst JR, et al. Long-term erythromycin therapy is associated with decreased chronic obstructive pulmonary disease exacerbations. Am J Respir Crit Care Med 2008;178(11):1139–47.

85. Li YJ, Azuma A, Usuki J, et al. EM703 improves bleomycin-induced pulmonary fibrosis in mice by the inhibition of TGF-beta signaling in lung fibroblasts. Respir Res 2006;7:16.

86. Sethi S, Jones PW, Theron MS, et al. Pulsed moxifloxacin for the prevention of exacerbations of chronic obstructive pulmonary disease: a randomized controlled trial. Respir Res 2010;11:10.

87. Varkey JB, Varkey B. Viral infections in patients with chronic obstructive pulmonary disease. Curr Opin Pulm Med 2008;14(2):89–94.

88. Brownlee JW, Turner RB. New developments in the epidemiology and clinical spectrum of rhinovirus infections. Curr Opin Pediatr 2008;20(1):67–71.
89. Patel IS, Roberts NJ, Lloyd-Owen SJ, et al. Airway epithelial inflammatory responses and clinical parameters in COPD. Eur Respir J 2003;22(1):94–9.
90. Baines KJ, Hsu AC, Tooze M, et al. Novel immune genes associated with excessive inflammatory and antiviral responses to rhinovirus in COPD. Respir Res 2013;14:15.
91. Klune JR, Dhupar R, Cardinal J, et al. HMGB1: endogenous danger signaling. Mol Med 2008;14(7–8):476–84.
92. Ramaswamy M, Groskreutz DJ, Look DC. Recognizing the importance of respiratory syncytial virus in chronic obstructive pulmonary disease. COPD 2009; 6(1):64–75.
93. Sikkel MB, Quint JK, Mallia P, et al. Respiratory syncytial virus persistence in chronic obstructive pulmonary disease. Pediatr Infect Dis J 2008;27(Suppl 10):S63–70.
94. Olszewska W, Openshaw P. Emerging drugs for respiratory syncytial virus infection. Expert Opin Emerg Drugs 2009;14(2):207–17.
95. Novel Swine-Origin Influenza A (H1N1) Virus Investigation Team, Dawood FS, Jain S, et al. Emergence of a novel swine-origin influenza A (H1N1) virus in humans. N Engl J Med 2009;360:2605–15.
96. Glezen WP. Clinical practice. Prevention and treatment of seasonal influenza. N Engl J Med 2008;359(24):2579–85.
97. Hayden F. Developing new antiviral agents for influenza treatment: what does the future hold? Clin Infect Dis 2009;48(Suppl 1):S3–13.
98. Sarir H, Henricks PA, van Houwelingen AH, et al. Cells, mediators and Toll-like receptors in COPD. Eur J Pharmacol 2008;585(2–3):346–53.
99. Raymond T, Schaller M, Hogaboam CM, et al. Toll-like receptors, Notch ligands, and cytokines drive the chronicity of lung inflammation. Proc Am Thorac Soc 2007;4(8):635–41.
100. O'Neill LA. The interleukin-1 receptor/Toll-like receptor superfamily: 10 years of progress. Immunol Rev 2008;226:10–8.
101. Kumar H, Kawai T, Akira S. Pathogen recognition in the innate immune response. Biochem J 2009;420(1):1–16.
102. Paul-Clark MJ, McMaster SK, Sorrentino R, et al. Toll-like receptor 2 is essential for the sensing of oxidants during inflammation. Am J Respir Crit Care Med 2009;179(4):299–306.
103. Williams AS, Leung SY, Nath P, et al. Role of TLR2, TLR4, and MyD88 in murine ozone-induced airway hyperresponsiveness and neutrophilia. J Appl Physiol 2007;103(4):1189–95.
104. Doz E, Noulin N, Boichot E, et al. Cigarette smoke-induced pulmonary inflammation is TLR4/MyD88 and IL-1R1/MyD88 signaling dependent. J Immunol 2008; 180(2):1169–78.
105. Foell D, Wittkowski H, Roth J. Mechanisms of disease: a 'DAMP' view of inflammatory arthritis. Nat Clin Pract Rheumatol 2007;3(7):382–90.
106. Bianchi ME. DAMPs, PAMPs and alarmins: all we need to know about danger. J Leukoc Biol 2007;81(1):1–5.
107. Areschoug T, Gordon S. Scavenger receptors: role in innate immunity and microbial pathogenesis. Cell Microbiol 2009;11(8):1160–9.
108. Ramasamy R, Yan SF, Schmidt AM. RAGE: therapeutic target and biomarker of the inflammatory response–the evidence mounts. J Leukoc Biol 2009;86(3): 505–12.

109. Sukkar MB, Xie S, Khorasani NM, et al. Toll-like receptor 2, 3, and 4 expression and function in human airway smooth muscle. J Allergy Clin Immunol 2006; 118(3):641–8.
110. O'Neill LA, Bryant CE, Doyle SL. Therapeutic targeting of toll-like receptors for infectious and inflammatory diseases and cancer. Pharmacol Rev 2009;61(2): 177–97.
111. Shirey KA, Lai W, Scott AJ, et al. The TLR4 antagonist Eritoran protects mice from lethal influenza infection. Nature 2013;497(7450):498–502.
112. Chaudhuri N, Whyte MK, Sabroe I. Reducing the toll of inflammatory lung disease. Chest 2007;131(5):1550–6.
113. Kenny EF, O'Neill LA. Signalling adaptors used by Toll-like receptors: an update. Cytokine 2008;43(3):342–9.
114. O'Connor BJ, Leaker BR, Barnes PJ, et al. Inhibition of LPS-induced neutrophilic inflammation in healthy volunteers. Eur Respir J 2007;30(Suppl 51):1294.
115. Holz O, Khalilieh S, Ludwig-Sengpiel A, et al. SCH527123, a novel CXCR2 antagonist, inhibits ozone-induced neutrophilia in healthy subjects. Eur Respir J 2010;35(3):564–70.
116. Kerstjens HA, Bjermer L, Eriksson L, et al. Tolerability and efficacy of inhaled AZD4818, a CCR1 antagonist, in moderate to severe COPD patients. Respir Med 2010;104(9):1297–303.
117. Norman P. DP(2) receptor antagonists in development. Expert Opin Investig Drugs 2010;19(8):947–61.
118. Seggev JS, Thornton WH Jr, Edes TE. Serum leukotriene B4 levels in patients with obstructive pulmonary disease. Chest 1991;99(2):289–91.
119. Beeh KM, Kornmann O, Buhl R, et al. Neutrophil chemotactic activity of sputum from patients with COPD: role of interleukin 8 and leukotriene B4. Chest 2003; 123(4):1240–7.
120. Snelgrove RJ, Jackson PL, Hardison MT, et al. A critical role for LTA4H in limiting chronic pulmonary neutrophilic inflammation. Science 2010;330(6000):90–4.
121. Watz H, Bock D, Meyer M, et al. Inhaled pan-selectin antagonist Bimosiamose attenuates airway inflammation in COPD. Pulm Pharmacol Ther 2012;26(2): 265–70.
122. Bedard PW, Kaila N. Selectin inhibitors: a patent review. Expert Opin Ther Pat 2010;20(6):781–93.
123. Currie GP, Butler CA, Anderson WJ, et al. Phosphodiesterase 4 inhibitors in chronic obstructive pulmonary disease: a new approach to oral treatment. Br J Clin Pharmacol 2008;65(6):803–10.
124. Giembycz MA. Can the anti-inflammatory potential of PDE4 inhibitors be realized: guarded optimism or wishful thinking? Br J Pharmacol 2008;155(3):288–90.
125. Sriskantharajah S, Hamblin N, Worsley S, et al. Targeting phosphoinositide 3-kinase delta for the treatment of respiratory diseases. Ann N Y Acad Sci 2013; 1280(1):35–9.
126. Rennard S, Knobil K, Rabe KF, et al. The efficacy and safety of cilomilast in COPD. Drugs 2008;68(Suppl 2):3–57.
127. Compton CH, Gubb J, Nieman R, et al. Cilomilast, a selective phosphodiesterase-4 inhibitor for treatment of patients with chronic obstructive pulmonary disease: a randomised, dose-ranging study. Lancet 2001;358(9278): 265–70.
128. Rennard SI, Schachter N, Strek M, et al. Cilomilast for COPD: results of a 6-month, placebo-controlled study of a potent, selective inhibitor of phosphodiesterase 4. Chest 2006;129(1):56–66.

129. Rabe KF, Bateman ED, O'Donnell D, et al. Roflumilast–an oral anti-inflammatory treatment for chronic obstructive pulmonary disease: a randomised controlled trial. Lancet 2005;366(9485):563–71.

130. Calverley PM, Sanchez-Toril F, McIvor A, et al. Effect of 1-year treatment with roflumilast in severe chronic obstructive pulmonary disease. Am J Respir Crit Care Med 2007;176(2):154–61.

131. Fabbri LM, Calverley PM, Izquierdo-Alonso JL, et al. Roflumilast in moderate-to-severe chronic obstructive pulmonary disease treated with longacting bronchodilators: two randomised clinical trials. Lancet 2009;374(9691):695–703.

132. Calverley PM, Rabe KF, Goehring UM, et al. Roflumilast in symptomatic chronic obstructive pulmonary disease: two randomised clinical trials. Lancet 2009; 374(9691):685–94.

133. Giembycz MA, Field SK. Roflumilast: first phosphodiesterase 4 inhibitor approved for treatment of COPD. Drug Des Devel Ther 2010;4:147–58.

134. Chong J, Poole P, Leung B, et al. Phosphodiesterase 4 inhibitors for chronic obstructive pulmonary disease. Cochrane Database Syst Rev 2011;(5):CD002309.

135. Calverley PM, Martinez FJ, Fabbri LM, et al. Does roflumilast decrease exacerbations in severe COPD patients not controlled by inhaled combination therapy? the REACT study protocol. Int J Chron Obstruct Pulmon Dis 2012;7:375–82.

136. Robichaud A, Stamatiou PB, Jin SL, et al. Deletion of phosphodiesterase 4D in mice shortens alpha(2)-adrenoceptor-mediated anesthesia, a behavioral correlate of emesis. J Clin Invest 2002;110(7):1045–52.

137. Seguin RM, Ferrari N. Emerging oligonucleotide therapies for asthma and chronic obstructive pulmonary disease. Expert Opin Investig Drugs 2009; 18(10):1505–17.

138. Barnes PJ. Corticosteroid resistance in patients with asthma and chronic obstructive pulmonary disease. J Allergy Clin Immunol 2013;131(3):636–45.

139. Simmons DL. Targeting kinases: a new approach to treating inflammatory rheumatic diseases. Curr Opin Pharmacol 2013;13(3):426–34.

140. Gaestel M, Kotlyarov A, Kracht M. Targeting innate immunity protein kinase signalling in inflammation. Nat Rev Drug Discov 2009;8(6):480–99.

141. Chung KF. p38 mitogen-activated protein kinase pathways in asthma and COPD. Chest 2011;139(6):1470–9.

142. Lomas DA, Lipson DA, Miller BE, et al. An oral inhibitor of p38 MAP kinase reduces plasma fibrinogen in patients with chronic obstructive pulmonary disease. J Clin Pharmacol 2012;52(3):416–24.

143. Langereis JD, Raaijmakers HA, Ulfman LH, et al. Abrogation of NF-kappaB signaling in human neutrophils induces neutrophil survival through sustained p38-MAPK activation. J Leukoc Biol 2010;88(4):655–64.

144. Caramori G, Casolari P, Adcock I. Role of transcription factors in the pathogenesis of asthma and COPD. Cell Commun Adhes 2013;20(1–2):21–40.

145. Patel S. Exploring novel therapeutic targets in gist: focus on the PI3K/Akt/mTOR pathway. Curr Oncol Rep 2013;15(4):386–95.

146. Marwick JA, Caramori G, Casolari P, et al. A role for phosphoinositol 3-kinase delta in the impairment of glucocorticoid responsiveness in patients with chronic obstructive pulmonary disease. J Allergy Clin Immunol 2010;125(5):1146–53.

147. Fung-Leung WP. Phosphoinositide 3-kinase delta (PI3Kdelta) in leukocyte signaling and function. Cell Signal 2011;23(4):603–8.

148. Fung-Leung WP. Phosphoinositide 3-kinase gamma in T cell biology and disease therapy. Ann N Y Acad Sci 2013;1280:40–3.

149. Doukas J, Eide L, Stebbins K, et al. Aerosolized phosphoinositide 3-kinase gamma/delta inhibitor TG100-115 [3-[2,4-diamino-6-(3-hydroxyphenyl)pteridin-7-yl]phenol] as a therapeutic candidate for asthma and chronic obstructive pulmonary disease. J Pharmacol Exp Ther 2009;328(3):758–65.
150. Shen Y, Chen L, Wang T, et al. PPARgamma as a potential target to treat airway mucus hypersecretion in chronic airway inflammatory diseases. PPAR Res 2012;2012:256874.
151. Onoue S, Sato H, Ogawa K, et al. Inhalable dry-emulsion formulation of cyclosporine A with improved anti-inflammatory effects in experimental asthma/COPD-model rats. Eur J Pharm Biopharm 2012;80(1):54–60.
152. Barnes PJ, Celli BR. Systemic manifestations and comorbidities of COPD. Eur Respir J 2009;33(5):1165–85.
153. Agusti A, Faner R. Systemic inflammation and comorbidities in chronic obstructive pulmonary disease. Proc Am Thorac Soc 2012;9(2):43–6.
154. Hunninghake DB. Cardiovascular disease in chronic obstructive pulmonary disease. Proc Am Thorac Soc 2005;2(1):44–9.
155. Barnes PJ. Future treatments for chronic obstructive pulmonary disease and its comorbidities. Proc Am Thorac Soc 2008;5(8):857–64.
156. Agusti A, Edwards LD, Rennard SI, et al. Persistent systemic inflammation is associated with poor clinical outcomes in COPD: a novel phenotype. PLoS One 2012;7(5):e37483.
157. Donaldson AV, Maddocks M, Martolini D, et al. Muscle function in COPD: a complex interplay. Int J Chron Obstruct Pulmon Dis 2012;7:523–35.
158. Steiner MC, Roubenoff R, Tal-Singer R, et al. Prospects for the development of effective pharmacotherapy targeted at the skeletal muscles in chronic obstructive pulmonary disease: a translational review. Thorax 2012;67(12):1102–9.
159. Jain MK, Ridker PM. Anti-inflammatory effects of statins: clinical evidence and basic mechanisms. Nat Rev Drug Discov 2005;4(12):977–87.
160. van Gestel YR, Hoeks SE, Sin DD, et al. Effect of statin therapy on mortality in patients with peripheral arterial disease and comparison of those with versus without associated chronic obstructive pulmonary disease. Am J Cardiol 2008;102(2):192–6.
161. Blamoun AI, Batty GN, DeBari VA, et al. Statins may reduce episodes of exacerbation and the requirement for intubation in patients with COPD: evidence from a retrospective cohort study. Int J Clin Pract 2008;62(9):1373–8.
162. Frost FJ, Petersen H, Tollestrup K, et al. Influenza and COPD mortality protection as pleiotropic, dose-dependent effects of statins. Chest 2007;131(4):1006–12.
163. Mancini GB, Etminan M, Zhang B, et al. Reduction of morbidity and mortality by statins, angiotensin-converting enzyme inhibitors, and angiotensin receptor blockers in patients with chronic obstructive pulmonary disease. J Am Coll Cardiol 2006;47(12):2554–60.
164. Soyseth V, Brekke PH, Smith P, et al. Statin use is associated with reduced mortality in COPD. Eur Respir J 2007;29(2):279–83.
165. Lahousse L, Loth DW, Joos GF, et al. Statins, systemic inflammation and risk of death in COPD: the Rotterdam study. Pulm Pharmacol Ther 2012;26(2):212–7.
166. van Gestel YR, Hoeks SE, Sin DD, et al. COPD and cancer mortality: the influence of statins. Thorax 2009;64(11):963–7.
167. Mak JC. Pathogenesis of COPD. Part II. Oxidative-antioxidative imbalance. Int J Tuberc Lung Dis 2008;12(4):368–74.

168. Kovacic P, Somanathan R. Pulmonary toxicity and environmental contamination: radicals, electron transfer, and protection by antioxidants. Rev Environ Contam Toxicol 2009;201:41–69.

169. Kirkham P, Rahman I. Antioxidant therapeutic strategies. In: Hansel TT, Barnes PJ, editors. New drugs and targets for respiratory diseases. London: Thomson-Reuters; 2009.

170. Rahman I, MacNee W. Antioxidant pharmacological therapies for COPD. Curr Opin Pharmacol 2012;12(3):256–65.

171. Wood JG, Rogina B, Lavu S, et al. Sirtuin activators mimic caloric restriction and delay ageing in metazoans. Nature 2004;430(7000):686–9.

172. Sharma G, Hanania NA, Shim YM. The aging immune system and its relationship to the development of chronic obstructive pulmonary disease. Proc Am Thorac Soc 2009;6(7):573–80.

173. Ito K, Barnes PJ. COPD as a disease of accelerated lung aging. Chest 2009; 135(1):173–80.

174. Harman D. Free radical theory of aging: an update: increasing the functional life span. Ann N Y Acad Sci 2006;1067:10–21.

175. Kumar V, Kumar S, Hassan M, et al. Novel chalcone derivatives as potent Nrf2 activators in mice and human lung epithelial cells. J Med Chem 2011;54(12):4147–59.

176. Rubio ML, Martin-Mosquero MC, Ortega M, et al. Oral N-acetylcysteine attenuates elastase-induced pulmonary emphysema in rats. Chest 2004;125(4): 1500–6.

177. Stey C, Steurer J, Bachmann S, et al. The effect of oral N-acetylcysteine in chronic bronchitis: a quantitative systematic review. Eur Respir J 2000;16(2): 253–62.

178. Decramer M, Rutten-van Molken M, Dekhuijzen PN, et al. Effects of N-acetylcysteine on outcomes in chronic obstructive pulmonary disease (Bronchitis Randomized on NAC Cost-Utility Study, BRONCUS): a randomised placebo-controlled trial. Lancet 2005;365(9470):1552–60.

179. Zheng JP, Kang J, Huang SG, et al. Effect of carbocisteine on acute exacerbation of chronic obstructive pulmonary disease (PEACE Study): a randomised placebo-controlled study. Lancet 2008;371(9629):2013–8.

180. Li L, Salto-Tellez M, Tan CH, et al. GYY4137, a novel hydrogen sulfide-releasing molecule, protects against endotoxic shock in the rat. Free Radic Biol Med 2009;47(1):103–13.

181. Rogers DF. Mucoactive agents for airway mucus hypersecretory diseases. Respir Care 2007;52(9):1176–93.

182. Foreman MG, DeMeo DL, Hersh CP, et al. Polymorphic variation in surfactant protein B is associated with COPD exacerbations. Eur Respir J 2008;32(4):938–44.

183. Hudson TJ. Dornase in treatment of chronic bronchitis. Ann Pharmacother 1996; 30:674–5.

184. Kueppers F. The role of augmentation therapy in alpha-1 antitrypsin deficiency. Curr Med Res Opin 2011;27(3):579–88.

185. Hunninghake GM, Cho MH, Tesfaigzi Y, et al. MMP12, lung function, and COPD in high-risk populations. N Engl J Med 2009;361(27):2599–608.

186. Korkmaz B, Horwitz MS, Jenne DE, et al. Neutrophil elastase, proteinase 3, and cathepsin G as therapeutic targets in human diseases. Pharmacol Rev 2010; 62(4):726–59.

187. Stevens T, Ekholm K, Granse M, et al. AZD9668: pharmacological characterization of a novel oral inhibitor of neutrophil elastase. J Pharmacol Exp Ther 2011; 339(1):313–20.

188. Vogelmeier C, Aquino TO, O'Brien CD, et al. A randomised, placebo-controlled, dose-finding study of AZD9668, an oral inhibitor of neutrophil elastase, in patients with chronic obstructive pulmonary disease treated with tiotropium. COPD 2012;9(2):111–20.
189. Brown RA, Lever R, Jones NA, et al. Effects of heparin and related molecules upon neutrophil aggregation and elastase release in vitro. Br J Pharmacol 2003;139(4):845–53.
190. Churg A, Zhou S, Wright JL. Series "matrix metalloproteinases in lung health and disease": matrix metalloproteinases in COPD. Eur Respir J 2012;39(1):197–209.
191. Bramhall SR, Hallissey MT, Whiting J, et al. Marimastat as maintenance therapy for patients with advanced gastric cancer: a randomised trial. Br J Cancer 2002;86(12):1864–70.
192. Magnussen H, Watz H, Kirsten A, et al. Safety and tolerability of an oral MMP-9 and -12 inhibitor, AZD1236, in patients with moderate-to-severe COPD: a randomised controlled 6-week trial. Pulm Pharmacol Ther 2011;24(5):563–70.
193. Dahl R, Titlestad I, Lindqvist A, et al. Effects of an oral MMP-9 and -12 inhibitor, AZD1236, on biomarkers in moderate/severe COPD: a randomised controlled trial. Pulm Pharmacol Ther 2012;25(2):169–77.
194. du Bois RM. Strategies for treating idiopathic pulmonary fibrosis. Nat Rev Drug Discov 2010;9(2):129–40.
195. Fernandez IE, Eickelberg O. New cellular and molecular mechanisms of lung injury and fibrosis in idiopathic pulmonary fibrosis. Lancet 2012;380(9842):680–8.
196. Sivakumar P, Ntolios P, Jenkins G, et al. Into the matrix: targeting fibroblasts in pulmonary fibrosis. Curr Opin Pulm Med 2012;18(5):462–9.
197. Datta A, Scotton CJ, Chambers RC. Novel therapeutic approaches for pulmonary fibrosis. Br J Pharmacol 2011;163(1):141–72.
198. Wuyts WA, Agostini C, Antoniou KM, et al. The pathogenesis of pulmonary fibrosis: a moving target. Eur Respir J 2013;41(5):1207–18.
199. Lee SB, Kalluri R. Mechanistic connection between inflammation and fibrosis. Kidney Int Suppl 2010;(119):S22–6.
200. Chilosi M, Poletti V, Rossi A. The pathogenesis of COPD and IPF: distinct horns of the same devil? Respir Res 2012;13:3.
201. Wilson MS, Wynn TA. Pulmonary fibrosis: pathogenesis, etiology and regulation. Mucosal Immunol 2009;2(2):103–21.
202. Laurent GJ, McAnulty RJ, Hill M, et al. Escape from the matrix: multiple mechanisms for fibroblast activation in pulmonary fibrosis. Proc Am Thorac Soc 2008;5(3):311–5.
203. Scotton CJ, Chambers RC. Molecular targets in pulmonary fibrosis: the myofibroblast in focus. Chest 2007;132(4):1311–21.
204. Krueger GG, Langley RG, Leonardi C, et al. A human interleukin-12/23 monoclonal antibody for the treatment of psoriasis. N Engl J Med 2007;356(6):580–92.
205. Milara J, Peiro T, Serrano A, et al. Epithelial to mesenchymal transition is increased in patients with COPD and induced by cigarette smoke. Thorax 2013;68(5):410–20.
206. Leung SY, Niimi A, Noble A, et al. Effect of transforming growth factor-beta receptor I kinase inhibitor 2,4-disubstituted pteridine (SD-208) in chronic allergic airway inflammation and remodeling. J Pharmacol Exp Ther 2006;319(2):586–94.

207. Suissa S, Ernst P, Hudson M. TNF-alpha antagonists and the prevention of hospitalisation for chronic obstructive pulmonary disease. Pulm Pharmacol Ther 2008;21(1):234–8.

208. Rennard SI, Fogarty C, Kelsen S, et al. The safety and efficacy of infliximab in moderate to severe chronic obstructive pulmonary disease. Am J Respir Crit Care Med 2007;175(9):926–34.

209. Barnes PJ. Unexpected failure of anti-tumor necrosis factor therapy in chronic obstructive pulmonary disease. Am J Respir Crit Care Med 2007;175(9):866–7.

210. Loza MJ, Watt R, Baribaud F, et al. Systemic inflammatory profile and response to anti-tumor necrosis factor therapy in chronic obstructive pulmonary disease. Respir Res 2012;13:12.

211. Wenzel SE, Barnes PJ, Bleecker ER, et al. A randomized, double-blind, placebo-controlled study of TNF-alpha blockade in severe persistent asthma. Am J Respir Crit Care Med 2009;179:549–58.

212. Paul-Pletzer K. Tocilizumab: blockade of interleukin-6 signaling pathway as a therapeutic strategy for inflammatory disorders. Drugs Today (Barc) 2006; 42(9):559–76.

213. Dhimolea E. Canakinumab. MAbs 2010;2(1):3–13.

214. Ivanov S, Linden A. Targeting interleukin-17 in the lungs. In: Hansel TT, Barnes PJ, editors. New drugs and targets for respiratory diseases. London: Thomson-Reuters; 2009.

215. Prause O, Bossios A, Silverpil E, et al. IL-17-producing T lymphocytes in lung tissue and in the bronchoalveolar space after exposure to endotoxin from Escherichia coli in vivo–effects of anti-inflammatory pharmacotherapy. Pulm Pharmacol Ther 2009;22(3):199–207.

216. Zijlstra GJ, ten Hacken NH, Hoffmann RF, et al. Interleukin-17A induces glucocorticoid insensitivity in human bronchial epithelial cells. Eur Respir J 2012; 39(2):439–45.

217. Leonardi C, Matheson R, Zachariae C, et al. Anti-interleukin-17 monoclonal antibody ixekizumab in chronic plaque psoriasis. N Engl J Med 2012;366(13): 1190–9.

218. Papp KA, Leonardi C, Menter A, et al. Brodalumab, an anti-interleukin-17-receptor antibody for psoriasis. N Engl J Med 2012;366(13):1181–9.

219. Ito K, Colley T, Mercado N. Geroprotectors as a novel therapeutic strategy for COPD, an accelerating aging disease. Int J Chron Obstruct Pulmon Dis 2012; 7:641–52.

220. Yao H, Rahman I. Perspectives on translational and therapeutic aspects of SIRT1 in inflammaging and senescence. Biochem Pharmacol 2012;84(10):1332–9.

221. Beauharnois JM, Bolivar BE, Welch JT. Sirtuin 6: a review of biological effects and potential therapeutic properties. Mol Biosyst 2013;9(7):1789–806.

222. Agusti A, MacNee W, Donaldson K, et al. Hypothesis: does COPD have an autoimmune component? Thorax 2003;58(10):832–4.

223. Lee SH, Goswami S, Grudo A, et al. Antielastin autoimmunity in tobacco smoking-induced emphysema. Nat Med 2007;13(5):567–9.

224. Feghali-Bostwick CA, Gadgil AS, Otterbein LE, et al. Autoantibodies in patients with chronic obstructive pulmonary disease. Am J Respir Crit Care Med 2008; 177(2):156–63.

225. Checkley W, West KP Jr, Wise RA, et al. Maternal vitamin A supplementation and lung function in offspring. N Engl J Med 2010;362(19):1784–94.

226. Butler JP, Loring SH, Patz S, et al. Evidence for adult lung growth in humans. N Engl J Med 2012;367(3):244–7.

227. Rennard SI, Wachenfeldt K. Rationale and emerging approaches for targeting lung repair and regeneration in the treatment of chronic obstructive pulmonary disease. Proc Am Thorac Soc 2011;8(4):368–75.
228. Hind M, Maden M. Is a regenerative approach viable for the treatment of COPD? Br J Pharmacol 2011;163(1):106–15.
229. Kubo H. Concise review: clinical prospects for treating chronic obstructive pulmonary disease with regenerative approaches. Stem Cells Transl Med 2012; 1(8):627–31.
230. Massaro GD, Massaro D. Retinoic acid treatment abrogates elastase-induced pulmonary emphysema in rats. Nat Med 1997;3(6):675–7.
231. Roth MD, Connett JE, D'Armiento JM, et al. Feasibility of retinoids for the treatment of emphysema study. Chest 2006;130(5):1334–45.
232. Stolk J, Stockley RA, Stoel BC, et al. Randomised controlled trial for emphysema with a selective agonist of the gamma-type retinoic acid receptor. Eur Respir J 2012;40(2):306–12.
233. Rankin S. Mesenchymal stem cells. Thorax 2012;67(6):565–6.
234. Weiss DJ, Casaburi R, Flannery R, et al. A placebo-controlled, randomized trial of mesenchymal stem cells in COPD. Chest 2013;143(6):1590–8.
235. Badylak SF, Weiss DJ, Caplan A, et al. Engineered whole organs and complex tissues. Lancet 2012;379(9819):943–52.

Collaborative Self-Management and Behavioral Change

Kathryn Rice, MD[a],*, Jean Bourbeau[b], Roderick MacDonald, MS[a],
Timothy J. Wilt, MD, MPH[a]

KEYWORDS

- Chronic obstructive pulmonary disease • Collaborative self-management
- Behavioral change • Pulmonary rehabilitation

KEY POINTS

- Behavioral change is critical for improving health outcomes in patients with chronic obstructive pulmonary disease.
- An educational approach alone is insufficient; effective collaborative self-management (CSM) to promote adaptive behaviors is necessary.
- CSM should be integrated with pulmonary rehabilitation programs, one of the main goals of which is to induce long-term changes in behavior.
- More research is needed to evaluate the effectiveness of assimilating CSM into primary care, patient-centered medical homes, and palliative care teams.

INTRODUCTION

According to the World Health Organization (WHO), chronic noncommunicable medical conditions, including chronic obstructive pulmonary disease (COPD), comprise more than half of the total global burden of disease. People who suffer from chronic diseases have complex medical, emotional, and social needs during the changing trajectory of their illnesses. These needs cannot be met by education alone; changes in behavior, especially the acquisition of self-care skills, are also required.[1] Chronic disease management, also termed collaborative self-management (CSM), is defined by the Disease Management Association of America as "a system of coordinated health care interventions and communications for populations with conditions in which patient self-care efforts are significant."[2] There is mounting evidence that embedding CSM within existing health care systems provides an effective model to meet these

This article originally appeared in *Clinics in Chest Medicine*, Volume 35, Issue 2, June 2014.
[a] Minneapolis VA Health Care System, One Veterans Drive, Minneapolis, MN 55417, USA;
[b] Montreal Chest Institute, McGill University Health Centre, Montréal, Québec, Canada
* Corresponding author.
E-mail address: kathryn.rice@va.gov

needs. The Joint Commission on Patient Safety and Quality in the United States has recently set out an evidence-based framework to improve self-management support for people with chronic conditions.[3] For people suffering from COPD, CSM is a multi-component model of health care delivery that guides self-management behaviors to help patients lead lives that are as healthy and functional as possible.

Regarding COPD, the first Cochrane review in 2003 found insufficient evidence to demonstrate the effectiveness of CSM.[4] The next Cochrane review of 14 randomized controlled trials (RCTs) reported that COPD CSM improved dyspnea scores and reduced respiratory-related hospitalizations.[5] In 2013, a new Cochrane review of 26 RCTs found that COPD CSM not only improved disease-specific health status and exercise capacity but also reduced hospital admissions and hospital days per person.[6] This meta-analysis found no difference in mortality, although more recent studies were not included. There was insufficient evidence to either refute or confirm the long-term effectiveness of COPD CSM.

CHALLENGES TO PROVIDING HIGH-QUALITY COPD CARE

Health care systems face major challenges in reducing the burden of illness and improving the functional status of people with chronic health problems.[7] Challenges for patients include the complexity of behavioral changes they are asked to make, communication problems, such as the fear of asking questions or "white-coat silence,"[8] a lack understanding of the disease and the severity of its symptoms, and nonadherence to medication.[9] Provider challenges include knowledge deficits and pessimism about COPD,[9–14] and acquiring the skills needed to guide behavioral changes. Challenges to health care systems are the availability of resources, including sufficient provider time to elicit and answer questions and ensure understanding[8]; role clarity for members of the health care team[15]; and systematic evaluation of the effectiveness of interventions.

Team-based models of care such as COPD CSM provide a framework for overcoming many of these challenges. The theoretical frameworks for these systems have been previously described in some detail.[16] CSM is based on Wagner's Chronic Care Model as shown in **Fig. 1**,[17] which emphasizes patient self-efficacy and behavior change. An additional framework for behavioral change is provided by the precede-proceed model.[18] According to this model, it is important to identify participants' learning needs based on the evaluation of factors that can influence their behavior, as follows. (1) The predisposing factors that refer to existing health-related knowledge, beliefs, attitudes, and values, and expected changes in behavior; in addition, the level of self-efficacy is an important predisposing factor to behavioral change. (2) The facilitating factors or barriers that are based on patients' past life experiences, knowledge, and skills already acquired, and the accessibility to services and financial resources. (3) The reinforcing factors that depend on patients' social support network and their successful past life experiences. Behavioral interventions must be planned in relation to identified learning needs that are meaningful for the patient and applied through methods enhancing self-efficacy to achieve the expected behavioral changes and outcomes.

Evidence supports the integration of CSM into routine health care for several chronic diseases, including congestive heart failure (CHF),[19,20] diabetes,[21] depression[22] and asthma.[23] In a systematic review of CSM for patients with COPD, a multi-component, as opposed to single-component, CSM intervention was required for success.[24] Specifically, the inclusion of 2 or more of the following components were associated with better clinical outcomes: (1) self-management, (2) advanced access

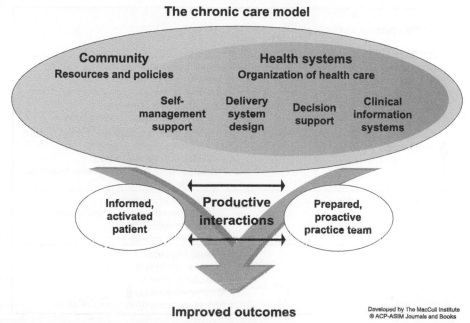

Improved outcomes   Developed by The MacColl Institute
® ACP-ASIM Journals and Books

Fig. 1. The Chronic Care Model. Notes: The Improving Chronic Illness Care Program is supported by The Robert Wood Johnson Foundation, with direction and technical assistance provided by Group Health Cooperative of Puget Sound's MacColl Institute for Healthcare Innovation, and its relationship to the Patient-Centered Medical Home. (*From* Wagner EH. Chronic disease management: what will it take to improve care for chronic illness? Eff Clin Pract 1998;1(1):2–4; with permission.)

care delivery, (3) decision support, and (4) clinical information systems. Categories of these components and specific examples of the types of care in COPD CSM are shown in **Tables 1** and **2**. Support for multicomponent COPD CSM was also provided in another systematic review, which found that successful interventions included all of the following dimensions: patient-related, professional-directed, and organizational.[23]

The primary aim of COPD CSM is to help patients deal with the spectrum of their condition, including both the "good days" and the "bad days"; that is, acute exacerbation of COPD (AECOPD). This goal is accomplished by providing careful and continuous communication with a case manager, fostering disease-specific knowledge and skills guided by a mutually understood care plan, and encouraging patient self-efficacy behaviors.

COPD CSM FOR THE "GOOD DAYS"

Behavioral change and psychological components of COPD CSM are aimed at helping patients lead as functional and as healthy a life (with as many "good days") as possible throughout the course of their condition. CSM enhances patients' knowledge and understanding of the disease, and, more importantly, encourages self-efficacious behavioral lifestyle changes. This self-management includes goal-setting, increased physical activity, adherence to exercise programs after completion of pulmonary rehabilitation, and coping with breathlessness, anxiety, and depression. Preventive behaviors include vaccination, smoking cessation, diet, good hand hygiene, and adherence to respiratory medication.

Table 1	
COPD CSM structure and examples	
Categories of Care	**Examples**
Self-management	Ongoing education behavioral support
	Prevention (vaccination, smoking)
	Motivation, self-efficacy, and goal-setting
	Physical activity programs
	Disease exacerbation action plans
	Team training in cognitive behavior change
Advanced access care delivery	24/7 plan for care accessibility
	Shared/group appointments
	Nonappointment care/telephone follow-up
	Home tele-care
Decision support	Integration of guidelines
	Specialty expertise and ongoing input
	Barrier identification
	Performance review
Clinical information system	Disease registries
	Provider reminders
	Provider feedback
	Quality improvement
	Risk management/resource utilization

Adapted from Adams SG, Smith PK, Allan PF, et al. Systematic review of the chronic care model in chronic obstructive pulmonary disease prevention and management. Arch Intern Med 2007;167(6):551–61.

Knowledge and Understanding

Although education alone in COPD CSM is insufficient to accomplish the myriad goals of managing this chronic condition throughout its course, it does provide an informational framework for shared decision making and correcting common misperceptions.[25] For example, a lack of understanding by patients and providers about correct inhalational techniques and the benefits of controller medications[11,12,14] can result in poor adherence. Likewise, because adherence to long-term oxygen treatment (LTOT) is often suboptimal,[26] patients should understand that improved survival, not merely immediate symptom relief, is the ultimate goal of LTOT.[27] There are many educational resource materials for COPD CSM, such as "Living Well with COPD" by the American College of Chest Physicians (2012), and the Canadian program for patients "Living Well with COPD" (www.livingwellwithcopd.com) and health professional guide "Krames On-Demand" (www.kramesstaywell.com).[28] Evidence that COPD CSM improves patient understanding of the disease is compelling. Knowledge informs the patient of the probable consequences and outcomes of their choices. Six of 7 RCTs that have reported this outcome have found a benefit.[29–35] Although new knowledge inspires individuals to consider changes in behavior, empirical evidence has shown that it is insufficient for generating sustained behavioral change.

Self-Efficacy Behaviors for Healthy Living

Few trials have reported on the direct effect of COPD CSM on measures of self-efficacy: whereas self-efficacy scores improved in one study,[36] another found no impact of COPD CSM on self-efficacy overall, although a post hoc analysis did find a reduction in COPD admissions and deaths in the subset of successful self-managers, who also had had lower baseline self-efficacy scores.[37] A qualitative

Table 2
Self-management skills and healthy behaviors for self-management of COPD

Healthy Behavior	Self-Management Skill (Strategy)
Live in a smoke-free environment	Quit smoking and remain nonsmoker, and avoid secondhand smoke
Comply with your medication	Take medication as prescribed on a regular basis and use proper inhalation techniques
Manage your breathing	Use according to directives: • The pursed-lip breathing technique • The forward body positions • The coughing techniques
Conserve your energy	Prioritize your activities, plan your schedule, and pace yourself
Manage your stress and anxiety	Use your relaxation and breathing techniques, try to solve one problem at a time, talk about your problems, and do not hesitate to ask for help and maintain a positive attitude
Prevent and manage aggravations of your symptoms (exacerbations)	Get your flu shot every year and your vaccine for pneumonia Identify and avoid factors that can make your symptoms worse Use your Plan of Action according to the directives (recognition of symptoms deterioration and actions to perform) Contact your resource person when needed
Maintain an active life	Maintain physical activities (activities of daily living, walking, climbing stairs, etc) Exercise regularly (according to a prescribed home exercise program)
Keep a healthy diet	Maintain a healthy weight, eat food high in protein, and eat smaller meals more often (5–6 meals/day)
Have good sleep habits	Maintain a routine, avoid heavy meals and stimulants before bedtime, and relax before bedtime
Maintain a satisfying sex life	Use positions that require less energy Share your feelings with your partner Do not limit yourself to intercourse, create a romantic atmosphere Use your breathing, relaxation, and coughing techniques
Get involved in leisure activities	Choose leisure activities that you enjoy Choose environments where your symptoms will not be aggravated Pace yourself through the activities while using your breathing techniques Respect your strengths and limitations

Adapted from Bourbeau J, Nault D. Self-management strategies in chronic obstructive pulmonary disease. Clin Chest Med 2007;28(3):617–28; with permission.

analysis embedded in another RCT showed that 59% of the CSM patients felt more self-confident and more secure.[38] Self-efficacy is lower in patients with low compliance to a maintenance exercise program than in patients with high compliance to maintenance exercise,[29,30] a finding that concurs with health behavior theory.[39] Specific disease-related self-efficacy goals for healthy living are discussed in subsequent sections.

Physical activity
Lower levels of physical activity in COPD are linked to a vicious circle of exertional dyspnea causing avoidance of activity, resulting in deconditioning, thereby exacerbating

exertional dyspnea and ultimately leading to a loss of self-confidence about the ability to perform activities of daily living.[40] Although COPD CSM differs somewhat from pulmonary rehabilitation in emphasis and approach, guiding patient behavior to increase regular physical activity is a core component of both.[25,41] Clinical trials of COPD CSM have mainly focused on exercise and physical capacity and not on physical activity. Earlier trials that did not include a structured or supervised exercise program found no significant effect on exercise capacity.[5,42-46] An a posteriori qualitative study[38] of a small sample of patients who received CSM showed an increase in activities of daily living and regular exercise. Although the results of this qualitative study may have relevance, further quantitative studies are needed.

Health status, psychological well-being, and dyspnea

Several recent studies of COPD CSM have found significant and clinically meaningful improvements in health status, as measured by the St George's Respiratory Questionnaire (SGRQ)[47] or the Chronic Respiratory Questionnaire (CRQ).[31,48-51] Other studies have reported no overall difference in health status,[29,34,36,44,45,52-56] but several of them reported improvements in selected domains, including the symptom and impact subscales of the SGRQ,[33,37,42] and the fatigue and mastery components of the CRQ.[46] The 2007 Cochrane analysis found a statistically significant difference in overall SGRQ scores, but it did not achieve the accepted minimal clinically important difference (MCID).[5] The most recent Cochrane update found a pooled mean difference on the SGRQ total score of -3.71 in favor of CSM that approached the MCID of -4 points.[6]

Psychological components of well-being are strong determinants of health status. Studies of the effect of COPD CSM on anxiety and depression are mixed, whereas the impact on subjective dyspnea scales has been generally positive. A study that compared cognitive-behavioral therapy for depression/anxiety with self-efficacy behavior education in COPD patients found that both interventions sustainably improved depression and health status.[50] By contrast, 2 RCTs of CSM found no differences in anxiety or depression scores.[36,37]

By providing ongoing team support, promoting self-efficacy, and teaching breathing-related behavioral skills, CSM can help break the vicious cycle of dyspnea, inactivity, deconditioning, and resulting worsening dyspnea. The 2007 Cochrane analysis of CSM in COPD found significant improvements in dyspnea scores,[5] and 3 of the 4 RCTs since 2006 that reported dyspnea scores also reported improvement.[57-60]

Preventive behaviors

Advice and assistance on smoking cessation is a standard component of COPD CSM,[5] although the few studies that examined its effect on smoking status reported mixed results.[31,33,43,46] Vaccination for respiratory infection is also a component of COPD CSM, although information is lacking about its efficacy of COPD CSM in increasing respiratory vaccination rates and health outcomes.[61-63] Good hand hygiene behavior, which reduces respiratory infections in patients at risk for influenza,[64] is also recommended in COPD CSM,[61] and was a core component in at least one successful trial.[51] Optimal nutrition is important for everyone's health, including those with COPD. An abnormally low body mass index is associated with increased mortality in patients with COPD,[65] and increased fruit intake in COPD patients is associated with decreased mortality.[66] A dietary intervention for patients with COPD improved exercise capacity in one study.[67] As a component of COPD CSM,[61] patients are encouraged to eat a healthy, balanced diet and are taught potentially beneficial eating techniques including multiple small meals, adequate fluid intake, and eating slowly. There is a dedicated diet module in the Canadian CSM Living Well with COPD[61] that has recently been developed by a team of dietitians. Despite the importance of this topic, information is lacking on the effect of COPD CSM on improving dietary habits.

Adherence to inhaled controller medications can maximize the number of "good days" for COPD patients by reducing dyspnea and by decreasing the frequency of exacerbations.[68,69] Studies that have measured the impact of COPD CSM on adherence to maintenance medications have generally been positive,[33,51,70] with the exceptions of 2 smaller trials.[46,71]

Change in Provider Behavior

The ultimate success in dealing with the current primary care crisis in providing chronic care hinges on establishing trust between providers and patients, developing team relationships, and promoting essential skills, including active listening and motivational interviewing.[72] However, there is a paucity of information about the effect of CSM on provider behavior. Successful implementation of the Chronic Care Model may provide a surrogate measure in this regard. The establishment of team-based medical homes has been shown to reduce physician burnout and improve patient experience ratings without increasing costs.[73] More specific insight about the effect on providers is provided by a study which found that health care workers who participated in COPD CSM developed a new sense of cooperation, and began to enjoy working with their patients.[58]

COPD CSM FOR THE "BAD DAYS"
Action Plans for AECOPD

AECOPD is a major negative determinant of health status: health status is worse in frequent exacerbators and contributes to the decline in pulmonary function.[74,75] Early recognition and treatment of AECOPD is associated with more rapid recovery, and failure to treat is associated with worse health status and increased emergency hospitalizations.[76] Reliance on traditional models of health care delivery to identify and treat AECOPD is suboptimal: half of all episodes go unreported to health care providers, and both reported and unreported exacerbations are associated with declines in health status.[77]

Most COPD CSM programs have included action plans for self-management of AECOPD, and adherence to written action plans for prompt treatment of AECOPD is associated with more rapid recovery times.[78] A retrospective study of a relatively small cohort of 89 patients found that action plans increased the use of prednisone and antibiotics without decreasing unplanned visits.[79] A systematic review of 5 RCTs that compared the provision of action plans for AECOPD (with minimal or no self-management education) versus usual care found that the former improved patients' ability to respond appropriately to COPD exacerbation symptoms but had no effect on health care utilization.[80] These results suggest that action plans should generally be used in the setting of a more comprehensive intervention, such as COPD CSM. Individually tailored action plans provide instructions on what the exacerbation is and what to do about it. This approach typically includes refillable prescriptions for antibiotics and short courses of oral corticosteroids to be initiated at onset of exacerbation symptoms, and emergency and follow-up information. Close follow-up, including regular communication with a case manager, is important. Action plans should also include instructions for patients to report exacerbations requiring prednisone or antibiotics to the CSM team, as well as any exacerbation not responding to action-plan medications. Patients must have a thorough understanding of the appropriate use of action plans so as to avoid delays or failure to initiate treatment, in addition to the potential dangers of excessive use of action plans, including adverse effects from frequent or prolonged systemic steroids, antibiotic resistance, and *Clostridium difficile* infections.[79] Another potential benefit of action plans may be to encourage patients to restrict oral corticosteroid exposure to short-term use only.[40] Patients must also learn how to recognize life-threatening symptoms that require prompt professional medical treatment. Even patients with a high burden of disease can achieve appropriate self-management behaviors in this setting, and this behavior may reduce health care utilization.[81]

In COPD, studies evaluating the effectiveness of action plans in exacerbation outcomes have had mixed results. In one study, adherence to action plans was strongly associated with a reduction in the number of days to total recovery from AECOPD.[36,52] Other studies reported that use of the action plan resulted in earlier identification and treatment of AECOPD.[44,70] However, a large Veterans Affairs (VA) Cooperative trial of CSM (centered on an action plan) versus usual care found no difference in self-reported exacerbations and no difference in the time from onset of symptoms to initiation of treatment.[36] Furthermore, although CSM patients were instructed to call the case manager in the event of an exacerbation, very few patients did indeed call. These data suggest that the CSM plan in this trial failed in its intent to provide timely care for patients with worsening symptoms of an exacerbation, and underlines the importance of following up and measuring the intended behavioral changes associated with COPD self-management.

Effect of CSM on Hospitalizations for AECOPD

Although hospitalizations for AECOPD are costly and burdensome to patients and society, there is a relative dearth of published information on CSM in this area.[82] One meta-analysis found that CSM decreased hospitalizations, but concluded that there was insufficient information about which components of CSM contribute the most benefit.[83] Although the most recent Cochrane review found reductions in respiratory-related hospital admissions over 12 months,[6] information is lacking on how to tailor this intervention to the heterogeneous population of patients with COPD; more specifically, it is not known why CSM reduces health care utilization in some patients and not in others.

COPD CSM RCTs that decreased hospitalizations

A relatively intense model of COPD CSM (education, 7–8 in-home sessions with nurses, respiratory therapists, or physiotherapists) in 191 patients previously hospitalized for AECOPD in Quebec, Canada, resulted in decreased respiratory-related hospitalizations (39.8%), and hospitalizations unrelated to COPD (57.1%).[42] A moderately intense COPD CSM intervention (tailored care plan including self-medication option, monthly nurse clinic visits, and general practice clinic visits every month for 1 year) in 135 outpatients in New Zealand with moderate to severe COPD decreased respiratory-related admissions, with an apparent reduction in all-cause admissions and a reduction in length of stay.[46] Another CSM study in Spain and Belgium (individually tailored care plans, a 2-hour education at discharge including strategies for future exacerbations, a home visit by a physician, nurse, and social worker, followed by telephone calls weekly for 1 month, 3 months, and 9 months) of 155 patients who were previously admitted for AECOPD resulted in a 45% reduction in hospitalizations.[43] The largest RCT to date (a single group session, customized action plans with refillable medication, and monthly phone contact with respiratory therapy disease managers) included 743 patients in the Midwest United States VA health care system at high risk for hospitalization for COPD.[51] Compared with usual care, CSM decreased respiratory-related hospitalizations by 30%, and all-cause hospitalizations or emergency department (ED) visits by 27%. Of note, cardiac and non-COPD hospitalizations also decreased by 32% in this study. One potential reason for this finding is that non-COPD cardiorespiratory admissions such as CHF are often preceded by pneumonia or another primary respiratory process.[84]

Other RCTs that have demonstrated reductions in hospitalizations include a study in 122 LTOT patients, which found that home-based visits every 3 months and monthly calls decreased hospital admissions by more than 50%[54]; a study of 50 patients in Germany with mild to very severe COPD that reported decreased hospitalizations[85]; a study of a relatively simplified model in 173 patients in Northern Ireland[33]; and an RCT of 85 patients in Japan of 6 months of tailored education with an action plan.[60] All the individual trials that have shown these benefits have in common a CSM intervention that included an AECOPD action plan embedded in an integrated health care system coordinated by a case manager, with regular communication (monthly visits or telephone calls) to reinforce patient empowerment.

COPD CSM RCTs that did not decrease hospitalizations

Several relatively large studies of COPD CSM have not demonstrated reductions in hospitalizations. One RCT of CSM (4 weekly group sessions for a total of 10 hours, a feedback session 3 months later, an action plan, a 2-year physical training program, and no scheduled follow-up calls or contacts) versus usual care in 248 outpatients with moderately severe COPD who were not otherwise at high risk for hospitalization[44] showed an apparent trend in decreased hospitalizations; however, in a subsequent economic analysis this was not considered cost-effective.[45] The VA Cooperative trial of CSM (the BREATH trial) (four 90-minute educational sessions, a group reinforcement session, action plans, and follow-up phone calls once a month for 3 months, then every 3 months thereafter) versus usual care had to be prematurely discontinued for safety concerns (increased mortality in the treatment group) after enrollment of 426 patients out of an anticipated 960.[36] At the time of discontinuation, the investigators found no suggestion of a reduction in COPD-related hospitalizations or hospitalizations for any cause. In contrast to other studies, the intervention did not change patient behaviors related to AECOPD. The times between the onset of AECOPD symptoms and self-treatment did not differ between the groups (1 week), and the difference in the use of action-plan medications was much lower than that reported in the other VA study.[51] Finally, the Glasgow-supported self-management trial (GSuST) of 464 high-risk patients found no overall effect on hospitalizations, although a post hoc analysis found reduction in COPD hospitalizations and deaths in the 40% of patients who were successful self-managers.[37]

Why some RCTs may have been successful while others were not

Determining why some COPD CSM programs succeed while others fail is challenging, but of considerable importance. Possible reasons for negative studies include: (1) lack of statistical power, as many studies enrolled fewer than 200 patients[29,32,52,53,55,56,86]; (2) inclusion of patients who were not at high risk for hospitalization (ie, the ceiling effect)[34,44,52,53,55]; and (3) follow-up for less than 1 year.[32,49,53] In addition, failure to empower patients to appropriately manage AECOPDs by not providing an action plan with refillable home prescriptions[32,53,55,87] or insufficient ongoing communication to reinforce patients' empowerment to change behavior could explain negative results in some studies.[34,36]

The aforementioned large, apparently well-designed, but ultimately negative, VA and Glasgow trials merit further discussion.[36,37] Although both were based on a successful CSM model,[42] there may have been discrepancies between the intent of the CSM programs and their actual administration; that is, "the devil is in the details." Possible discrepancies might have been ensuring sufficient background and training for disease managers, or heterogeneity in the delivery of the educational content. The main focus may have been on education and not on promoting and supporting adaptive behaviors. Key messages about self-management might have been lost amid the complexity of the educational content, particularly among patients who were too recently ill to receive information and participate collaboratively. In addition, the educational content delivered might have made some patients overly confident about their ability to self-manage, and unable to recognize an urgent need for professional medical attention.

Mortality and safety concerns in COPD CSM

The benefits of COPD CSM must be carefully balanced against potential harms. Concerns about the safety of COPD CSM were recently raised when the BREATH study (see earlier discussion) had to be stopped prematurely because of increased all-cause and respiratory deaths in the CSM group in comparison with the usual care group (28 vs 10 deaths, $P = .003$).[36] In this study, the investigators made an extensive effort to collect and analyze complete information about the deaths, but could find no explanation for the excess mortality. Aside from the possibility of actual harm from COPD CSM, one potential explanation for the increased deaths is random chance, as discussed in the accompanying editorial.[88] Apparent, albeit small, imbalances in the distribution of baseline characteristics such as marital status, ethnicity, and cardiac comorbidities could conceivably have resulted in an imbalance in mortality.

Three meta-analyses of mortality from COPD CSM versus usual care are currently available. Although the trials included in each analysis varied slightly, they all concluded that there was no statistically significant difference in mortality between groups, at both short-term and long-term follow-up,[6,89] and in patients who were enrolled after a COPD hospitalization and those who were not (**Table 3**). Despite these encouraging data, safety must never be underestimated. CSM programs should be properly adapted to respond to patient needs, taking into account disease severity and comorbidities. It may not be realistic or safe for some patients to make independent medical decisions without proper support and communication with a health care professional.

INTEGRATION OF COPD CSM AND PULMONARY REHABILITATION

Although studies with a primary focus on pulmonary rehabilitation were excluded from Cochrane reviews of COPD CSM, the integration of COPD CSM with pulmonary rehabilitation provides a natural, evidence-based health care delivery model for managing COPD patients of all degrees of severity. It allows the inclusion of patients with more severe disease, more comorbidities, inability to exercise, or limited ability to attend multiple sessions.[41,81] Both COPD CSM and pulmonary rehabilitation share similar holistic and systematic approaches, and both can rapidly adapt their practices in the face of new evidence. Pulmonary rehabilitation, with its strong emphasis on formal exercise training, is the best intervention to improve exercise capacity, with a primary objective of relieving disability by decreasing dyspnea and improving the ability to perform activities of daily living.[90] However, improvements in exercise capacity do not automatically equate with increases in physical activity. In other words, pulmonary rehabilitation provides patients the "can do," whereas CSM provides patients the "will

Table 3
All-cause mortality: randomized controlled trials for COPD CDM

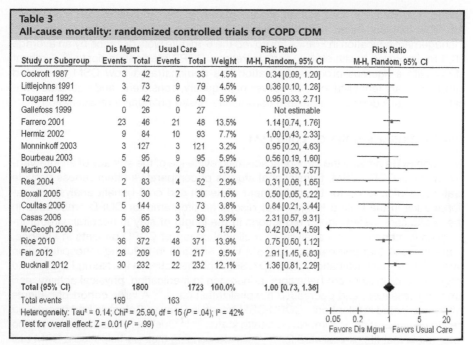

Study or Subgroup	Dis Mgmt Events	Total	Usual Care Events	Total	Weight	Risk Ratio M-H, Random, 95% CI
Cockroft 1987	3	42	7	33	4.5%	0.34 [0.09, 1.20]
Littlejohns 1991	3	73	9	79	4.5%	0.36 [0.10, 1.28]
Tougaard 1992	6	42	6	40	5.9%	0.95 [0.33, 2.71]
Gallefoss 1999	0	26	0	27		Not estimable
Farrero 2001	23	46	21	48	13.5%	1.14 [0.74, 1.76]
Hermiz 2002	9	84	10	93	7.7%	1.00 [0.43, 2.33]
Monninkoff 2003	3	127	3	121	3.2%	0.95 [0.20, 4.63]
Bourbeau 2003	5	95	9	95	5.9%	0.56 [0.19, 1.60]
Martin 2004	9	44	4	49	5.5%	2.51 [0.83, 7.57]
Rea 2004	2	83	4	52	2.9%	0.31 [0.06, 1.65]
Boxall 2005	1	30	2	30	1.6%	0.50 [0.05, 5.22]
Coultas 2005	5	144	3	73	3.8%	0.84 [0.21, 3.44]
Casas 2006	5	65	3	90	3.9%	2.31 [0.57, 9.31]
McGeogh 2006	1	86	2	73	1.5%	0.42 [0.04, 4.59]
Rice 2010	36	372	48	371	13.9%	0.75 [0.50, 1.12]
Fan 2012	28	209	10	217	9.5%	2.91 [1.45, 5.83]
Bucknall 2012	30	232	22	232	12.1%	1.36 [0.81, 2.29]
Total (95% CI)		1800		1723	100.0%	1.00 [0.73, 1.36]
Total events	169		163			

Heterogeneity: Tau² = 0.14; Chi² = 25.90, df = 15 (P = .04); I² = 42%
Test for overall effect: Z = 0.01 (P = .99)

Favors Dis Mgmt   Favors Usual Care

Courtesy of Roderick MacDonald, MS and Timothy Wilt, MD, Center for Chronic Disease Outcomes Research, Minneapolis Veterans Affairs Health Care System, Minneapolis, MN.

do." Pulmonary rehabilitation is too often restricted to an acute care time frame (6–12 weeks). Integrating pulmonary rehabilitation with ongoing CSM provides a longer-term, day-to-day approach to change and maintain behavior, including adherence to exercise programs and increases in day-to-day physical activity. In the most recent American Thoracic Society/European Respiratory Society Statement on Pulmonary Rehabilitation,[41] behavioral changes and CSM are emphasized as essential components of pulmonary rehabilitation: "Health behavior change is vital to optimization and maintenance of benefits from any intervention in chronic care, and pulmonary rehabilitation has taken a lead in implementing strategies to achieve this goal."

Several recent studies have successfully combined pulmonary rehabilitation with components of COPD CSM. A nurse-led study of home-based pulmonary rehabilitation combined with patient education in Turkey improved lung function, health status, dyspnea, and functional capacity.[91] An RCT of 4 months of multidisciplinary rehabilitation followed by 20 months of maintenance support with comprehensive COPD CSM education in the Netherlands improved health status and exercise capacity.[59] A study of personalized physical activity training, continuous self-management education including personal goal-setting, optimization of medications, action plans, and adherence monitoring in 2 towns in the Netherlands improved health status and dyspnea scores.[58] Another study of postpulmonary rehabilitation maintenance, education, and psychosocial support intervention embedded within a health care network in France improved health status and exercise capacity.[92] An RCT of home pulmonary rehabilitation, education, and promotion of healthy behaviors in Egypt improved exercise capacity and health status.[93] An RCT of pulmonary rehabilitation, self-management education, action plans, monthly telephone calls, and home visits in

London reported improved self-management of AECOPD and decreased mortality.[94] An RCT that combined hospital-based, supervised exercise sessions with self-management education in France improved the 6-minute walk distance by an average 50.5 m, improved health status, and decreased COPD medication costs.[95] A recent study with a rigorous process evaluation has demonstrated how CSM integrated into pulmonary rehabilitation can deliver high-quality, consistent, and equitable education sessions during hospital and community-based pulmonary rehabilitation.[96]

TRANSLATIONAL STUDIES OF COPD CSM

Although RCTs provide the strongest scientific evidence of the efficacy of an intervention such as COPD CSM, translational studies of comparative effectiveness provide real-world information for the betterment of health and cost-benefit analysis. A national audit in the United Kingdom of discharge programs for COPD embedded in the health care system found reductions in the length of stay in hospital without increases in mortality.[97] An analysis of a clinical cohort of COPD patients in Quebec, Canada found that participation in CSM was effective in reducing rehospitalization rates.[92] A pre-post evaluation of COPD CSM implementation in the Netherlands found improvements in self-care behaviors, adherence to medication, physical activity, and smoking cessation, and decreased hospitalization rates.[98] A large cohort of patients who participated in telephonic COPD CSM based in Denver, Colorado had decreased health care utilization and improved health status.[99] In Quebec, Canada, patients who returned to real-life clinical care for 2 years after ending their participation a CSM trial had sustained reductions in all-cause hospitalizations and ED visits.[42,100] The same group of investigators recently published another study of a cohort of patients with more severe COPD than patients in the original 2003 RCT.[81] In real-life practice, COPD CSM was effective in sustaining healthy self-management behavior and reducing health care utilization.

Costs

In addition to direct benefits to patient health, translating COPD CSM into practice has the potential to help control rising health care costs through reducing expensive health care utilization and promoting healthy behaviors. Reports of the impact of CSM in reducing medical expenditures are mixed. An early systematic review[101] and several other studies found no significant cost savings.[45,49,98,102] However, other trials have suggested that health service utilization and associated costs can be decreased.[54,86,103–106]

INTEGRATION OF COPD CSM INTO CLINICAL PRACTICE
Medical Home Model

The integration of COPD CSM into the patient-centered medical home (PCMH) model provides an opportunity to change the focus from a pessimistic, reactive, rescue approach to proactive, collaborative management. By teaching patients the behavioral skills required to implement disease-specific regimens, CSM can serve as a link between primary care and secondary care. Incorporating COPD CSM into the PCMH model can improve access to care, allow team members to practice at the "top of their license," establish continuity with other providers and community resources, and use health information technology to more efficiently manage care and assess quality improvement, risk-management performance, and resource utilization.[107]

Qualification and Training of COPD CSM Managers

The chronic disease manager is the linchpin of the CSM team, and the importance of his or her experience, training, and skills cannot be overemphasized.[81] CSM team members should have up-to-date training in cognitive-behavioral therapy (CBT) and motivational interviewing. CBT has proved to be effective in inducing behavioral change in patients with chronic respiratory disease such as COPD.[108] CBT offers relatively simple and structured techniques that can be incorporated by the members of a multidisciplinary team, for example in pulmonary rehabilitation. Successful implementation depends on interprofessional training and the development of team relationships and skills, such as active listening and motivational interviewing,[72] and adapting CSM to fit local health care delivery systems.[82]

The professional qualifications of successful COPD CSM managers vary according to the health care systems in which they are embedded. Successful trials have employed nurses,[42,109] respiratory therapists,[42,51] pharmacists,[110] and physiotherapists.[42] Employing lay community care guides as members of the CSM team is another recent innovation reported in a study of patients with the chronic metabolic syndrome.[111] As suggested in the accompanying editorial, the success of this strategy might be attributable to the concept that "knowing just the basics may have its advantages—what people don't know is less likely to distract them."[112]

The COPD CSM case manager should be a facilitator agent with skills in COPD content and CBT, and the ability to evaluate patients' learning outcomes, for example, patients' achievement of changes in behavior. The COPD CSM case manager should also be a resource person and, above all, he or she should have good communication skills and a nonjudgmental approach. Reference guides are available to help COPD CSM case managers implement programs (www.livingwellwithcopd.com). However, studies are needed that better define the expertise and validate the training required by the COPD CSM managers.

Frequency and Intensity of Contacts

COPD CSM is founded on collaboration between patients and care team members, which, by definition, is ongoing. The amount of ongoing CSM contact has been correlated with positive outcomes.[51] Successful approaches have used 1-on-1 or group sessions, streamlined education and behavioral change sessions with follow-up telephone reinforcement,[33,51,58,59] or more numerous and comprehensive sessions.[42]

While effective CSM interventions do exist, the implementation rate of such interventions is lagging behind the increasing burden of chronic disease on an already strained health care system, with shortages in case managers who have the expertise to deliver such interventions. As a result, facets of communication, monitoring, reinforcement, and the intensity of the intervention for COPD CSM may vary among health care systems, although they ideally should be matched to patients' needs. Health information technology is another approach to provide effective, timely, and sustained patient support. Home tele-care presents an innovative tool for CSM that provides targeted "automated hovering."[113] An automated tele-care platform has been reported to help patients successfully identify AECOPDs.[57] Combining education with home tele-care can reduce ED visits and hospitalizations, improve health status, increase exercise capacity and BODE (Body mass index, airflow Obstruction, Dyspnea, Exercise capacity) index, and reduce smoking rates.[114] A recent Cochrane review of 10 RCTs of tele-care for COPD confirmed reductions in health care utilization, but noted that more research is needed to determine how this fits into more complex CSM delivery models.[115]

Patient Selection for COPD CSM

Uncertainty exists regarding which patients should be targeted for COPD CSM. To avoid a ceiling effect, many, but not all, successful COPD CSM interventions have focused on patients with advanced disease. A more proactive approach in patients who are less sick may be justified, however, if resources can be efficiently applied. Evidence for inclusion of patients with less severe COPD is suggested by the 2007 Cochrane review, which found reductions in hospitalizations in both low-risk and high-risk patients.[5] Whether to include or exclude patients with various comorbidities is also unclear. Patients with severe comorbidities, especially CHF,[43] have been excluded from some studies, presumably because of the difficulty in distinguishing the cause of symptoms. A recent study[36] suggests that CSM may increase mortality in patients with severe disease and cardiac comorbidities. Such patients, therefore, may not be good candidates for CSM that includes medical self-management.

Other studies, reflecting the real-world clinical setting, have not excluded these types of patients.[42,46,51] Targeting patients who are more likely to adopt successful behavioral change is also a consideration, as suggested by one study in which COPD admissions and deaths decreased in the subset of successful self-managers.[37] However, it is unclear how these patients might be identified in advance. Conversely, enrollment of patients with psychiatric disorders, a history of nonadherence, or other behavioral problems was actively encouraged in the Midwest VA study,[51] in reflection of real-world clinical needs.

THE CONTINUUM OF DISEASE: ADVANCE CARE PLANNING AND PALLIATIVE CARE

As COPD patients continue along the trajectory of their illness, strategies of care delivery must be adjusted to continue supporting the goal of providing the best possible quality of life, including relief of physical and psychological suffering. Achieving these goals requires coordination between primary care providers, the CSM team, and the palliative care team. COPD patients experience inadequacies in discussing details about the progression of illness, prognosis, and dying in traditional health care systems.[116] The inclusion of the palliative care team at earlier stages of any serious chronic illness not only addresses suffering but also assists patients in understanding the likely outcomes of their illness and in setting realistic goals.[117]

SUMMARY

Patients with COPD have complex medical, emotional, and social needs throughout the changing course of their disease. COPD CSM is based on the principle that guiding individual behavioral changes is the key to meeting these complex changing needs. Many models of multicomponent, team-based COPD CSM have been shown to improve outcomes, such as health status and health care utilization, in rigorously designed RCTs. However, self-management may not suit all patients. Patient care and medical decisions may need to be assumed by health professionals at certain points in the disease trajectory that pose an unacceptable risk of mortality; that is, severe disease instability or comorbidities that interfere with decision-making capacity. Ideally, integrated systems of care such as CSM should adapt and adjust to these changing patient needs.

More importance must be lent to the training of the CSM team members in CBT and motivational interviewing. There is still a lot to learn, such as how to make sure that the CSM team members are qualified to properly guide the patients on their behavior-modification process; for example, helping them to set realistic goals and improve their motivation and self-efficacy. Furthermore, various evaluation methods need to be better defined and standardized so as to assess patients' readiness and progress at each intervention point. These issues will need to be incorporated into future trials, and adapted for use in clinical practice.

Larger, high-quality, longer-term studies using customized, well-described self-management interventions aimed at behavioral change are needed to evaluate real-world effectiveness, safety, and costs of integrating COPD CSM with pulmonary rehabilitation, the PCMH model, and palliative care teams. Finally, new technological communication interfaces are promising additions to the management of chronic diseases including COPD, and further studies that incorporate them with COPD CSM are needed.

ACKNOWLEDGMENTS

The authors would like to thank Louise Auclair and Esther Tomkee for their clerical work.

REFERENCES

1. Bourbeau J. Clinical decision processes and patient engagement in self-management. Dis Manag Health Outcome 2008;16(5):327–33.
2. Windham BG, Bennett RG, Gottlieb S. Care management interventions for older patients with congestive heart failure. Am J Manag Care 2003;9(6):447–59.
3. Battersby M, Von KM, Schaefer J, et al. Twelve evidence-based principles for implementing self-management support in primary care. Jt Comm J Qual Patient Saf 2010;36(12):561–70.
4. Monninkhof E, van der Valk P, van der Palen J, et al. Self-management education for patients with chronic obstructive pulmonary disease: a systematic review. Thorax 2003;58(5):394–8.
5. Effing T, Monninkhof E, van der Valk PD, et al. Self-management education for patients with chronic obstructive pulmonary disease. Cochrane Database Syst Rev 2007;(4):CD002990.
6. Kruis AL, Smidt N, Assendelft WJ, et al. Integrated disease management interventions for patients with chronic obstructive pulmonary disease. Cochrane Database Syst Rev 2013;(10):CD009437.
7. Schoen C, Osborn R, How SK, et al. In chronic condition: experiences of patients with complex health care needs, in eight countries, 2008. Health Aff (Millwood) 2009;28(1):w1–16.
8. Judson TJ, Detsky AS, Press MJ. Encouraging patients to ask questions: how to overcome "white-coat silence". JAMA 2013;309(22):2325–6.
9. Cooke CE, Sidel M, Belletti DA, et al. Review: clinical inertia in the management of chronic obstructive pulmonary disease. COPD 2012;9(1):73–80.
10. Johnson DR, Nichol KL, Lipczynski K. Barriers to adult immunization. Am J Med 2008;121(7 Suppl 2):S28–35.
11. Melani AS, Canessa P, Coloretti I, et al. Inhaler mishandling is very common in patients with chronic airflow obstruction and long-term home nebuliser use. Respir Med 2012;106(5):668–76.
12. Mularski RA, Asch SM, Shrank WH, et al. The quality of obstructive lung disease care for adults in the United States as measured by adherence to recommended processes. Chest 2006;130(6):1844–50.

13. Rutschmann OT, Janssens JP, Vermeulen B, et al. Knowledge of guidelines for the management of COPD: a survey of primary care physicians. Respir Med 2004;98(10):932–7.
14. Solem CT, Lee TA, Joo MJ, et al. Complexity of medication use in newly diagnosed chronic obstructive pulmonary disease patients. Am J Geriatr Pharmacother 2012;10(2):110–22.
15. Johnston KN, Young M, Grimmer-Somers KA, et al. Why are some evidence-based care recommendations in chronic obstructive pulmonary disease better implemented than others? Perspectives of medical practitioners. Int J Chron Obstruct Pulmon Dis 2011;6:659–67.
16. Bourbeau J, Nault D. Self-management strategies in chronic obstructive pulmonary disease. Clin Chest Med 2007;28(3):617–28.
17. Wagner EH. Chronic disease management: what will it take to improve care for chronic illness? Eff Clin Pract 1998;1(1):2–4.
18. Green LW, Kreuter MW. Health promotion planning: an educational and environmental approach. 3rd edition. London: Mayfield Publishing Company; 1999.
19. McAlister FA, Lawson FM, Teo KK, et al. A systematic review of randomized trials of disease management programs in heart failure. Am J Med 2001;110(5):378–84.
20. Weintraub A, Gregory D, Patel AR, et al. A multicenter randomized controlled evaluation of automated home monitoring and telephonic disease management in patients recently hospitalized for congestive heart failure: the SPAN-CHF II trial. J Card Fail 2010;16(4):285–92.
21. Pimouguet C, Le GM, Thiebaut R, et al. Effectiveness of disease-management programs for improving diabetes care: a meta-analysis. CMAJ 2011;183(2):E115–27.
22. Kates N, Mach M. Chronic disease management for depression in primary care: a summary of the current literature and implications for practice. Can J Psychiatry 2007;52(2):77–85.
23. Lemmens KM, Nieboer AP, Huijsman R. A systematic review of integrated use of disease-management interventions in asthma and COPD. Respir Med 2009; 103(5):670–91.
24. Adams SG, Smith PK, Allan PF, et al. Systematic review of the chronic care model in chronic obstructive pulmonary disease prevention and management. Arch Int Med 2007;167:551–61.
25. Nici L, Donner C, Wouters E, et al. American Thoracic Society/European Respiratory Society statement on pulmonary rehabilitation. Am J Respir Crit Care Med 2006;173(12):1390–413.
26. Lacasse Y, Lecours R, Pelletier C, et al. Randomised trial of ambulatory oxygen in oxygen-dependent COPD. Eur Respir J 2005;25(6):1032–8.
27. Stuart-Harris CH, Bishop JM, Clark TJ, et al. Long term domiciliary oxygen therapy in chronic hypoxic cor pulmonale complicating chronic bronchitis and emphysema: report of the Medical Research Council Working Party. Lancet 1981;1(8222):681–6.
28. Huang L. Krames on-demand (KOD). J Med Libr Assoc 2006;94(2):234–5.
29. Cockcroft A, Bagnall P, Heslop A, et al. Controlled trial of respiratory health worker visiting patients with chronic respiratory disability. Br Med J (Clin Res Ed) 1987;294(6566):225–8.
30. Hill K, Mangovski-Alzamora S, Blouin M, et al. Disease-specific education in the primary care setting increases the knowledge of people with chronic obstructive pulmonary disease: a randomized controlled trial. Patient Educ Couns 2010; 81(1):14–8.

31. Efraimsson EO, Hillervik C, Ehrenberg A. Effects of COPD self-care management education at a nurse-led primary health care clinic. Scand J Caring Sci 2008;22(2):178–85.
32. Hermiz O, Comino E, Marks G, et al. Randomised controlled trial of home based care of patients with chronic obstructive pulmonary disease. BMJ 2002; 325(7370):938–42.
33. Khdour MR, Kidney JC, Smyth BM, et al. Clinical pharmacy-led disease and medicine management programme for patients with COPD. Br J Clin Pharmacol 2009;68(4):588–98.
34. McGeoch GR, Willsman KJ, Dowson CA, et al. Self-management plans in the primary care of patients with chronic obstructive pulmonary disease. Respirology 2006;11(5):611–8.
35. Sashima S, Takahashi I, Nakazawa K. Identification and characterization of beta-D-galactosyl-transferase in chick corneas. Jpn J Ophthalmol 2002;46(6): 607–15.
36. Fan VS, Gaziano JM, Lew R, et al. A comprehensive care management program to prevent chronic obstructive pulmonary disease hospitalizations: a randomized, controlled trial. Ann Intern Med 2012;156(10):673–83.
37. Bucknall CE, Miller G, Lloyd SM, et al. Glasgow supported self-management trial (GSuST) for patients with moderate to severe COPD: randomised controlled trial. BMJ 2012;344:e1060.
38. Bourbeau J, Nault D, Dang-Tan T. Self-management and behaviour modification in COPD. Patient Educ Couns 2004;52(3):271–7.
39. Bandura A. Social cognitive theory: an agentic perspective. Annu Rev Psychol 2001;52:1–26.
40. Tiep B. Disease management of COPD with pulmonary rehabilitation. Chest 1997;112(6):1630–56.
41. Spruit MA, Singh SJ, Garvey C, et al. An official American Thoracic Society/European Respiratory Society statement: key concepts and advances in pulmonary rehabilitation. Am J Respir Crit Care Med 2013;188(8):e13–64.
42. Bourbeau J, Julien M, Maltais F, et al. Reduction of hospital utilization in patients with chronic obstructive pulmonary disease: a disease-specific self-management intervention. Arch Intern Med 2003;163(5):585–91.
43. Casas A, Troosters T, Garcia-Aymerich J, et al. Integrated care prevents hospitalisations for exacerbations in COPD patients. Eur Respir J 2006;28(1):123–30.
44. Monninkhof E, van der Valk P, van der Palen J, et al. Effects of a comprehensive self-management programme in patients with chronic obstructive pulmonary disease. Eur Respir J 2003;22(5):815–20.
45. Monninkhof E, van der Valk P, Schermer T, et al. Economic evaluation of a comprehensive self-management programme in patients with moderate to severe chronic obstructive pulmonary disease. Chron Respir Dis 2004;1(1):7–16.
46. Rea H, McAuley S, Stewart A, et al. A chronic disease management programme can reduce days in hospital for patients with chronic obstructive pulmonary disease. Intern Med J 2004;34(11):608–14.
47. Jones PW, Quirk FH, Baveystock CM, et al. A self-complete measure of health status for chronic airflow limitation. The St. George's Respiratory Questionnaire. Am Rev Respir Dis 1992;145(6):1321–7.
48. Guyatt GH, Berman LB, Townsend M, et al. A measure of quality of life for clinical trials in chronic lung disease. Thorax 1987;42(10):773–8.
49. Koff PB, Jones RH, Cashman JM, et al. Proactive integrated care improves quality of life in patients with COPD. Eur Respir J 2009;33(5):1031–8.

50. Kunik ME, Veazey C, Cully JA, et al. COPD education and cognitive behavioral therapy group treatment for clinically significant symptoms of depression and anxiety in COPD patients: a randomized controlled trial. Psychol Med 2008; 38(3):385–96.

51. Rice KL, Dewan N, Bloomfield HE, et al. Disease management program for chronic obstructive pulmonary disease: a randomized controlled trial. Am J Respir Crit Care Med 2010;182(7):890–6.

52. Bischoff EW, Akkermans R, Bourbeau J, et al. Comprehensive self management and routine monitoring in chronic obstructive pulmonary disease patients in general practice: randomised controlled trial. BMJ 2012;345:e7642.

53. Coultas D, Frederick J, Barnett B, et al. A randomized trial of two types of nurse-assisted home care for patients with COPD. Chest 2005;128(4):2017–24.

54. Farrero E, Escarrabill J, Prats E, et al. Impact of a hospital-based home-care program on the management of COPD patients receiving long-term oxygen therapy. Chest 2001;119(2):364–9.

55. Littlejohns P, Baveystock C, Parnell H, et al. Randomised controlled trial of the effectiveness of a respiratory health worker in reducing impairment, disability, and handicap due to chronic airflow limitation. Thorax 1991;46(8):559–64.

56. Martin IR, McNamara D, Sutherland FR, et al. Care plans for acutely deteriorating COPD: a randomized controlled trial. Chron Respir Dis 2004;1(4): 191–5.

57. Bischoff EW, Boer LM, Molema J, et al. Validity of an automated telephonic system to assess COPD exacerbation rates. Eur Respir J 2012;39:1090–6.

58. Chavannes NH, Schermer TR, Wouters EF, et al. Predictive value and utility of oral steroid testing for treatment of COPD in primary care: the COOPT study. Int J Chron Obstruct Pulmon Dis 2009;4:431–6.

59. van Wetering CR, Hoogendoorn M, Mol SJ, et al. Short- and long-term efficacy of a community-based COPD management programme in less advanced COPD: a randomised controlled trial. Thorax 2010;65(1):7–13.

60. Wakabayashi R, Motegi T, Yamada K, et al. Efficient integrated education for older patients with chronic obstructive pulmonary disease using the Lung Information Needs Questionnaire. Geriatr Gerontol Int 2011;11(4):422–30.

61. Living well with COPD. Available at: http://livingwellwithcopd.com. 2013. Accessed March 17, 2014.

62. Nichol KL, Baken L, Nelson A. Relation between influenza vaccination and outpatient visits, hospitalization, and mortality in elderly persons with chronic lung disease. Ann Intern Med 1999;130(5):397–403.

63. Nichol KL, Nordin JD, Nelson DB, et al. Effectiveness of influenza vaccine in the community-dwelling elderly. N Engl J Med 2007;357(14):1373–81.

64. Godoy P, Castilla J, Gado-Rodriguez M, et al. Effectiveness of hand hygiene and provision of information in preventing influenza cases requiring hospitalization. Prev Med 2012;54(6):434–9.

65. Landbo C, Prescott E, Lange P, et al. Prognostic value of nutritional status in chronic obstructive pulmonary disease. Am J Respir Crit Care Med 1999; 160(6):1856–61.

66. Walda IC, Tabak C, Smit HA, et al. Diet and 20-year chronic obstructive pulmonary disease mortality in middle-aged men from three European countries. Eur J Clin Nutr 2002;56(7):638–43.

67. Slinde F, Gronberg AM, Engstrom CR, et al. Individual dietary intervention in patients with COPD during multidisciplinary rehabilitation. Respir Med 2002;96(5): 330–6.

68. Calverley PM, Anderson JA, Celli B, et al. Salmeterol and fluticasone propionate and survival in chronic obstructive pulmonary disease. N Engl J Med 2007; 356(8):775–89.
69. Tashkin DP, Celli B, Senn S, et al. A 4-year trial of tiotropium in chronic obstructive pulmonary disease. N Engl J Med 2008;359(15):1543–54.
70. Garcia-Aymerich J, Hernandez C, Alonso A, et al. Effects of an integrated care intervention on risk factors of COPD readmission. Respir Med 2007;101(7):1462–9.
71. Gallefoss F, Bakke PS. How does patient education and self-management among asthmatics and patients with chronic obstructive pulmonary disease affect medication? Am J Respir Crit Care Med 1999;160(6):2000–5.
72. Frolkis JP. A piece of my mind. The Columbo phenomenon. JAMA 2013;309(22): 2333–4.
73. Reid RJ, Fishman PA, Yu O, et al. Patient-centered medical home demonstration: a prospective, quasi-experimental, before and after evaluation. Am J Manag Care 2009;15(9):e71–87.
74. Donaldson GC, Seemungal TA, Bhowmik A, et al. Relationship between exacerbation frequency and lung function decline in chronic obstructive pulmonary disease. Thorax 2002;57(10):847–52.
75. Seemungal TA, Donaldson GC, Paul EA, et al. Effect of exacerbation on quality of life in patients with chronic obstructive pulmonary disease. Am J Respir Crit Care Med 1998;157(5 Pt 1):1418–22.
76. Wilkinson TM, Donaldson GC, Hurst JR, et al. Early therapy improves outcomes of exacerbations of chronic obstructive pulmonary disease. Am J Respir Crit Care Med 2004;169(12):1298–303.
77. Langsetmo L, Platt RW, Ernst P, et al. Underreporting exacerbation of chronic obstructive pulmonary disease in a longitudinal cohort. Am J Respir Crit Care Med 2008;177(4):396–401.
78. Bischoff EW, Hamd DH, Sedeno M, et al. Effects of written action plan adherence on COPD exacerbation recovery. Thorax 2011;66(1):26–31.
79. Beaulieu-Genest L, Chretien D, Maltais F, et al. Self-administered prescriptions of oral steroids and antibiotics in chronic obstructive pulmonary disease: are we doing more harm than good? Chron Respir Dis 2007;4(3):143–7.
80. Walters JA, Turnock AC, Walters EH, et al. Action plans with limited patient education only for exacerbations of chronic obstructive pulmonary disease. Cochrane Database Syst Rev 2010;(5):CD005074.
81. Bourbeau J, Saad N, Joubert A, et al. Making collaborative self-management successful in COPD patients with high disease burden. Respir Med 2013; 107(7):1061–5.
82. Burke RE, Coleman EA. Interventions to decrease hospital readmissions: keys for cost-effectiveness. JAMA Intern Med 2013;173(8):695–8.
83. Peytremann-Bridevaux I, Staeger P, Bridevaux PO, et al. Effectiveness of chronic obstructive pulmonary disease-management programs: systematic review and meta-analysis. Am J Med 2008;121(5):433–43.
84. Fonarow GC, Abraham WT, Albert NM, et al. Factors identified as precipitating hospital admissions for heart failure and clinical outcomes: findings from OPTIMIZE-HF. Arch Intern Med 2008;168(8):847–54.
85. Bosch D, Feierabend M, Becker A. COPD outpatient education programme (ATEM) and BODE index. Pneumologie 2007;61(10):629–35 [in German].
86. Chuang C, Levine SH, Rich J. Enhancing cost-effective care with a patient-centric chronic obstructive pulmonary disease program. Popul Health Manag 2011;14(3):133–6.

87. Cockburn J, Gibberd RW, Reid AL, et al. Determinants of non-compliance with short term antibiotic regimens. Br Med J (Clin Res Ed) 1987;295(6602):814–8.
88. Pocock SJ. Ethical dilemmas and malfunctions in clinical trials research. Ann Intern Med 2012;156(10):746–7.
89. Hurley J, Gerkin RD, Fahy B, et al. Meta-analysis of self-management education for patients with chronic obstructive pulmonary disease. Southwest J Pulm Crit Care 2012;4:194–202.
90. Puhan MA, Gimeno-Santos E, Scharplatz M, et al. Pulmonary rehabilitation following exacerbations of chronic obstructive pulmonary disease. Cochrane Database Syst Rev 2011;(10):CD005305.
91. Akinci AC, Olgun N. The effectiveness of nurse-led, home-based pulmonary rehabilitation in patients with COPD in Turkey. Rehabil Nurs 2011;36(4):159–65.
92. Moullec G, Lavoie KL, Rabhi K, et al. Effect of an integrated care programme on re-hospitalization of patients with chronic obstructive pulmonary disease. Respirology 2012;17(4):707–14.
93. Ghanem M, Elaal EA, Mehany M, et al. Home-based pulmonary rehabilitation program: effect on exercise tolerance and quality of life in chronic obstructive pulmonary disease patients. Ann Thorac Med 2010;5(1):18–25.
94. Sridhar M, Taylor R, Dawson S, et al. A nurse led intermediate care package in patients who have been hospitalised with an acute exacerbation of chronic obstructive pulmonary disease. Thorax 2008;63(3):194–200.
95. Ninot G, Moullec G, Picot MC, et al. Cost-saving effect of supervised exercise associated to COPD self-management education program. Respir Med 2011; 105(3):377–85.
96. Cosgrove D, Macmahon J, Bourbeau J, et al. Facilitating education in pulmonary rehabilitation using the living well with COPD programme for pulmonary rehabilitation: a process evaluation. BMC Pulm Med 2013;13:50.
97. Kastelik JA, Lowe D, Stone RA, et al. National audit of supported discharge programmes for management of acute exacerbations of chronic obstructive pulmonary disease 2008. Thorax 2012;67(4):371–3.
98. Steuten L, Vrijhoef B, van Merode F, et al. Evaluation of a regional disease management programme for patients with asthma or chronic obstructive pulmonary disease. Int J Qual Health Care 2006;18(6):429–36.
99. Tinkelman D, Corsello P, McClure D, et al. One-year outcomes from a disease management program for chronic obstructive pulmonary disease. Dis Manag Health Outcome 2003;11:49–59.
100. Gadoury MA, Schwartzman K, Rouleau M, et al. Self-management reduces both short- and long-term hospitalisation in COPD. Eur Respir J 2005;26(5):853–7.
101. Ofman JJ, Badamgarav E, Henning JM, et al. Does disease management improve clinical and economic outcomes in patients with chronic diseases? A systematic review. Am J Med 2004;117(3):182–92.
102. Dewan N, Rice K, Caldwell M, et al. Economic evaluation for a disease management program for chronic obstructive pulmonary disease. COPD 2011;8(3):153–9.
103. Gallefoss F, Bakke P. Patient satisfaction with healthcare in asthmatics and patients with COPD before and after patient education. Respir Med 2000;94(11):1057–64.
104. Tougaard L, Krone T, Sorknaes A, et al. Economic benefits of teaching patients with chronic obstructive pulmonary disease about their illness. The PASTMA Group. Lancet 1992;339(8808):1517–20.
105. Zajac B. Measuring outcomes of a chronic obstructive pulmonary disease management program. Dis Manag 2002;5(1):9–23.

106. Bourbeau J, Collet JP, Schwartzman K, et al. Economic benefits of self-management education in COPD. Chest 2006;130:1704–11.
107. Ortiz G, Fromer L. Patient-Centered Medical Home in chronic obstructive pulmonary disease. J Multidiscip Healthc 2011;4:357–65.
108. Fritzsche A, Clamor A, von Leupoldt A. Effects of medical and psychological treatment of depression in patients with COPD—a review. Respir Med 2011; 105(10):1422–33.
109. Taylor SJ, Candy B, Bryar RM, et al. Effectiveness of innovations in nurse led chronic disease management for patients with chronic obstructive pulmonary disease: systematic review of evidence. BMJ 2005;331(7515):485–8.
110. Gourley G, Portner T, Gourley D, et al. Humanistic outcomes in the hypertension and COPD arms of a multicenter outcomes study. J Am Pharm Assoc (Wash) 1998;38(5):586–97.
111. Adair R, Wholey DR, Christianson J, et al. Improving chronic disease care by adding laypersons to the primary care team: a parallel randomized trial. Ann Intern Med 2013;159(3):176–84.
112. Santa J, Lipman MM. Knowledge and ignorance in the care of chronic disease. Ann Intern Med 2013;159(3):225–6.
113. Asch DA, Muller RW, Volpp KG. Automated hovering in health care—watching over the 5000 hours. N Engl J Med 2012;367(1):1–3.
114. Linderman DJ, Koff PB, Freitag TJ, et al. Effect of integrated care on advanced chronic obstructive pulmonary disease in high-mortality rural areas. Arch Intern Med 2011;171(22):2059–61.
115. McClean S, Nurmatov U, Liu JL, et al. Telehealthcare for chronic obstructive pulmonary disease [review]. Cochrane Database Syst Rev 2011;(7). CD007718. Available at: http://onlinelibrary.wiley.com/doi/10.1002/14651858.CD007718.pub2/pdf.
116. Au DH, Udris EM, Engelberg RA, et al. A randomized trial to improve communication about end-of-life care among patients with COPD. Chest 2012;141(3): 726–35.
117. Strand JJ, Kamdar MM, Carey EC. Top 10 things palliative care clinicians wished everyone knew about palliative care. Mayo Clin Proc 2013;88(8):859–65.

Strategies to Enhance the Benefits of Exercise Training in the Respiratory Patient

Kylie Hill, PhD[a,b,c,*], Anne E. Holland, PhD[d,e,f]

KEYWORDS

- Chronic obstructive pulmonary disease • Exercise training • Heliox
- Neuromuscular electrical stimulation • Noninvasive ventilation • Rollators
- Supplemental oxygen

KEY POINTS

- In people with chronic obstructive pulmonary disease, exercise training offered as part of pulmonary rehabilitation has strong evidence for increasing exercise capacity, reducing symptoms of dyspnea and fatigue, and improving health-related quality of life.
- Nevertheless, there is a proportion of people referred to pulmonary rehabilitation who achieve minimal gains, most likely because of profound ventilatory limitation during exercise or the presence of comorbid conditions that limit participation in exercise training.
- Several adjuncts or strategies have been explored to optimize the proportion of people referred to pulmonary rehabilitation who achieve significant and meaningful gains on program completion.

INTRODUCTION

Pulmonary rehabilitation has been defined as a comprehensive intervention that follows a thorough patient assessment and includes therapies such as exercise training

This article originally appeared in *Clinics in Chest Medicine*, Volume 35, Issue 2, June 2014.
Disclosure and Conflict of Interest Statement: Neither author has any conflict of interest with the content of this article.
[a] School of Physiotherapy and Exercise Science, Faculty of Health Science, Curtin University, GPO Box U1987, Perth, Western Australia 6845, Australia; [b] Lung Institute of Western Australia, Centre for Asthma, Allergy and Respiratory Research, University of Western Australia, Hospital Avenue, Nedlands, Western Australia 6009, Australia; [c] Physiotherapy Department, Royal Perth Hospital, Wellington Street, Perth, Western Australia 6000, Australia; [d] Department of Physiotherapy, La Trobe University, Level 4, The Alfred Centre, 99 Commercial Road, Melbourne, Victoria 3004, Australia; [e] Department of Physiotherapy, Alfred Health, Commercial Road, Melbourne, Victoria 3004, Australia; [f] Institute for Breathing and Sleep, Studley Road, Heidelberg, Victoria 3084, Australia
* Corresponding author. School of Physiotherapy and Exercise Science, Faculty of Health Science, Curtin University, GPO Box U1987, Perth, Western Australia 6845, Australia.
E-mail address: k.hill@curtin.edu.au

and education.[1] The aim of pulmonary rehabilitation is to improve the physical and psychological condition of people with chronic respiratory disease as well as promote long-term adherence to health-enhancing behaviors.[1] Exercise training is the cornerstone of an effective pulmonary rehabilitation program. Most studies examining the effect of pulmonary rehabilitation have been conducted in people with chronic obstructive pulmonary disease (COPD).[2] In this population, there is strong evidence that pulmonary rehabilitation, which includes exercise training, confers significant and important improvements in exercise capacity, symptoms such as dyspnea and fatigue, and health-related quality of life as well as reductions in health care use.[2–4] These effects are seen in people with stable disease as well as during or immediately after an acute exacerbation of their condition.[2,5] The mechanism of improvement relates largely to conditioning the muscles of locomotion, namely the quadriceps.[6,7] After rehabilitation, the changes in muscle morphology and biochemistry optimize the capacity of the quadriceps to meet the demands of exercise using aerobic energy systems.[6,7] This process in turn reduces the early reliance on anaerobic energy systems, delays the onset of blood lactate accumulation, and decreases the ventilatory load and sensation of dyspnea at submaximal exercise intensities.[6,7]

Although the evidence for pulmonary rehabilitation is strong, there are a proportion of people who do not achieve meaningful gains in exercise capacity.[8,9] These so called "nonresponders" seem to be characterized by more severe airflow obstruction and profound ventilatory limitation during exercise.[8,9] This situation may preclude the person from reaching an exercise intensity that constitutes an adequate stimulus to induce a training adaptation in the peripheral muscles. Furthermore, at least half of all people referred to pulmonary rehabilitation have 1 or more comorbid conditions, including musculoskeletal disorders, which compromise the training dose that can be achieved.[10] This situation has led to an interest in the role of adjuncts or alternative strategies, implemented during an exercise training program, to increase the load borne by the muscles of locomotion. Some of these strategies are commonplace and may be perceived by clinicians as easy to implement, such as the use of (1) supplemental oxygen, (2) rollators or wheeled walkers, (3) water-based exercise modalities, and (4) inspiratory muscle training (IMT). Others are less commonly used and may be perceived by clinicians as more difficult to implement, such as the use of (1) heliox (a helium-oxygen mixture), (2) noninvasive ventilation (NIV), (3) neuromuscular electrical stimulation (NMES), and (4) partitioning the exercising muscle mass. These approaches are described in this article.

SUPPLEMENTAL OXYGEN

Exercise-induced oxyhemoglobin desaturation is common in pulmonary rehabilitation participants. In 572 people with COPD undertaking a 6-minute walk test (6MWT), most of whom were entering a pulmonary rehabilitation program, desaturation of 4% or greater to less than 90% occurred in 47% of tests.[11] Although there are no strong data regarding the adverse effects of transient oxyhemoglobin desaturation during exercise, supplemental oxygen improves exercise performance and reduces dyspnea in people with COPD.[12] This finding is primarily related to a reduction in ventilation for a given exercise workload, leading to a delay in dynamic hyperinflation and prolonged exercise time.[13] These effects have been shown both in desaturators[13] and nondesaturators.[14] The reduction in ventilation at submaximal workloads may be associated with a slower increase in blood lactate as a result of better oxygen delivery to peripheral muscle[15] or direct chemoreceptor inhibition.[14] These acute effects of supplemental oxygen may facilitate training of the locomotor muscles at a higher intensity, or for a longer duration, to enhance training benefits.

There are now 7 randomized controlled trials (RCTs) that have evaluated the impact of supplemental oxygen during exercise training in COPD (**Table 1**). Despite the good physiologic rationale underpinning this intervention, 5 of the 7 trials found no beneficial effect on pulmonary rehabilitation outcomes.[16–20] Another trial measured exercise outcomes on the assigned gas, so it was unclear whether the benefits seen in the oxygen trained participants were related to the training program or the acute effects of the gas on exercise performance.[21] One well-designed trial that included participants who did not desaturate during exercise showed significantly increased endurance time during a constant power cycle ergometry test in the group who trained on supplemental oxygen compared with the air trained group after 7 weeks.[22] The oxygen group trained at a higher work rate, which progressed more rapidly over the course of the program, consistent with the hypothesis that the benefits of supplemental oxygen are attributable to a higher training intensity. It is unclear whether application of supplemental oxygen in previous trials had facilitated higher training workloads, which may explain the lack of positive findings in these studies. A Cochrane review[23] including 5 of these trials has concluded that there are small effects of supplemental oxygen during training on endurance time at the end of the program (mean improvement in exercise time compared with room air 2.69 minutes, 95% confidence interval 0.07–5.28 minutes, 2 trials with 53 participants) and Borg dyspnea score at the end of the endurance test (mean reduction in dyspnea 1.22 points, 95% confidence interval 0.06–2.39 points, 2 trials with 53 participants). There were no data to support effects on health-related quality of life or longer-term clinical outcomes.

Recent guidelines for pulmonary rehabilitation reflect both the uncertainty arising from this body of literature and the common use of supplemental oxygen in clinical practice. The British Thoracic Society guidelines for pulmonary rehabilitation state that supplemental oxygen should not be used routinely, but should be offered to those who fulfill the criteria for long-term oxygen therapy or ambulatory oxygen therapy.[24] The American Thoracic Society/European Respiratory Society statement on pulmonary rehabilitation suggests that individualized oxygen titration trials should be used to identify those people with COPD who may respond to oxygen supplementation during exercise testing.[1] Given the potent effects of oxygen supplementation in reducing operating lung volumes and evidence of its usefulness to increase training intensity, a trial of supplemental oxygen may be justified in both desaturators and non-desaturators if dynamic hyperinflation or severe dyspnea limit the progression of exercise intensity or duration.

ROLLATORS (WHEELED WALKERS)

Most clinicians who work in the area of pulmonary rehabilitation have had their patients tell them they find it easier to walk in shopping centers where they can use a trolley or a cart. There are now data of people with COPD showing that the provision of a rollator (or wheeled walker) increases the distance achieved during the 6MWT and reduces dyspnea on test completion.[25,26] This effect was most evident in those with marked functional limitation (ie, 6-minute walk distance <300 m).[25] The mechanisms underpinning these improvements are likely to be multifactorial and include an increased capacity to use the accessory muscles of respiration when the arms are fixed, as well as the greater pressure-generating capacity of the inspiratory muscles in the forward lean position.[27,28] Further, it may relate to a reduction in the metabolic cost of walking.[29] Taken together, these factors serve to optimize the capacity of the respiratory system to meet the ventilatory demands imposed during walking-based exercise and offset the sensation of dyspnea.[30]

Table 1
Effect of supplemental oxygen during exercise training on exercise outcomes in COPD RCTs

Study	Included Participants	Exercise Program (wk, times/wk)	Treatment Group			Control Group			Between Group Difference in Exercise Capacity After Training
			Sample Size	FEV_1 (% pred)	Oxygen	Sample Size	FEV_1 (% pred)	Comparator Treatment	
Rooyackers, 1997	Desaturators	10, 5	12	29 ± 7	4 L/min	12	38 ± 11	Room air	No difference Wmax No difference 6MWD
Fichter, 1999	Moderate to severe COPD	4, 5	5	—	Fio_2 35%	5	—	Room air	No difference Wmax
Garrod, 2000	Desaturators	6, 3	12	35 ± 10	4 L/min	13	29 ± 10	Compressed air 4 L/min	No difference ISWT
Wadell, 2001	Desaturators	8, 3	10	39[a]	5 L/min	10	52[a]	Compressed air 5 L/min	No difference 6MWD
Emtner, 2003	Nondesaturators	7, 3	14	35 ± 10	3 L/min	15	38 ± 8	Compressed air 3 L/min	↑ endurance time in oxygen group
Scorsone, 2010	Desaturators	8, 3	10	47 ± 10	Fio_2 40%	10	50 ± 12	Room air	No difference Wmax No difference endurance time
Dyer, 2012	Desaturators, ↑ ESWT at least 10% on oxygen	6–7, 2	24	39 ± 16	2–6 L/min	23	44 ± 11	Room air	↑ ESWT in oxygen group Each group performed ESWT on allocated gas

Data are mean ± standard deviation, except [a]median.

Abbreviations: 6MWD, 6-minute walk distance; ESWT, endurance shuttle walk test; FEV_1 (% pred), forced expiratory volume in first second expressed as a percentage of the predicted value; Fio_2, fraction of inspired oxygen; ISWT, incremental shuttle walk test; Wmax, maximum workload on cycle ergometer.

Despite these effects being shown on completion of walking tasks, no study has explored the effect of using a rollator to optimize walking-based exercise training in the context of pulmonary rehabilitation. The use of rollators as part of pulmonary rehabilitation is likely to increase given the predominance of comorbid conditions, including musculoskeletal disorders among people who are referred to pulmonary rehabilitation.[10] In contrast with many of the other approaches described in this article, there are data to show that rollators, when prescribed for use by an appropriately trained health care professional, are used frequently in the home environment, and people report a high level of satisfaction with them.[31] Specifically, rollators seem to promote walking outdoors[31] and may therefore increase participation in physical activity on completion of pulmonary rehabilitation.

WATER-BASED EXERCISE

Given the high prevalence of comorbid conditions in people who have been referred to a pulmonary rehabilitation program,[10] studies have explored alternative training modalities to traditional land-based exercise, such as water-based exercise. Three RCTs have compared the effects of land-based exercise, water-based exercise, and a control group.[32–34] The first group comprised water-based or land-based training, performed 3 times per week, for 45 minutes per session, over 12 weeks. Compared with both the control group and the group who underwent land-based exercise, those who completed the water-based training achieved greater gains in endurance walking capacity measured via the endurance shuttle walk test.[32] The second study included participants with 1 or more physical comorbidities, defined as obesity, musculoskeletal disorders, peripheral vascular disease, or neurologic conditions. Compared with a group who received usual care, or land-based exercise, those who underwent water-based training 3 times a week, for 60 minutes per session, over 8 weeks achieved greater gains in exercise capacity, measured via the incremental and endurance shuttle walk tests. Similar results were shown for the fatigue domain of a health-related quality-of-life questionnaire.[34] The results of a third RCT[33] also showed gains in exercise capacity, measured via the 6MWT on completion of a water-based training program, conducted 3 times a week, for 90 minutes per session, over 8 weeks. However, these gains were not of greater magnitude than those seen in a group that completed land-based training.

Studies in this area have reported no serious adverse events and high levels of acceptability of water-based exercise as an alternative training modality.[32–35] In addition to the effect that buoyancy has on unloading of peripheral and spinal joints, the hydrostatic force on the chest wall associated with water immersion may assist in reducing lung volumes during exercise[36]; an effect similar to that reported in obese people with COPD.[37] In turn, these effects may serve to increase the training dose that can be tolerated and thus optimize the magnitude of any physiologic training adaptation. Therefore, for people with COPD, especially those who have difficulty participating in land-based exercise because of comorbid conditions, consideration should be given to implementing a water-based exercise training program.

INSPIRATORY MUSCLE TRAINING

In people with COPD, pulmonary hyperinflation serves to shorten and flatten the diaphragm, reducing its mechanical advantage and pressure-generating capacity.[38] This reduction in pressure-generating capacity has been associated with the severity of dyspnea and also with impairments in exercise capacity.[39,40] Traditional exercise training, such as walking and cycling, does not impose sufficient load on the inspiratory muscles to induce a training adaptation. This situation has led to an interest in the role of specifically loading the inspiratory muscles, with the goal of improving their function as a way to ameliorate dyspnea and optimize exercise tolerance. The results of early studies in this area were confounded by limitations of resistive loading devices.[41] Studies that used a resistive device to load the inspiratory muscles without constraining the breathing pattern were unlikely to have imposed a load that was of sufficient magnitude to induce a training adaptation.[42] However, since that time, several robust RCTs have examined the effects of IMT applied in isolation and combined with exercise training. Meta-analyses of these trials provide strong evidence that IMT improves inspiratory muscle function (strength and endurance) and reduces dyspnea.[43] There is some evidence that IMT improves exercise capacity and health-related quality of life.[43] However, the effects are less convincing when the meta-analyses were restricted to those RCTs that specifically explored the role of IMT as an adjunct to a program of exercise training. In these studies, gains were reported in inspiratory muscle strength, but not exercise tolerance, symptoms, or health-related quality of life.[43,44]

The role of IMT in the rehabilitation of people with COPD is often debated.[45,46] Proponents of this approach support its use in those people with marked inspiratory muscle weakness.[47] Further, there is evidence that as little as 5 weeks of high-intensity IMT is capable of inducing changes in respiratory muscle morphology.[48] Based on current evidence, it seems reasonable to offer IMT to those people who continue to experience intractable dyspnea despite completion of a comprehensive pulmonary rehabilitation program.

NON-INVASIVE VENTILATION

The use of NIV during exercise is an alternative strategy to counter the deleterious effects of dynamic hyperinflation on respiratory muscle function. Whereas IMT aims to strengthen the respiratory muscles, the aim of NIV during exercise is to unload the respiratory muscles, thus reducing the oxygen cost of breathing and delaying the onset of intolerable dyspnea. Within a single exercise session, NIV has been shown to decrease inspiratory muscle effort, increase inspiratory and expiratory flows, increase minute ventilation, and improve gas exchange compared with exercise without ventilatory support.[49–51] There is a significant reduction in dyspnea at equivalent exercise workloads, the extent of which is proportional to degree of respiratory muscle unloading achieved with NIV.[49] As a result of these acute changes in physiology and symptoms, exercise tolerance is increased. A systematic review and meta-analysis including 7 trials of NIV versus unassisted breathing during cycling or walking in COPD found that NIV increased endurance time by an average of 3.3 minutes (55%).[52] Similarly, NIV during lower limb resistance exercise has been shown to delay the onset of quadriceps fatigue.[53] An increase in blood flow to the locomotor muscles may contribute to these findings, possibly as a result of redirection of the available cardiac output from respiratory muscles that are unloaded under NIV.[54]

Use of NIV during an entire 6-week to 8-week exercise training program has consistently been associated with improved exercise outcomes in people with advanced COPD. Compared with training on room air or oxygen, NIV-assisted training confers greater gains in maximum exercise performance,[55,56] functional exercise capacity,[57] and endurance exercise capacity.[56] These benefits are likely related to training at a higher intensity.[55,56,58] No studies have evaluated whether these benefits persist over the longer-term. Whether the increase in exercise capacity with NIV can be translated into greater improvements in symptoms and health-related quality of life when compared with unassisted training is not yet clear, because studies have not been powered to assess these outcomes.[57] No additional benefits of NIV were seen in an RCT in which participants had less severe disease.[59]

Current evidence indicates that NIV may be a useful adjunct to exercise training in carefully selected individuals. As well as potential application during outpatient pulmonary rehabilitation, consideration should be given to use of NIV to facilitate early exercise training in hospitalized patients recovering from acute exacerbations of COPD, in whom it has been shown to increase walking time, improve oxyhemoglobin saturation, and reduce dyspnea.[60] However, only a few people are suitable, and it may not be an acceptable treatment to those who are not using NIV.[61]

Use of NIV during training requires consideration of equipment and technique. Acute improvements in exercise endurance are more consistent when using inspiratory pressure support than other ventilatory modes.[52] This evidence, together with its ready availability and ease of use, suggests that inspiratory pressure support is the first choice for NIV-assisted training. Higher levels of inspiratory pressure support, in the region of 8 to 12 cm H_2O, give rise to better training outcomes than lower pressure levels.[62] A systematic review showed that positive effects of NIV-assisted training are seen in RCTs in which the mean FEV_1 (forced expiratory volume in 1 second) was less than 40% predicted, confirming that this technique is useful only in advanced disease.[62] Some studies have shown significant dropout rates during NIV-assisted training, with several citing discomfort related to the mask or ventilator.[62] For people to successfully use NIV during exercise, rehabilitation clinicians must have sufficient time and expertise in its implementation and titration, which is likely to limit this adjunct to a few centers.

HELIOX/HELIUM-HYPEROXIA

Heliox is formed when the nitrogen in air is replaced by helium, resulting in a gas that is 79% helium and 21% oxygen. Because helium has a lower density than nitrogen, heliox has a density nearly 3 times lower than air. As a result, the inhalation of heliox results in significantly lower turbulence and a greater tendency toward laminar flow, with an overall decrease in airway resistance. The beneficial effects of inhaling heliox during a single session of submaximal exercise in COPD have been well described, including reduced dynamic hyperinflation,[63–65] reduced respiratory muscle loading,[66,67] increased exercise endurance time,[63,64] less dyspnea,[63,66] and less leg fatigue.[66] Increasing the concentration of oxygen in the inhaled gas (eg, 40% oxygen, 70% helium), known as helium-hyperoxia, may have even greater effects on dynamic hyperinflation and exercise endurance than either normoxic helium or hyperoxia alone, with additive and independent effects of each gas on the work of breathing.[68–70] Physiologic benefits of inhaling helium gas mixtures are most evident in those with more severe airflow obstruction.[68]

Recent studies have shown that heliox results in increased locomotor muscle oxygen delivery in people with moderate to severe COPD,[64,66,67] as a result of improvements in both systemic oxygen delivery and locomotor muscle blood flow.[66] This finding suggests a potential role for helium gas mixtures in optimizing the effects of exercise training on locomotor muscles during pulmonary rehabilitation. Three RCTs have investigated the effects of heliox during exercise training in COPD (**Table 2**), with conflicting results. A single study showed a greater increase in endurance time in participants trained on helium-hyperoxia compared with training on room air,[71] whereas 2 others have shown no benefits of either heliox[72] or helium-hyperoxia.[20] These disparate results are likely a result of the training stimulus applied. The first

Table 2
RCTs that have investigated the effects of heliox or helium-hyperoxia during exercise training in COPD

Study	Program Details	Treatment Group			Control Groups			Between Group Differences After Exercise Training
		Sample Size	FEV$_1$ (% pred)	Intervention	Sample Size	FEV$_1$ (% pred)	Comparators	
Johnson, 2002	6 wk, twice weekly, 20 min treadmill training and education	11	34 ± 13	Heliox	13 15	31 ± 11 32 ± 9	Humidified air NIV during training, EPAP 2 cm H$_2$O, IPAP 8–12 cm H$_2$O	No difference in total exercise time on treadmill between groups
Eves, 2009	6 wk, thrice weekly, 30 min exercise and education	19	47 ± 19	HH 60% helium, 40% oxygen	19	46 ± 14	Air	Greater change in constant load exercise time in HH group Greater change in SGRQ total score in HH group but no difference in domain scores
Scorsone, 2010	8 wk, thrice weekly, 30 min cycle ergometer	10	49 ± 12	HH 60% helium, 40% oxygen	10 10	47 ± 10 50 ± 12	Supplemental oxygen 40% Humidified air	No difference in constant load exercise time between groups

Data are mean ± standard deviation.
Abbreviations: EPAP, expiratory positive airway pressure; FEV$_1$ (% pred), forced expiratory volume in first second expressed as a percentage of the predicted value; HH, helium-hyperoxia; IPAP, inspiratory positive airway pressure; SGRQ, St George's Respiratory Questionnaire.

study commenced training at a higher absolute workload in the helium-hyperoxia group than the air group, with regular increments thereafter.[71] In the other 2 studies,[20,72] the training intensity achieved with helium gas mixtures did not exceed the training intensity achieved in the control groups. This finding suggests that the benefits of breathing helium gas mixtures during exercise training may be apparent only if this intervention allows a higher training load to be applied. No studies have directly assessed the effects of exercise training using helium gas mixtures on adaptations in the muscles of locomotion.

The complex nature of applying helium gas mixtures during exercise training, together with the added expense and lack of conclusive clinical benefits, suggests that this therapy does not have a routine role in pulmonary rehabilitation for COPD. Further studies are required to establish whether heliox or helium-hyperoxia can augment the effects of exercise training in selected people with COPD, with sustained benefits after the training period.

NEUROMUSCULAR ELECTRICAL STIMULATION

NMES involves applying an intermittent electrical current to a superficial peripheral muscle using electrodes and a stimulator.[70] The electrical current serves to trigger an action potential and depolarize the motor nerve to elicit an involuntary muscle contraction.[74] Although any superficial peripheral muscle can be stimulated to contract in this way, most studies have focused on stimulating the quadriceps femoris. The stimulator can be programmed to elicit contractions that are more likely to favor gains in strength or endurance. Strength protocols involve relatively few contractions, using high-frequency stimulation, at the highest current that can be tolerated.[73] A short duty cycle, characterized by a long contraction period followed by an even longer rest period, may be advantageous.[75] In contrast, endurance protocols involve multiple contractions over prolonged periods (often hours), using low-frequency stimulation and a moderate current with relatively short contractions followed by short rest periods.[76] Electrical stimulation is an attractive option to train the peripheral muscles in people characterized by profound ventilatory limitation, because it evokes minimal ventilatory response and therefore minimal experience of dyspnea.[77] This situation is true for high-frequency and low-frequency stimulation parameters.[77]

The RCTs that have investigated NMES, in isolation from other therapies, in people with COPD are summarized in **Table 3**.[78–82] All have reported consistent changes in muscle function, including gains in force-generating capacity, endurance, cross-sectional area, and upregulation of pathways involved in muscle anabolism. Most have also reported gains in exercise capacity. These studies were conducted in participants characterized by moderate to severe disease, and 2 were conducted in participants who were hospitalized with an acute exacerbation. In contrast to these RCTs, 2 randomized crossover studies of NMES applied in isolation from exercise training have failed to show any gains in muscle force-generating capacity or exercise capacity.[83,84] Both of these studies recruited participants with less severe lung disease ($FEV_1 \sim 50\%$ predicted), which may have contributed to the lack of effect. Earlier work[82,84] has reported that the capacity of the person to tolerate a progressive increase in current is a consistent predictor of response to NMES. Higher currents are associated with greater gains in muscle function,[81,82] and men may be more likely to tolerate the sensation associated with high currents.[81]

Two RCTs have investigated the effects of adding NMES to a program of exercise.[85,86] Both were conducted among inpatients, characterized by severe functional limitation and muscle atrophy, who were receiving rehabilitation after a period of

Table 3
RCTs that have investigated the effects of NMES in patients with COPD

Study	Setting	Sample Size	FEV₁ (% pred)	Muscles Stimulated	Stimulation Frequency (Hz)	Initial Duty Cycle	Program Details	Sample Size	FEV₁ (% pred)	Sham Protocol	Between Group Differences After Intervention
		Treatment Group						Control Group			
Bourjeily-Habr, 2002	Outpatient training	9	36 ± 4	Quadriceps, hamstrings and calves	50	200 ms on: 1500 ms off	20 min, 3 × per wk, 6 wk	9	41 ± 4	Yes	↑ quadriceps and hamstring strength, ↑ exercise capacity
Neder, 2002	Home-based training	9	38 ± 10	Quadriceps	50	2 s on: 18 s off	15 min increased to 30 min after first wk, 5 × per wk, 6 wk	6	40 ± 13	No	↑ Vo₂peak, ↑ exercise time, ↑ quadriceps strength, ↓ quadriceps fatigue
Abdellaoui, 2011	Inpatient	9	15 [17]	Quadriceps and hamstrings	35	Not stated	60 min, 5 × per wk, 6 wk	6	25 [24]	Yes	↑ quadriceps strength, ↑ exercise capacity, change in proportion of muscle fibers
Giavendoni, 2012	Inpatient	11	41 ± 6	Quadriceps (dominant leg only)	50	8 s on: 20 s off	30 min daily sessions for 14 d	11	41 ± 6	No stimulation of nondominant leg	↑ quadriceps strength
Vivodtzev, 2012	Home-based training	12	30 ± 4	Quadriceps and calves	50	6 s on: 16 s off	5 × per wk, 60 min per session, for 6 wk	12	34 ± 3	Yes	↑ muscle CSA, ↑ quadriceps strength and endurance, ↑ muscle signaling pathways favoring anabolism

Data are mean ± standard deviation or median [interquartile range].
Abbreviations: CSA, cross-sectional area; FEV₁ (% pred), forced expiratory volume in first second expressed as a percentage of the predicted value; Vo₂peak, peak rate of oxygen consumption.

Table 4
RCTs that have investigated the effects of 1-leg cycling in patients with COPD

Study	Program Details	Treatment Group			Control Group			Between Group Differences After Training
		Sample Size	FEV$_1$ (% pred)	Training Intensity	Sample Size	FEV$_1$ (% pred)	Training Intensity	
Dolmage, 2008	Supervised 30 min sessions, 3 × a wk, 7 wk	9	37 ± 8	50% of peak power achieved during CPET	9	40 ± 23	70% of peak power achieved during CPET	↑Vo$_{2peak}$ ↑ peak power, ↑Vco$_{2peak}$ ↑V$_{Epeak}$ ↓ minute ventilation and heart rate at submaximal Vo$_2$
Bjorgen, 2009	Supervised, 16 min, 3 × a wk, 8 wk	12	41 ± 10	Interval training: 4 × 4 min exercise at 85%–95% HRmax (measured during 1-leg CPET) Each 4 min exercise period alternated between the 2 legs, giving a total of 8 intervals	7	45 ± 8	Interval training: 4 × 4 min exercise at 85%–95% HRmax (measured during 2-leg CPET), interspersed with 3 min active rest (60%–70% HRmax)	↑Vo$_{2peak}$ ↑ peak power, ↑Vco$_{2peak}$ and ↑V$_{Epeak}$

Data are mean ± standard deviation.
Abbreviations: CPET, cardiopulmonary exercise test; FEV$_1$ (% pred), forced expiratory volume in first second expressed as a percentage of the predicted value; HRmax, maximum heart rate; Vco$_{2peak}$, peak rate of carbon dioxide production; V$_{Epeak}$, peak rate of minute ventilation; Vo$_{2peak}$, peak rate of oxygen consumption.

serious illness. Many participants in these studies were essentially bedbound, and exercise training comprised active or active-assisted limb movements and treadmill walking when able. Compared with the group who underwent exercise training alone, the grouped who received NMES in addition to exercise training achieved benefits in muscle force-generating capacity, measures of dyspnea during activities of daily living, and the capacity to undertake functional tasks. Further work is needed to determine whether offering NMES confers additional benefits among those people who are referred to outpatient pulmonary rehabilitation.

PARTITIONING EXERCISING MUSCLE MASS

The ventilatory load imposed during exercise is related to the intensity and duration of exercise as well as the volume of exercising muscle mass. During pulmonary rehabilitation, for those people who are unable to cope with high-intensity exercise, the ventilatory load is often reduced by reducing exercise intensity.[87] Such an approach may compromise the effectiveness of the training program and reduce the likelihood of any physiologic adaptation in the exercising muscles.[6] In 1999, Richardson and colleagues[88] reported that partitioning the exercise muscle mass served to reduce the ventilatory load associated with exercise and, in turn, optimize the muscle-specific work rate. This concept was suggested as a training strategy by Dolmage and colleagues,[89] who reported that, compared with cycling using both legs, cycling at the same relevant intensity using only 1 leg increased constant power exercise time by a factor of 3.6. Since this time, there have been 2 studies that have compared the effect of completing a cycle-based exercise training program, using 2 legs simultaneously versus training each leg independently.[90,91] These studies are summarized in **Table 4**. Both studies have shown that a protocol of 1-leg versus 2-leg cycling conferred greater gains in the peak power and peak rate of oxygen uptake measured on completion of the training program. This approach seems to be readily translated into clinical practice.[92]

SUMMARY

Several exercise training adjuncts can be used to maximize benefit through increasing the load on the locomotor muscles during pulmonary rehabilitation programs. This article has presented several strategies for which there is a strong physiologic rationale for their use in patients with COPD. However, most are suitable for only a carefully selected subgroup of individuals attending pulmonary rehabilitation, and in many cases, their long-term effects have not been examined. Clinicians should consider the judicious use of training adjuncts such as these to optimize training intensity and maximize the number of people who achieve meaningful improvements in outcomes that are important to patients after pulmonary rehabilitation.

REFERENCES

1. Spruit MA, Singh S, Garvey C, et al. An official American Thoracic Society/European Respiratory Society statement: key concepts and advances in pulmonary rehabilitation–an executive summary. Am J Respir Crit Care Med 2013;188(8):e13–64.
2. Lacasse Y, Goldstein R, Lasserson TJ, et al. Pulmonary rehabilitation for chronic obstructive pulmonary disease. Cochrane Database Syst Rev 2006;(4):CD003793.
3. Raskin J, Spiegler P, McCusker C, et al. The effect of pulmonary rehabilitation on healthcare utilization in chronic obstructive pulmonary disease: the Northeast Pulmonary Rehabilitation Consortium. J Cardiopulm Rehabil 2006;26(4):231–6.

4. Cecins N, Geelhoed E, Jenkins SC. Reduction in hospitalisation following pulmonary rehabilitation in patients with COPD. Aust Health Rev 2008;32(3):415–22.
5. Puhan MA, Gimeno-Santos E, Scharplatz M, et al. Pulmonary rehabilitation following exacerbations of chronic obstructive pulmonary disease. Cochrane Database Syst Rev 2011;(10):CD005305.
6. Casaburi R, Patessio A, Ioli F, et al. Reductions in exercise lactic acidosis and ventilation as a result of exercise training in patients with obstructive lung disease. Am Rev Respir Dis 1991;143(1):9–18.
7. Maltais F, LeBlanc P, Simard C, et al. Skeletal muscle adaptation to endurance training in patients with chronic obstructive pulmonary disease. Am J Respir Crit Care Med 1996;154(2 Pt 1):442–7.
8. Troosters T, Gosselink R, Decramer M. Exercise training in COPD: how to distinguish responders from nonresponders. J Cardiopulm Rehabil 2001;21(1):10–7.
9. Scott AS, Baltzan MA, Fox J, et al. Success in pulmonary rehabilitation in patients with chronic obstructive pulmonary disease. Can Respir J 2010;17(5): 219–23.
10. Crisafulli E, Costi S, Luppi F, et al. Role of comorbidities in a cohort of patients with COPD undergoing pulmonary rehabilitation. Thorax 2008;63(6).487–92.
11. Jenkins S, Cecins N. Six-minute walk test: observed adverse events and oxygen desaturation in a large cohort of patients with chronic lung disease. Intern Med J 2011;41(5):416–22.
12. Dean NC, Brown JK, Himelman RB, et al. Oxygen may improve dyspnea and endurance in patients with chronic obstructive pulmonary disease and only mild hypoxemia. Am Rev Respir Dis 1992;146(4):941–5.
13. O'Donnell DE, D'Arsigny C, Webb KA. Effects of hyperoxia on ventilatory limitation during exercise in advanced chronic obstructive pulmonary disease. Am J Respir Crit Care Med 2001;163(4):892–8.
14. Somfay A, Porszasz J, Lee SM, et al. Dose-response effect of oxygen on hyperinflation and exercise endurance in nonhypoxaemic COPD patients. Eur Respir J 2001;18(1):77–84.
15. O'Donnell DE, Bain DJ, Webb KA. Factors contributing to relief of exertional breathlessness during hyperoxia in chronic airflow limitation. Am J Respir Crit Care Med 1997;155(2):530–5.
16. Rooyackers JM, Dekhuijzen PN, Van Herwaarden CL, et al. Training with supplemental oxygen in patients with COPD and hypoxaemia at peak exercise. Eur Respir J 1997;10(6):1278–84.
17. Fichter J, Fleckenstein J, Stahl C, et al. Effect of oxygen (FIO2: 0.35) on the aerobic capacity in patients with COPD. Pneumologie 1999;53(3):121–6 [in German].
18. Garrod R, Paul EA, Wedzicha JA. Supplemental oxygen during pulmonary rehabilitation in patients with COPD with exercise hypoxaemia. Thorax 2000;55(7): 539–43.
19. Wadell K, Henriksson-Larsen K, Lundgren R. Physical training with and without oxygen in patients with chronic obstructive pulmonary disease and exercise-induced hypoxaemia. J Rehabil Med 2001;33(5):200–5.
20. Scorsone D, Bartolini S, Saporiti R, et al. Does a low-density gas mixture or oxygen supplementation improve exercise training in COPD? Chest 2010;138(5): 1133–9.
21. Dyer F, Callaghan J, Cheema K, et al. Ambulatory oxygen improves the effectiveness of pulmonary rehabilitation in selected patients with chronic obstructive pulmonary disease. Chron Respir Dis 2012;9(2):83–91.

22. Emtner M, Porszasz J, Burns M, et al. Benefits of supplemental oxygen in exercise training in nonhypoxemic chronic obstructive pulmonary disease patients. Am J Respir Crit Care Med 2003;168(9):1034–42.

23. Nonoyama ML, Brooks D, Lacasse Y, et al. Oxygen therapy during exercise training in chronic obstructive pulmonary disease. Cochrane Database Syst Rev 2007;(2):CD005372.

24. Bolton CE, Bevan-Smith EF, Blakey JD, et al. British Thoracic Society guideline on pulmonary rehabilitation in adults. Thorax 2013;68(Suppl 2):ii1–30.

25. Solway S, Brooks D, Lau L, et al. The short-term effect of a rollator on functional exercise capacity among individuals with severe COPD. Chest 2002;122(1):56–65.

26. Probst VS, Troosters T, Coosemans I, et al. Mechanisms of improvement in exercise capacity using a rollator in patients with COPD. Chest 2004;126(4):1102–7.

27. O'Neill S, McCarthy DS. Postural relief of dyspnoea in severe chronic airflow limitation: relationship to respiratory muscle strength. Thorax 1983;38(8):595–600.

28. Cavalheri V, Camillo CA, Brunetto AF, et al. Effects of arm bracing posture on respiratory muscle strength and pulmonary function in patients with chronic obstructive pulmonary disease. Rev Port Pneumol 2010;16(6):887–91.

29. Hill K, Dolmage TE, Woon LJ, et al. Rollator use does not consistently change the metabolic cost of walking in people with chronic obstructive pulmonary disease. Arch Phys Med Rehabil 2012;93(6):1077–80.

30. Parshall MB, Schwartzstein RM, Adams L, et al. An official American Thoracic Society statement: update on the mechanisms, assessment, and management of dyspnea. Am J Respir Crit Care Med 2012;185(4):435–52.

31. Hill K, Goldstein R, Gartner EJ, et al. Daily utility and satisfaction with rollators among persons with chronic obstructive pulmonary disease. Arch Phys Med Rehabil 2008;89(6):1108–13.

32. Wadell K, Sundelin G, Henriksson-Larsen K, et al. High intensity physical group training in water–an effective training modality for patients with COPD. Respir Med 2004;98(5):428–38.

33. de Souto Araujo ZT, de Miranda Silva Nogueira PA, Cabral EE, et al. Effectiveness of low-intensity aquatic exercise on COPD: a randomized clinical trial. Respir Med 2012;106(11):1535–43.

34. McNamara RJ, McKeough ZJ, McKenzie DK, et al. Water-based exercise in COPD with physical comorbidities: a randomised controlled trial. Eur Respir J 2013;41(6):1284–91.

35. Rae S, White P. Swimming pool-based exercise as pulmonary rehabilitation for COPD patients in primary care: feasibility and acceptability. Prim Care Respir J 2009;18(2):90–4.

36. Girandola RN, Wiswell RA, Mohler JG, et al. Effects of water immersion on lung volumes: implications for body composition analysis. J Appl Physiol Respir Environ Exerc Physiol 1977;43(2):276–9.

37. Ora J, Laveneziana P, Wadell K, et al. Effect of obesity on respiratory mechanics during rest and exercise in COPD. J Appl Physiol (1985) 2011;111(1):10–9.

38. Smith J, Bellemare F. Effect of lung volume on in vivo contraction characteristics of human diaphragm. J Appl Physiol (1985) 1987;62(5):1893–900.

39. Hamilton AL, Killian KJ, Summers E, et al. Symptom intensity and subjective limitation to exercise in patients with cardiorespiratory disorders. Chest 1996;110(5):1255–63.

40. Gosselink R, Troosters T, Decramer M. Peripheral muscle weakness contributes to exercise limitation in COPD. Am J Respir Crit Care Med 1996;153(3):976–80.

41. Smith K, Cook D, Guyatt GH, et al. Respiratory muscle training in chronic airflow limitation: a meta-analysis. Am Rev Respir Dis 1992;145(3):533–9.
42. Belman MJ, Thomas SG, Lewis MI. Resistive breathing training in patients with chronic obstructive pulmonary disease. Chest 1986;90(5):662–9.
43. Gosselink R, De Vos J, van den Heuvel SP, et al. Impact of inspiratory muscle training in patients with COPD: what is the evidence? Eur Respir J 2011;37(2): 416–25.
44. O'Brien K, Geddes EL, Reid WD, et al. Inspiratory muscle training compared with other rehabilitation interventions in chronic obstructive pulmonary disease: a systematic review update. J Cardiopulm Rehabil Prev 2008;28(2):128–41.
45. Ambrosino N. The case for inspiratory muscle training in COPD. For. Eur Respir J 2011;37(2):233–5.
46. Polkey MI, Moxham J, Green M. The case against inspiratory muscle training in COPD. Against. Eur Respir J 2011;37(2):236–7.
47. Charususin N, Gosselink R, Decramer M, et al. Inspiratory muscle training protocol for patients with chronic obstructive pulmonary disease (IMTCO study): a multicentre randomised controlled trial. BMJ Open 2013;3(8).
48. Ramirez-Sarmiento A, Orozco-Levi M, Guell R, et al. Inspiratory muscle training in patients with chronic obstructive pulmonary disease: structural adaptation and physiologic outcomes. Am J Respir Crit Care Med 2002; 166(11):1491–7.
49. Maltais F, Reissmann H, Gottfried SB. Pressure support reduces inspiratory effort and dyspnea during exercise in chronic airflow obstruction. Am J Respir Crit Care Med 1995;151(4):1027–33.
50. Kyroussis D, Polkey MI, Hamnegard CH, et al. Respiratory muscle activity in patients with COPD walking to exhaustion with and without pressure support. Eur Respir J 2000;15(4):649–55.
51. Dreher M, Storre JH, Windisch W. Noninvasive ventilation during walking in patients with severe COPD: a randomised cross-over trial. Eur Respir J 2007; 29(5):930–6.
52. van 't Hul A, Kwakkel G, Gosselink R. The acute effects of noninvasive ventilatory support during exercise on exercise endurance and dyspnea in patients with chronic obstructive pulmonary disease: a systematic review. J Cardiopulm Rehabil 2002;22(4):290–7.
53. Borghi-Silva A, Di Thommazo L, Pantoni CB, et al. Non-invasive ventilation improves peripheral oxygen saturation and reduces fatigability of quadriceps in patients with COPD. Respirology 2009;14(4):537–44.
54. Borghi-Silva A, Oliveira CC, Carrascosa C, et al. Respiratory muscle unloading improves leg muscle oxygenation during exercise in patients with COPD. Thorax 2008;63(10):910–5.
55. Reuveny R, Ben-Dov I, Gaides M, et al. Ventilatory support during training improves training benefit in severe chronic airway obstruction. Isr Med Assoc J 2005;7(3):151–5.
56. van 't Hul A, Gosselink R, Hollander P, et al. Training with inspiratory pressure support in patients with severe COPD. Eur Respir J 2006;27(1):65–72.
57. Borghi-Silva A, Mendes RG, Toledo AC, et al. Adjuncts to physical training of patients with severe COPD: oxygen or noninvasive ventilation? Respir Care 2010; 55(7):885–94.
58. Hawkins P, Johnson LC, Nikoletou D, et al. Proportional assist ventilation as an aid to exercise training in severe chronic obstructive pulmonary disease. Thorax 2002;57(10):853–9.

59. Bianchi L, Foglio K, Porta R, et al. Lack of additional effect of adjunct of assisted ventilation to pulmonary rehabilitation in mild COPD patients. Respir Med 2002; 96(5):359–67.

60. Menadue C, Alison JA, Piper AJ, et al. Bilevel ventilation during exercise in acute on chronic respiratory failure: a preliminary study. Respir Med 2010;104(2): 219–27.

61. Dyer F, Flude L, Bazari F, et al. Non-invasive ventilation (NIV) as an aid to rehabilitation in acute respiratory disease. BMC Pulm Med 2011;11:58.

62. Corner E, Garrod R. Does the addition of non-invasive ventilation during pulmonary rehabilitation in patients with chronic obstructive pulmonary disease augment patient outcome in exercise tolerance? A literature review. Physiother Res Int 2010;15(1):5–15.

63. Palange P, Valli G, Onorati P, et al. Effect of heliox on lung dynamic hyperinflation, dyspnea, and exercise endurance capacity in COPD patients. J Appl Physiol (1985) 2004;97(5):1637–42.

64. Chiappa GR, Queiroga F Jr, Meda E, et al. Heliox improves oxygen delivery and utilization during dynamic exercise in patients with chronic obstructive pulmonary disease. Am J Respir Crit Care Med 2009;179(11):1004–10.

65. Laveneziana P, Valli G, Onorati P, et al. Effect of heliox on heart rate kinetics and dynamic hyperinflation during high-intensity exercise in COPD. Eur J Appl Physiol 2011;111(2):225–34.

66. Vogiatzis I, Habazettl H, Aliverti A, et al. Effect of helium breathing on intercostal and quadriceps muscle blood flow during exercise in COPD patients. Am J Physiol Regul Integr Comp Physiol 2011;300(6):R1549–59.

67. Louvaris Z, Zakynthinos S, Aliverti A, et al. Heliox increases quadriceps muscle oxygen delivery during exercise in COPD patients with and without dynamic hyperinflation. J Appl Physiol (1985) 2012;113(7):1012–23.

68. Laude EA, Duffy NC, Baveystock C, et al. The effect of helium and oxygen on exercise performance in chronic obstructive pulmonary disease: a randomized crossover trial. Am J Respir Crit Care Med 2006;173(8):865–70.

69. Eves ND, Petersen SR, Haykowsky MJ, et al. Helium-hyperoxia, exercise, and respiratory mechanics in chronic obstructive pulmonary disease. Am J Respir Crit Care Med 2006;174(7):763–71.

70. Queiroga F Jr, Nunes M, Meda E, et al. Exercise tolerance with helium-hyperoxia versus hyperoxia in hypoxaemic patients with COPD. Eur Respir J 2013;42(2): 362–70.

71. Eves ND, Sandmeyer LC, Wong EY, et al. Helium-hyperoxia: a novel intervention to improve the benefits of pulmonary rehabilitation for patients with COPD. Chest 2009;135(3):609–18.

72. Johnson JE, Gavin DJ, Adams-Dramiga S. Effects of training with heliox and noninvasive positive pressure ventilation on exercise ability in patients with severe COPD. Chest 2002;122(2):464–72.

73. Maffiuletti NA. Physiological and methodological considerations for the use of neuromuscular electrical stimulation. Eur J Appl Physiol 2010;110(2):223–34.

74. Vivodtzev I, Lacasse Y, Maltais F. Neuromuscular electrical stimulation of the lower limbs in patients with chronic obstructive pulmonary disease. J Cardiopulm Rehabil Prev 2008;28(2):79–91.

75. Filipovic A, Kleinoder H, Dormann U, et al. Electromyostimulation–a systematic review of the influence of training regimens and stimulation parameters on effectiveness in electromyostimulation training of selected strength parameters. J Strength Cond Res 2011;25(11):3218–38.

76. Nuhr MJ, Pette D, Berger R, et al. Beneficial effects of chronic low-frequency stimulation of thigh muscles in patients with advanced chronic heart failure. Eur Heart J 2004;25(2):136–43.
77. Sillen MJ, Wouters EF, Franssen FM, et al. Oxygen uptake, ventilation, and symptoms during low-frequency versus high-frequency NMES in COPD: a pilot study. Lung 2011;189(1):21–6.
78. Bourjeily-Habr G, Rochester CL, Palermo F, et al. Randomised controlled trial of transcutaneous electrical muscle stimulation of the lower extremities in patients with chronic obstructive pulmonary disease. Thorax 2002;57(12):1045–9.
79. Neder JA, Sword D, Ward SA, et al. Home based neuromuscular electrical stimulation as a new rehabilitative strategy for severely disabled patients with chronic obstructive pulmonary disease (COPD). Thorax 2002;57(4):333–7.
80. Abdellaoui A, Prefaut C, Gouzi F, et al. Skeletal muscle effects of electrostimulation after COPD exacerbation: a pilot study. Eur Respir J 2011;38(4):781–8.
81. Giavedoni S, Deans A, McCaughey P, et al. Neuromuscular electrical stimulation prevents muscle function deterioration in exacerbated COPD: a pilot study. Respir Med 2012;106(10):1429–34.
82. Vivodtzev I, Debigare R, Gagnon P, et al. Functional and muscular effects of neuromuscular electrical stimulation in patients with severe COPD: a randomized clinical trial. Chest 2012;141(3):716–25.
83. Dal Corso S, Napolis L, Malaguti C, et al. Skeletal muscle structure and function in response to electrical stimulation in moderately impaired COPD patients. Respir Med 2007;101(6):1236–43.
84. Napolis LM, Dal Corso S, Neder JA, et al. Neuromuscular electrical stimulation improves exercise tolerance in chronic obstructive pulmonary disease patients with better preserved fat-free mass. Clinics (Sao Paulo) 2011;66(3):401–6.
85. Zanotti E, Felicetti G, Maini M, et al. Peripheral muscle strength training in bed-bound patients with COPD receiving mechanical ventilation: effect of electrical stimulation. Chest 2003;124(1):292–6.
86. Vivodtzev I, Pepin JL, Vottero G, et al. Improvement in quadriceps strength and dyspnea in daily tasks after 1 month of electrical stimulation in severely deconditioned and malnourished COPD. Chest 2006;129(6):1540–8.
87. Maltais F, LeBlanc P, Jobin J, et al. Intensity of training and physiologic adaptation in patients with chronic obstructive pulmonary disease. Am J Respir Crit Care Med 1997;155(2):555–61.
88. Richardson RS, Sheldon J, Poole DC, et al. Evidence of skeletal muscle metabolic reserve during whole body exercise in patients with chronic obstructive pulmonary disease. Am J Respir Crit Care Med 1999;159(3):881–5.
89. Dolmage TE, Goldstein RS. Response to one-legged cycling in patients with COPD. Chest 2006;129(2):325–32.
90. Dolmage TE, Goldstein RS. Effects of one-legged exercise training of patients with COPD. Chest 2008;133(2):370–6.
91. Bjorgen S, Hoff J, Husby VS, et al. Aerobic high intensity one and two legs interval cycling in chronic obstructive pulmonary disease: the sum of the parts is greater than the whole. Eur J Appl Physiol 2009;106(4):501–7.
92. Evans RA, Dolmage TE, Mangovski-Alzamora S, et al. One-legged cycling for chronic obstructive pulmonary disease (COPD): knowledge translation to pulmonary rehabilitation. Am J Respir Crit Care Med 2013;A2574.

Current Drug Treatment, Chronic and Acute

Peter Calverley, DSc, FMedSc

KEYWORDS

• Bronchodilators • Inhaled corticosteroids • COPD and exacerbations

KEY POINTS

- Increasing the dose or number of bronchodilators together with a short course of oral corticosteroids reduces the severity of chronic obstructive pulmonary disease (COPD) exacerbation.
- Supplementary methylxanthine treatment adds nothing to exacerbation management except risk for patients.
- Long-acting antimuscarinics should be given once daily as a first-line treatment of COPD, although new once daily long-acting beta-agonists may prove equally effective.
- Adding inhaled corticosteroids to a long-acting beta agonist prevents exacerbations in severe disease and seems to be effective in some once daily combination treatments.
- Pneumonia is seen with all treatments containing fluticasone-related drugs, but appears to be less evident with budesonide. Once-daily tiotropium seems safe when given as a dry power, but there are concerns about its use when inhaled from a soft mist system.

INTRODUCTION

The appropriate management of chronic obstructive pulmonary disease (COPD) involves more than taking prescription medicines. The key components have been set out in detail in many treatment guidelines, both national and international.[1-3] They include the avoidance of identified risk factors, especially tobacco smoking, and the optimization of daily physical activity, topics covered elsewhere in this volume.

For a few patients with severe disease, noninvasive ventilation can be a lifesaving treatment in the acute episode,[4] although not all patients benefit.[5] There is a role for long-term domiciliary oxygen treatment, which is widely used in the United States and can reduce mortality and even improve exercise performance.[6,7] However, the effectiveness of ambulatory oxygen has been challenged[8]; the use of oxygen to relieve breathlessness after exercise having been shown to be ineffective when compared

This article originally appeared in *Clinics in Chest Medicine*, Volume 35, Issue 1, March 2014.
Respiratory Research, Clinical Sciences Department, Institute of Ageing & Chronic Diseases, University Hospital Aintree, Lower Lane, Liverpool L9 7AL, UK
E-mail address: pmacal@liverpool.ac.uk

Clinics Collections 6 (2015) 333–350
http://dx.doi.org/10.1016/j.ccol.2015.05.046

with room air.[9] These considerations do not seem to have dented the popularity of this treatment, with patients and their physicians indicating the limits of evidence-based clinical practice. However for many patients with COPD, a key part of their care remains the drugs their doctors prescribe and in recent years both the choice of treatment and the evidence for its effectiveness has improved.

This article reviews the key components of the pharmacologic treatment of COPD, both acute and chronic, with an emphasis on those recent studies, which are likely to change practice in the next few years.

DRUG TREATMENT IN ACUTE EXACERBATIONS

Acute exacerbations of COPD drive the morbidity and cost associated with this disease and the markers of an increased risk of dying, especially after the patients have been hospitalized.[10] In patients with more severe COPD and those attending the emergency department, breathlessness is the dominant symptom; there are good data showing that this results from a mixture of static and dynamic hyperinflation and consequent restriction on tidal volume.[11,12] Worsening lung mechanics leads to the deterioration in ventilation-perfusion matching and an increase in dead space, producing hypoxemia with or without hyperpnoea. Hence, the management of the acute episode focuses on reversing or limiting these physiologic abnormalities. The distress and ill health of the hospitalized patient makes the conduct of randomized control trials difficult or risky and so we have almost no clinical trial data to support the use of oxygen to either reduce breathlessness or improve outcomes in COPD. We do know that oxygen-induced hypercapnia can be dangerous,[13] but for physicians to take the opposite view and not prescribe oxygen to critically ill patients would seem to be perverse.

Similar considerations apply to drug treatment, but here there is at least some direct physiologic evidence of benefit resulting from studies conducted over the last decade.

Inhaled bronchodilators are the key components of management. For good practical reasons related to the speed of onset of action and the risk of adverse effects, the inhaled route is preferred for both acute and chronic treatment, and the main drug classes are beta-agonists (BA) and antimuscarinic (MA), which are also known as anticholinergic drugs.

There is little evidence for a dose-response effect with either BA or MA in COPD, although some data for unstable disease suggest a potential benefit of high doses of ipratropium.[14] However, many physicians prescribe nebulized BA, usually salbutamol in doses of 2.5 to 5.0 mg or MA such as ipratropium 250 to 500 mcg alone, or in combination with each other, to reduce symptoms in hospitalized patients with exacerbations. Adding ipratropium to salbutamol did not change the rate of recovery of forced expiratory volume in the first second of expiration (FEV_1) in one small UK study,[15] which did not examine other markers of lung mechanics or symptoms. However, there is evidence that even at high doses of BA, adding another drug of a different class can produce physiologically important reductions in end expiratory lung volumes,[16] changes similar to those observed after combination bronchodilators in acutely ill patients with COPD.[12]

There are no good studies to indicate when this high-dose treatment should be discontinued; this decision is usually an empiric one, made by the attending physician. Patients often think high-dose nebulized drugs during an exacerbation should be continued during their chronic care; but the evidence for this is lacking and is confused by the facial cooling effects of the nebulized mist, which can decrease acute breathlessness.[17] Other considerations related to the reimbursement of nebulized drugs may also be potent reasons why these agents are considered. The most common adverse events are tachycardia and palpitations with high doses of BA while hypokalemia is not a problem in normal clinical practice. MA drugs are well tolerated, although there is a risk of inducing glaucoma if mist from a facial mask enters the eyes of susceptible patients.

Intravenous aminophylline was used as the primary treatment of hospitalized acute COPD exacerbations long before safer inhaled bronchodilators were available, and it is still often added to the treatment of patients with severe breathlessness caused by acute COPD. However, xanthenes are weak bronchodilators and only effective at near-toxic doses.[18] Data from Rice and colleagues[19] suggested that it was ineffective when used acutely. This finding was confirmed in a large randomized controlled trial that showed that aminophylline reduced arterial carbon dioxide slightly but made no difference to the rate of recover, symptoms, lung function, or to the time spent in hospital.[20] Given the toxicity of this therapy, it should not be used in hospitalized patients with COPD. A trial of the acute effects of the phosphodiesterase IV inhibitor roflumilast in acute exacerbations of COPD is currently being conducted; but until these data are available, this drug is not recommended for acute use.

Acute exacerbations are characterized by an increase in inflammation,[21] triggered by infections and/or environmental insults, which produce the acute deterioration in lung mechanics noted earlier. Two therapies have been applied to reduce inflammation and shorten the acute episode.

High-dose enteral or parenteral corticosteroids have been tested in a limited number of studies. With one exception, patients were recruited from the emergency department (ED) or had been hospitalized; in these settings, corticosteroid treatment delayed the time to relapse (including relapses occurring within 30 days of an ED visit), reduced the number of treatment failures related to the primary event, and accelerated the rate at which lung function improved (**Fig. 1**), thereby reducing the hospital stay.[22–24] Lower doses of oral prednisolone (approximately 30 mg/d) were as effective as large doses of methylprednisolone. Although the large trials gave treatment for 10 to 14 days, most of the benefit accrues in the first week; one small study has shown that 10 days of treatment is better than 3 days.[25] Data on ambulatory output patient

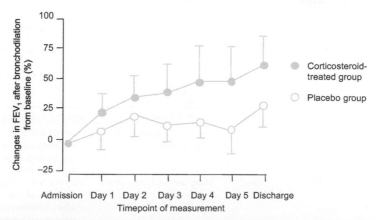

Fig. 1. Rate of recovery of FEV_1 in hospitalized patients with COPD treated with oral corticosteroids (*closed circles*) or placebo (*open circles*). (*Adapted from* Davies L, Angus RM, Calverley PM. Oral corticosteroids in patients admitted to hospital with exacerbations of chronic obstructive pulmonary disease: a prospective randomised controlled trial. Lancet 1999;354(9177):456–60; with permission.)

events are very limited, but arterial oxygen tension improved more rapidly in those patients given prednisolone.[26] This treatment is widely prescribed for exacerbations of COPD in the community, particularly in Western Europe. Hyperglycemia is somewhat more common in corticosteroid-treated COPD exacerbations, but the degree is as likely to be a marker of the severity of the insult as the use of short courses of corticosteroids per see. The major risk of oral corticosteroid treatment is that it is sustained and converted into chronic oral therapy, which is hazardous to patients, producing a host of undesirable complications, including marked muscle weakness and immobility.[27]

The alternative and potentially complementary method of modifying exacerbation-related inflammation is the prescription of antibiotics with courses normally lasting 5 to 7 days. The choice of treatment is best determined by local sensitivity patterns to *Haemophilus influenzae* and *Streptococcus pneumoniae*, the dominant causes of these episodes.[28] In practice, coverage of other pathogens likely to cause pneumonia is also sensible, given the difficulties of distinguishing pneumonias from COPD exacerbations.[29] Only a few studies have compared antibiotics with placebo in COPD exacerbations, most trials having been comparator studies of microbiological cure rates. However, one community-based randomized controlled trial in Dutch patients all treated with oral prednisolone is instructive. This study showed that patients who had a history of cough, sputum production, and breathlessness recovered more rapidly when randomized to antibiotic treatment than with placebo,[30] a finding that confirmed the observations by Anthonisen and colleagues[31] some 25 years earlier.[32] There is database evidence that patients in intensive care unit (ICU) with COPD exacerbations who receive antibiotics have better outcomes,[32] and so the threshold for prescription in hospitalized patients should probably be lower than in the community at large.

Table 1 summarizes the current approaches to drug treatment and the management of acute exacerbations of COPD.

Table 1
Pharmacologic management of COPD exacerbations

Drug	Setting	Route	Dose	Comment
Bronchodilator (SABA/SAMA)	OP	Inhaled	2 puffs 3–4/h	Frequency of use should decrease over 48 h or seek help
	IP	Inhaled	Salbutamol 2.5 or 5 mg and Ipratropium 500 mcg 6/h	Nebulized till symptoms resolve
Corticosteroids	OP and IP	Oral	Prednisolone 30 mg	Give for 7–10 d and stop
Antibiotics	OP	Oral	Drug with appropriate sensitivity	Give for 5–7 d in patients with worse cough and sputum and dyspnea
	IP	Oral	Drug with appropriate sensitivity	Give for 5–7 d if one or more of the aforementioned; parenteral route seldom needed

To be used with appropriate supportive care and subsequent preventive management.
Abbreviations: IP, hospitalized in-patient or ED attendee; OP, outpatient; SABA, short-acting beta-agonist; SAMA, short-acting anti-muscarinic agents.

DRUG TREATMENT IN CHRONIC MANAGEMENT

Management approaches to stable COPD still rely heavily on drug treatment, but the way in which patients are evaluated and in which treatments are used have recently changed. **Box 1** summarizes the principal goals of medical treatment, whereas **Figs.** 2 and 3 illustrate the preferred management approaches advocated by the Global Initiative in Obstructive Lung Disease (GOLD) and by the evidence-based UK National Institute of Health and Clinical Excellence's (NICE) guidelines.[33,34] Drug therapy is based on the use of long-acting inhaled bronchodilators, whereas shorter-acting inhaled treatments for rapid onset, usually salbutamol, are reserved for rescue treatment, when symptoms increase unexpectedly (eg, after exercise or during exacerbations). The efficacy of short-acting beta-agonists (SABA) treatment in reducing symptoms like this is not well established. Bronchodilators and phosphodiesterase 4 (PDE4) antagonists are considered in detail elsewhere; but before examining how these treatments are deployed, it is worth considering the current evidence for the use of inhaled corticosteroids (ICS) alone or in combination with other drugs.

ICS AND COPD

ICS have revolutionized the management of bronchial asthma for the first-line treatment of patients with persistent symptoms.[35] They decrease eosinophilic inflammation dramatically but have little, if any, effect on inflammation and COPD, at least over 6 weeks to 3 months of treatment,[36,37] although some effects, in some patients, have been reported over longer periods.[38] Given the observed benefits of high-dose corticosteroids during exacerbations, it was reasonable to assess whether ICS had any effects in stable patients with COPD.

After 10 years, the general consensus can be summarized as follows:

- ICS have no effect on the rate of decline of lung function in lung disease in patients with GOLD grade 1 and 2 disease who smoke and in patients with severe COPD.[39–42] The different views derived from post hoc meta-analysis[43] and patient level meta-analysis[44] about whether these conclusions are correct, are likely to say more about the methodology than the effect of ICS.
- Small but consistent increases in FEV_1 are observed, the degree differing with the initial severity of airflow obstruction. This finding likely reflects the patients studied because improvement with short-acting bronchodilators is greater in patients

---

Box 1
Goals of COPD Management

- Improve lung function
- Prevent disease progression
- Relieve symptoms
- Improve exercise tolerance
- Improve health status
- Prevent and treat exacerbations
- Prevent and treat complications
- Reduce mortality
- Minimize side effects from treatment

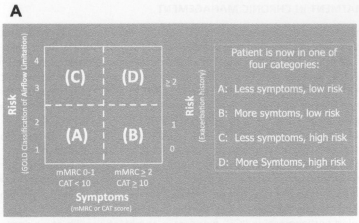

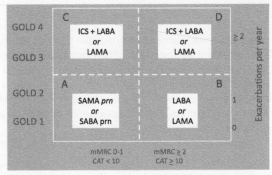

Fig. 2. Assessment by symptom severity and future risk as proposed by Vestbo and colleagues.[33] (*A*) Indicates groups in nonproportional quadrants, and (*B*) indicates the suggested initial treatment of patients in each quadrant. CAT, COPD Assessment Test; ICS, inhaled corticosteroids; LABA, long-acting beta-agonist; LAMA, long-acting anti-muscarinic agents; mMRC, modified Medical Research council breathlessness scale; prn, as needed; SABA, short-acting beta-agonist; SAMA, short-acting anti-muscarinic agents.

with moderate severity disease than those with severe problems.[45] At any given GOLD grade, the change in postbronchodilator lung function with ICS is similar to that seen with roflumilast.[46,47]

- There is a reduction in the number of exacerbations defined by the need for medical treatment in patients treated with ICS.[42,48] This reduction seems to be especially true for episodes treated with oral corticosteroids, even though the doctor is blind to the background preventative medication.[49]
- ICS is not associated with any change in mortality as compared with placebo, but neither is mortality likely to be reduced.[50] This finding is contrary to the initial impression based on the result of the database analysis whereby confounding by disease severity may have played a role.[51] By contrast, combining a long-acting beta-agonist (LABA) with an ICS produced a trend to improvement mortality relative to placebo and a significantly better mortality than what was seen with ICS alone in the TORCH (TOwards a Revolution in COPD Health) trial.[50]
- ICS have not been conclusively shown to increase the risk of osteoporosis or cataracts, at least over a 3-year study in a randomized controlled trial. The

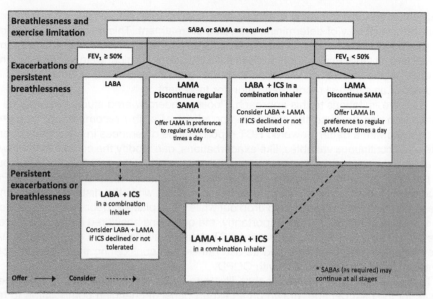

Fig. 3. Evidence-based treatment recommendations for patients with COPD as suggested by the UK National Institute for Clinical Excellence. ICS, inhaled corticosteroids; LABA, long-acting beta-agonist; LAMA, long-acting anti-muscarinic agents; SABA, short-acting beta-agonist; SAMA, short-acting anti-muscarinic agents. (*Adapted from* O'Reilly J, Jones MM, Parnham J, et al. Management of stable chronic obstructive pulmonary disease in primary and secondary care: summary of updated NICE guidance. BMJ 2010;340:c3134; with permission.)

background frequency with which these occur in patients with COPD makes it difficult to detect a small effect.[52] However, pneumonia, reported by physicians and subsequently confirmed radiologically, is more common in ICS-treated patients with COPD.[53] This effect is shown most clearly for fluticasone[49] and more recently for fluticasone furoate[54]; the signal with budesonide was smaller and did not reach statistical significance.[55] In the Investigating New Standards for Prophylaxis in Reduction of Exacerbations (INSPIRE) study, the excess of pneumonia events in patients treated with an ICS/LABA combination treatment was mainly caused by exacerbations that failed to resolve.[29] Patients treated with ICS have a higher airway bacterial load,[56] although whether this is a causal association and relates to the greater number of pneumonia events remains to be determined.

Based on these findings, there is consensus that ICS should not be used as the only regular treatment of COPD or combined with regular short-acting bronchodilators. Their role together with LABA is considered further later.

EVIDENCE-BASED THERAPY

The movement toward evidence-based therapy is both logical and desirable. Identifying areas where there is good evidence from randomized controlled trials (RCT) and other areas where practice is supported mainly by professional consensus is clinically helpful. However, some unintended consequences have arisen and effect the guidance in COPD care. Careful analysis of data, according to prespecified questions, with either systematic review or formal data pooling in a meta-analysis has become the preeminent way of determining the value of treatment. This method has reached its most sophisticated form in the GRADE (Grading Recommendations Assessment, Development and Evaluation) guideline methodology, which weighs data by the strength of the studies assessed on technical grounds and offers nuanced terms in support of an eventual recommendation for treatment.

There are limitations to this approach. Pooling underpowered studies to produce a conclusion can produce the disconcerting effect of a firm recommendation being overturned with a better-powered RCT report. Subtle differences in the a priori event rate of discontinuous variables, like exacerbations, can modify the conclusions drawn or at least the strength of the recommendations supporting them. Differential drop out in patients randomized to placebo treatment, a recurrent feature in recent COPD studies,[57,58] means that the study quality is penalized while the distorting effect and the loss of the sicker patients who drop out while using placebo decreases the chance of a positive outcome.[59] Most importantly, the questions answered by the guidelines are shrunk to ones for which sufficient RCT data are available; this often means that they focus on drug treatment and its use rather than considering the wider aspects relevant to the care of patients with COPD.

Two recent contrasting approaches illustrate these issues. The GOLD guidelines have, for the past decade, drawn on an expert panel of changing composition to review new data about COPD management, expanding the recommendations in its original report, by applying a standard methodology to consider important new data.[2] The 2011 version of the GOLD document changed its focus because the task of analyzing all of the recommendations using a grade approach has become prohibitively expensive.[33] Similar concerns have inhibited a full review of the previous American Thoracic Society/European Respiratory Society's (ATS/ERS) COPD guidelines. Instead, the new version of GOLD offers a management strategy with some preferred options for treatment. This version allows it to escape criticism as a guideline but means that its recommendations are less clearly evidenced based than in the past.

By contrast, the greater resources available to the American College of Physicians (ACP) (working jointly with the ERS and ATS) and to the UK government have allowed them to ask specific grade-based questions, producing focused recommendations.[34,60] The UK NICE updated a previous expert group approach and discovered a wider range of questions than did the ACP. Even so, many specific issues remain unanswered, particularly relating how long to continue with the specific treatment before it is changed, how best to assess the success of therapy, and how strong the evidence is in favor of one treatment rather than another.

As examples of these different approaches, the remainder of this review focuses on the similarities and differences brought up by these well-written, authoritative documents.

EVALUATING PATIENTS

For the last decade, there has been a strong emphasis on the need to monitor spirometry, preferably after a bronchodilator, to determine the disease severity in COPD. Treatment guidance has been closely anchored to this, by both the ATS/ERS' guidelines and in the NICE COPD revision. The current spirometric severity grades advocated by GOLD are as follows:

1. FEV_1 greater than 80% predicted: mild
2. FEV_1 79% to 50% predicted: moderate
3. FEV_1 49% to 30% predicted: severe

4. FEV_1 less than 30% predicted: very severe

Clinical trials have been aligned with these criteria and, hence, data on new drugs can be evaluated relative to their predecessors. However, patient well-being, expressed as either symptoms or health status, is only poorly related to FEV_1[61] and is significantly influenced by the number of COPD exacerbations.[62] To capture this component and make patient evaluation more clinically relevant, the 2011 GOLD revision separated patients into those with mild/moderate disease (GOLD grades 1 and 2) and severe/very severe disease (GOLD grades 3 and 4). In addition, the presence of symptoms evaluated by either an Medical Research Council (MRC) breathlessness score of 2 or greater or a COPD assessment test score of 10 or more was used to further subdivide patient groups.[63,64] FEV_1 was considered a marker of future risk, as was the number of exacerbations, with patients with a history of frequent exacerbations with 2 or more exacerbations forming a distinct phenotype[65] that predicted more future problems. The resulting matrix displayed in **Fig. 2** gives rise to 4 possible groups, A to D, each with a potentially different treatment approach.

The NICE approach also stratified patients with a cutoff point of an FEV_1 of 50% predicted and based initial treatment recommendations on the responses of patient groups defined spirometrically. However, they did consider the possibility that symptoms might be persistent or associated with recurrent exacerbations, despite treatment; therefore, they offered a follow-up treatment option for patients who had already received the first-line therapy but continued to have problems. This approach is somewhat closer to the one that operates in outpatient clinics and is helpful when spirometry is readily available. For many clinicians, the GOLD approach is attractive because it stresses not only spirometry but also the importance of symptoms and exacerbations.

The exact size of the patient population contained within each of the GOLD quadrants is open to debate and seems to depend on whether hospital-based or population-based cohorts are studied.[66] Impaired spirometry rather than simply high numbers of exacerbation seemed to determine the patients in groups C and D. There is some uncertainty about the equivalence of the MRC and the COPD Assessment Test (CAT) cut points, and it is hoped that this will be resolved.[67]

Ultimately, the GOLD proposal needs to be tested prospectively, both for its robustness and its clinical utility. Nonetheless, this new classification represents an important step forward in the way that patients with COPD are managed and treatment choices are evaluated.

INITIAL DRUG THERAPY

The preferred initial choices of drug treatment are shown in **Figs. 2B and 3** and are remarkably similar in both the GOLD and NICE approaches. Patients with well-preserved lung function and relatively few symptoms, which would equate to a CAT score of less than 10, can be tried on short-acting bronchodilators, with no clear preference between SABA or short-acting anti-muscarinic agents (SAMA). How effective such an approach might be has never been studied, and this recommendation remains largely consensus based.

If patients have an FEV_1 of more than 50% predicted, are more symptomatic, but have no exacerbation history, then either a long-acting anti-muscarinic agents (LAMA) or a long-acting beta-agonists (LABA) should be tried. Since the NICE evidence review, Vogelmeier and colleagues[68] have published convincing evidence that using once-daily tiotropium is more effective than twice-daily salmeterol in preventing COPD exacerbations, regardless of the background use of ICS. Whether the same would be true for once-daily LABA, such as indacaterol, is still to be established. Several studies have suggested that these drugs are at least equivalent in terms of their lung function and health status changes[69,70]; but to date, a direct comparison based on exacerbation frequency has not been presented.

For patients with more severe disease spirometrically, the first-line options are either an LAMA or an LABA/ICS combination. There are clear data to show that LABA/ICS is more effective than its components in reducing exacerbations, improving health status and lung function, and in exercise capacity.[50] Patients who would be included in the GOLD C group because of increased exacerbations rather than poor lung function (a small number in secondary care practice) also benefit from LABA/ICS treatment.[71] However, most patients with more substantial reductions in FEV_1 will also be symptomatic and have an exacerbation history; here the NICE data review suggests that either LAMA or a combination can be given with a slight preference for the combination based on data about secondary end points, such as hospitalization, study drop out, and health status, described in the INSPIRE study.[49] However, the primary outcome of that study was to show equivalence between the treatments in terms of preventing exacerbations.

ALTERNATIVE THERAPIES

Unlike GOLD, NICE makes explicit evidence-based recommendations for treatment when exacerbations remain frequent and/or breathlessness cannot be reduced to acceptable levels. For patients in GOLD grades 1 and 2, the suggestion is to add another long-acting bronchodilator of a different class to that used initially. Until recently, there has been only limited evidence of efficacy from this approach, with most of the data coming from the Canadian Optimal trial, with combination drugs performing disappointingly, relative to tiotropium therapy.[72] However, a recent 6-month study comparing once-daily indacaterol with the LAMA glycopyrronium in a combination inhaler showed that the combination was superior to either component alone in terms of improving lung function over 3 months. The changes in health status were rather more equivocal and no exacerbation data were presented.[73] However, the well-conducted SPARK study has shown in more severe disease a small but significant reduction in COPD exacerbation rates when these 2 bronchodilators are given compared with either agent alone, lending stronger support to the value of dual bronchodilator therapy.[74]

The next option for these patients with less severe spirometric impairment and the preferred second-line option for those with an FEV_1 of less than 50% predicted is to use the combination of LABA/LAMA and ICS. There are data to show that this triple therapy can reduce exacerbation and improve morning symptoms, at least then the budesonide-formoterol combination is used.[75] In practice, such a combined regimen has been widely adopted in patients with COPD or those at risk of hospitalization. This approach is supported by the GOLD guideline and may be a first-line choice for some patients.

The GOLD system also offers data about the PDE4 inhibitor roflumilast, which has been shown to prevent corticosteroid-treated exacerbations, in patients with a history of these events, who also have chronic bronchitis and an FEV_1 of less than 50% predicted.[76] It seems effective in patients who use ICS (but not LABA)[77] or those who use either LABA or LAMA (but not ICS).[47] It is most effective when the background exacerbation rate is high[78] and converts frequent exacerbators to infrequent exacerbators. Further studies investigating the effect of roflumilast on top of either LABA/ICS or triple therapy are currently ongoing.[79] However, the most common side effects seen with roflumilast are a pharmacologically predictable increase in nausea, diarrhea, and, more surprisingly, weight loss, which are likely to limit its use in some patients.

A range of other alternative treatments is suggested by GOLD, although not necessarily in any preferred order of use. Again, this represents expert preference because specific studies defining clinical effectiveness in comparable groups are lacking. GOLD also offers some options for cheaper treatment for more cash-limited health care systems, although the comparability of studies conducted when there is almost no background therapy, even with short-acting bronchodilators to trials whereby other effective agents were already deployed, is difficult to evaluate.[80]

EMERGING ISSUES

All of the aforementioned treatments have the potential for adverse effects as well as beneficial ones. As noted in the acute episodes, beta-agonists can produce troublesome tremor and palpitations, particularly in older patients, although the metabolic effects, including hypokalemia, are not troublesome. Patients with coexisting cardiac disease are common in COPD, although the evidence to date suggests that the use of beta-agonists alone or in combination with ICS is not associated with an increased mortality and may actually be beneficial.[81] LAMA drugs, such as tiotropium, are absorbed somewhat more readily than ipratropium; the use of these agents seems to be associated with more cases of urinary retention.[82,83] Dry mouth is not a major side effect and is reported less frequently with tiotropium than ipratropium. The twice-daily anticholinergic aclinidium does not seem to have this side effect.[84]

Initial concerns about an excess recurrence of cardiac deaths with LAMA treatments have been allayed by data from the follow-up of patients in the large randomized controlled Understanding the Potential Long term Improvement in Function with Tiotropium (UPLIFT) trial whereby overall fewer patients died if randomized to tiotropium treatment.[85] Recently, anxieties have been raised about the use of a soft-mist aerosol form of tiotropium, which is available in Western Europe. Greater numbers of deaths were reported on patients randomized to this treatment in the regulatory studies, which were not primarily designed to assess mortality risk.[86,87] This finding has led some to call for this delivery system to be discontinued and is unlikely to become available in the United States until these issues are resolved. Important information about this problem will come from the TIOtropium Safety and Performance in Respimat (TIOSPIR) study of more than 17,000 patients who are receiving either 2 different doses of tiotropium from the soft-mist inhaler or conventional tiotropium from the dry power device.[88]

A range of new drugs belonging to the LABA and LAMA classes given once or twice daily alone or in combination with each other or inhaled corticosteroids are in the process of development and registration. One such combination of the LABA vilanterol and the inhaled corticosteroid fluticasone furoate has received a favorable assessment at a Food and Drug Administration advisory panel.

At present, no new twice-daily LABA drugs have been evaluated; but twice-daily aclidinium bromide has been licensed for use in the United States and Western Europe, and studies combining this with formoterol are ongoing. Once-daily inhaled indacaterol has been combined with glycopyrronium, as noted earlier,[73,74] and is also being studied together with mometasone furoate, an ICS that can prove effective when given once daily.[89]

A new LABA, olodaterol, is being combined with tiotropium; but these studies have used the soft-mist delivery system discussed earlier, and their outcome will be influenced by the results of TIOSPIR. The vilanterol/fluticasone furoate combination has been investigated in several doses[90] and in replicate 1-year studies.[54] The inhaled steroid adds relatively little to the bronchodilator effect, but this is associated with fewer exacerbations than is seen with the LABA alone (**Fig. 4**). As with other fluticasone

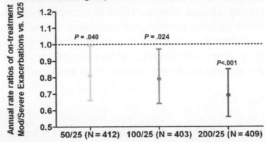

Fig. 4. Effect on exacerbation rate of adding the once-daily inhaled corticosteroid flutica-sone furoate to the long-acting inhaled beta-agonist vilanterol (VI) in a 1-year clinical trial. Note the improvement in exacerbation rate with the corticosteroid in the absence of significant differences in FEV₁. Mod, moderate. (*Adapted from* Dransfield MT, Bourbeau J, Jones PW, et al. Once-daily inhaled fluticasone furoate and vilanterol vs vilanterol only for prevention of exacerbations of COPD: two replicate double-blind, parallel-group, randomised controlled trials. Lancet Respir Med 2013;1:210–23; with permission.)

preparations, pneumonia was more common when the ICS was used; but overall, the combination of 25 mcg vilanterol and 200 mcg fluticasone furoate gave the most favorable benefit/risk profile.

Ultimately, the plethora of newer chemically and clinically similar entities will need a clear-sighted appraisal of the cost-effectiveness of treatment before these agents can be recommended in future treatment guidelines. The next generation of clinical trials will need to define not just whether the treatment works relative to a placebo comparator (an approach which seems to be increasingly unethical, given the established effects of treatment) but also how much benefit such treatment provides for the patients and payer. Defining when it is appropriate to add treatment to existing regimens or replace components of a current therapy will be our next challenge.

SUMMARY

Choosing the optimal drug therapy is a key component of the management of COPD. Acute exacerbation treatment, whether in the community or hospital, has changed little in recent years and involves increasing the frequency and/or dose of inhaled bronchodilators, giving a short (up to 10 days) course of oral prednisolone, having a low threshold for starting antibiotics of an appropriate spectrum to cover likely pathogens, and avoiding the use of methylxanthines.

Chronic treatment choices are influenced by baseline lung function, symptom intensity, and how often patients have exacerbated in the past. Short-acting reliever treatment with beta-agonists or antimuscarinics may be appropriate for patients with few symptoms and preserved lung function; but at present, long-acting antimuscarinic treatment is the first-line option when managing patients whose FEV₁ is more than 50% predicted. Those with more severe disease spirometrically and/or a history of 2 or more exacerbations per year gain benefits from either long-acting antimuscarinics but especially from combinations of LABA and ICS. These 3 treatment approaches can be combined if there are persistent problems, especially in patients who exacerbate often.

Other agents, such as PDE4 inhibitor roflumilast, can be considered as an alternative to ICS and may prove helpful in disease that is difficult to manage with triple treatment, although this has yet to be definitely established. Many other options exist, with once-daily combinations of bronchodilators and bronchodilator corticosteroids becoming available in the near future.

REFERENCES

1. Celli BR, MacNee W. Standards for the diagnosis and treatment of patients with COPD: a summary of the ATS/ERS position paper. Eur Respir J 2004;23(6): 932–46.
2. Rabe KF, Hurd S, Anzueto A, et al. Global strategy for the diagnosis, management, and prevention of chronic obstructive pulmonary disease: GOLD executive summary. Am J Respir Crit Care Med 2007;176(6):532–55.
3. National Collaborating Centre for Chronic Conditions. Chronic obstructive pulmonary disease. National clinical guideline on management of chronic obstructive pulmonary disease in adults in primary and secondary care. Thorax 2004; 59(Suppl 1):1–232.
4. Lightowler JV, Wedzicha JA, Elliott MW, et al. Non-invasive positive pressure ventilation to treat respiratory failure resulting from exacerbations of chronic obstructive pulmonary disease: cochrane systematic review and meta-analysis. BMJ 2003;326(7382):185.
5. Chakrabarti B, Angus RM, Agarwal S, et al. Hyperglycaemia as a predictor of outcome during non invasive ventilation in decompensated COPD. Thorax 2009;64(10):857–62.
6. Albert P, Calverley PM. Drugs (including oxygen) in severe COPD. Eur Respir J 2008;31(5):1114–24.
7. O'Donnell DE, D'Arsigny C, Webb KA. Effects of hyperoxia on ventilatory limitation during exercise in advanced chronic obstructive pulmonary disease. Am J Respir Crit Care Med 2001;163(4):892–8.
8. Lacasse Y, Lecours R, Pelletier C, et al. Randomised trial of ambulatory oxygen in oxygen-dependent COPD. Eur Respir J 2005;25(6):1032–8.
9. Stevenson NJ, Calverley PM. Effect of oxygen on recovery from maximal exercise in patients with chronic obstructive pulmonary disease. Thorax 2004;59(8): 668–72.
10. Suissa S, Dell'Aniello S, Ernst P. Long-term natural history of chronic obstructive pulmonary disease: severe exacerbations and mortality. Thorax 2012;67(11): 957–63.
11. Parker CM, Voduc N, Aaron SD, et al. Physiological changes during symptom recovery from moderate exacerbations of COPD. Eur Respir J 2005;26(3):420–8.
12. Stevenson NJ, Walker PP, Costello RW, et al. Lung mechanics and dyspnea during exacerbations of chronic obstructive pulmonary disease. Am J Respir Crit Care Med 2005;172(12):1510–6.
13. Austin MA, Wills KE, Blizzard L, et al. Effect of high flow oxygen on mortality in chronic obstructive pulmonary disease patients in prehospital setting: randomised controlled trial. BMJ 2010;341:c5462. http://dx.doi.org/10.1136/bmj. c5462.:c5462.
14. Gross NJ, Petty TL, Friedman M, et al. Dose response to ipratropium as a nebulized solution in patients with chronic obstructive pulmonary disease. A three-center study [see comments]. Am Rev Respir Dis 1989;139(5):1188–91.
15. Moayyedi P, Congleton J, Page RL, et al. Comparison of nebulised salbutamol and ipratropium bromide with salbutamol alone in the treatment of chronic obstructive pulmonary disease. Thorax 1995;50(8):834–7.

16. Hadcroft J, Calverley PM. Alternative methods for assessing bronchodilator reversibility in chronic obstructive pulmonary disease. Thorax 2001;56(9):713–20.

17. Parshall MB, Schwartzstein RM, Adams L, et al. An official American Thoracic Society statement: update on the mechanisms, assessment, and management of dyspnea. Am J Respir Crit Care Med 2012;185(4):435–52.

18. McKay SE, Howie CA, Thomson AH, et al. Value of theophylline treatment in patients handicapped by chronic obstructive lung disease. Thorax 1993;48(3):227–32.

19. Rice KL, Leatherman JW, Duane PG, et al. Aminophylline for acute exacerbations of chronic obstructive pulmonary disease. A controlled trial. Ann Intern Med 1987;107(3):305–9.

20. Duffy N, Walker P, Diamantea F, et al. Intravenous aminophylline in patients admitted to hospital with exacerbations of chronic obstructive pulmonary disease: a prospective randomised controlled trial. Thorax 2005;60(9):713–7.

21. Qiu Y, Zhu J, Bandi V, et al. Biopsy neutrophilia, neutrophil chemokine and receptor gene expression in severe exacerbations of chronic obstructive pulmonary disease. Am J Respir Crit Care Med 2003;168(8):968–75.

22. Niewoehner DE, Erbland ML, Deupree RH, et al. Effect of systemic glucocorticoids on exacerbations of chronic obstructive pulmonary disease. N Engl J Med 1999;340(25):1941–7.

23. Davies L, Angus RM, Calverley PM. Oral corticosteroids in patients admitted to hospital with exacerbations of chronic obstructive pulmonary disease: a prospective randomised controlled trial. Lancet 1999;354(9177):456–60.

24. Aaron SD, Vandemheen KL, Hebert P, et al. Outpatient oral prednisone after emergency treatment of chronic obstructive pulmonary disease. N Engl J Med 2003;348(26):2618–25.

25. Sayiner A, Aytemur ZA, Cirit M, et al. Systemic glucocorticoids in severe exacerbations of COPD [see comments]. Chest 2001;119(3):726–30.

26. Thompson WH, Nielson CP, Carvalho P, et al. Controlled trial of oral prednisone in outpatients with acute COPD exacerbation. Am J Respir Crit Care Med 1996; 154(2 Pt 1):407–12.

27. Decramer M, de Bock V, Dom R. Functional and histologic picture of steroid-induced myopathy in chronic obstructive pulmonary disease. Am J Respir Crit Care Med 1996;153(6 Pt 1):1958–64.

28. Wedzicha JA, Seemungal TA. COPD exacerbations: defining their cause and prevention. Lancet 2007;370(9589):786–96.

29. Calverley PM, Stockley RA, Seemungal TA, et al. Reported pneumonia in patients with COPD: findings from the INSPIRE study. Chest 2011;139(3):505–12.

30. Daniels JM, Snijders D, de Graaff CS, et al. Antibiotics in addition to systemic corticosteroids for acute exacerbations of chronic obstructive pulmonary disease. Am J Respir Crit Care Med 2010;181(2):150–7.

31. Anthonisen NR, Manfreda J, Warren CP, et al. Antibiotic therapy in exacerbations of chronic obstructive pulmonary disease. Ann Intern Med 1987;106(2):196–204.

32. Rothberg MB, Pekow PS, Lahti M, et al. Antibiotic therapy and treatment failure in patients hospitalized for acute exacerbations of chronic obstructive pulmonary disease. JAMA 2010;303(20):2035–42.

33. Vestbo J, Hurd SS, Agusti AG, et al. Global strategy for the diagnosis, management and prevention of chronic obstructive pulmonary disease, GOLD executive summary. Am J Respir Crit Care Med 2013;187(4):347–65.

34. O'Reilly J, Jones MM, Parnham J, et al. Management of stable chronic obstructive pulmonary disease in primary and secondary care: summary of updated NICE guidance. BMJ 2010;340:c3134. http://dx.doi.org/10.1136/bmj.c3134.:c3134.

35. Bateman ED, Hurd SS, Barnes PJ, et al. Global strategy for asthma management and prevention: GINA executive summary. Eur Respir J 2008;31(1):143–78.
36. Hattotuwa KL, Gizycki MJ, Ansari TW, et al. The effects of inhaled fluticasone on airway inflammation in chronic obstructive pulmonary disease: a double-blind, placebo-controlled biopsy study. Am J Respir Crit Care Med 2002;165(12):1592–6.
37. Bourbeau J, Christodoulopoulos P, Maltais F, et al. Effect of salmeterol/fluticasone propionate on airway inflammation in COPD: a randomised controlled trial. Thorax 2007;62(11):938–43.
38. Lapperre TS, Snoeck-Stroband JB, Gosman MM, et al. Effect of fluticasone with and without salmeterol on pulmonary outcomes in chronic obstructive pulmonary disease: a randomized trial. Ann Intern Med 2009;151(8):517–27.
39. Vestbo J, Sorensen T, Lange P, et al. Long-term effect of inhaled budesonide in mild and moderate chronic obstructive pulmonary disease: a randomised controlled trial. Lancet 1999;353(9167):1819–23.
40. Pauwels RA, Lofdahl CG, Laitinen LA, et al. Long-term treatment with inhaled budesonide in persons with mild chronic obstructive pulmonary disease who continue smoking. N Engl J Med 1999;340(25):1948–53.
41. The Lung Health Study Research Group. Effect of inhaled triamcinolone on the decline in pulmonary function in chronic obstructive pulmonary disease. N Engl J Med 2000;343:1902–9.
42. Burge PS, Calverley PM, Jones PW, et al. Randomised, double blind, placebo controlled study of fluticasone propionate in patients with moderate to severe chronic obstructive pulmonary disease: the ISOLDE trial. BMJ 2000;320(7245):1297–303.
43. Sutherland ER, Allmers H, Ayas NT, et al. Inhaled corticosteroids reduce the progression of airflow limitation in chronic obstructive pulmonary disease: a meta-analysis. Thorax 2003;58(11):937–41.
44. Soriano JB, Sin DD, Zhang X, et al. A pooled analysis of FEV1 decline in COPD patients randomized to inhaled corticosteroids or placebo. Chest 2007;131(3):682–9.
45. Albert P, Agusti A, Edwards L, et al. Bronchodilator responsiveness as a phenotypic characteristic of established chronic obstructive pulmonary disease. Thorax 2012;67(8):701–8.
46. Rabe KF, Bateman ED, O'donnell D, et al. Roflumilast–an oral anti-inflammatory treatment for chronic obstructive pulmonary disease: a randomised controlled trial. Lancet 2005;366(9485):563–71.
47. Fabbri LM, Calverley PM, Izquierdo-Alonso JL, et al. Roflumilast in moderate-to-severe chronic obstructive pulmonary disease treated with long acting bronchodilators: two randomised clinical trials. Lancet 2009;374(9691):695–703.
48. Kardos P, Wencker M, Glaab T, et al. Salmeterol/fluticasone propionate versus salmeterol on exacerbations in severe chronic obstructive pulmonary disease. Am J Respir Crit Care Med 2007;175(2):144–9.
49. Wedzicha JA, Calverley PM, Seemungal TA, et al. The prevention of chronic obstructive pulmonary disease exacerbations by salmeterol/fluticasone propionate or tiotropium bromide. Am J Respir Crit Care Med 2008;177(1):19–26.
50. Calverley PM, Anderson JA, Celli B, et al. Salmeterol and fluticasone propionate and survival in chronic obstructive pulmonary disease. N Engl J Med 2007;356(8):775–89.
51. Kiri VA, Pride NB, Soriano JB, et al. Inhaled corticosteroids in chronic obstructive pulmonary disease: results from two observational designs free of immortal time bias. Am J Respir Crit Care Med 2005;172(4):460–4.

52. Ferguson GT, Calverley PM, Anderson JA, et al. Prevalence and progression of osteoporosis in patients with COPD. Results from TORCH. Chest 2009;136(6): 1456–65.

53. Crim C, Calverley PM, Anderson JA, et al. Pneumonia risk in COPD patients receiving inhaled corticosteroids alone or in combination: TORCH study results. Eur Respir J 2009;34(3):641–7.

54. Dransfield MT, Bourbeau J, Jones PW, et al. Oncedaily inhaled fluticasone furoate and vilanterol versus vilanterol only for prevention of exacerbations of COPD: two replicate double-blind, parallel-group, randomised controlled trials. Lancet Respir Med 2013;1(30):210–23.

55. Sin DD, Tashkin D, Zhang X, et al. Budesonide and the risk of pneumonia: a meta-analysis of individual patient data. Lancet 2009;374(9691):712–9.

56. Garcha DS, Thurston SJ, Patel AR, et al. Changes in prevalence and load of airway bacteria using quantitative PCR in stable and exacerbated COPD. Thorax 2012;67(12):1075–80.

57. Vestbo J, Anderson JA, Calverley PM, et al. Bias due to withdrawal in long-term randomised trials in COPD: evidence from the TORCH study. Clin Respir J 2011; 5(1):44–9.

58. Kesten S, Plautz M, Piquette CA, et al. Premature discontinuation of patients: a potential bias in COPD clinical trials. Eur Respir J 2007;30(5):898–906.

59. Calverley PM, Rennard SI. What have we learned from large drug treatment trials in COPD? Lancet 2007;370(9589):774–85.

60. Qaseem A, Wilt TJ, Weinberger SE, et al. Diagnosis and management of stable chronic obstructive pulmonary disease: a clinical practice guideline update from the American College of Physicians, American College of Chest Physicians, American Thoracic Society, and European Respiratory Society. Ann Intern Med 2011;155(3):179–91.

61. Spencer S, Calverley PM, Burge PS, et al. Health status deterioration in patients with chronic obstructive pulmonary disease. Am J Respir Crit Care Med 2001; 163(1):122–8.

62. Spencer S, Calverley PM, Burge PS, et al. Impact of preventing exacerbations on deterioration of health status in COPD. Eur Respir J 2004;23(5):698–702.

63. Bestall JC, Paul EA, Garrod R, et al. Usefulness of the Medical Research Council (MRC) dyspnoea scale as a measure of disability in patients with chronic obstructive pulmonary disease. Thorax 1999;54(7):581–6.

64. Jones PW, Harding G, Berry P, et al. Development and first validation of the COPD assessment test. Eur Respir J 2009;34(3):648–54.

65. Hurst JR, Vestbo J, Anzueto A, et al. Susceptibility to exacerbation in chronic obstructive pulmonary disease. N Engl J Med 2010;363(12):1128–38.

66. Han MK, Muellerova H, Curran-Everett D, et al. GOLD 2011 disease severity classification in COPDGene: a prospective cohort study. Lancet Respir Med 2013;1:43–9.

67. Jones P, Adamek L, Nadeau G, et al. Comparisons of health status scores with MRC grades in a primary care COPD population: implications for the new GOLD 2011 classification. Eur Respir J 2013;42(3):647–54.

68. Vogelmeier C, Hederer B, Glaab T, et al. Tiotropium versus salmeterol for the prevention of exacerbations of COPD. N Engl J Med 2011;364(12):1093–103.

69. Jones PW, Barnes N, Vogelmeier C, et al. Efficacy of indacaterol in the treatment of patients with COPD. Prim Care Respir J 2011;20(4):380–8.

70. Donohue JF, Fogarty C, Lotvall J, et al. Once-daily bronchodilators for chronic obstructive pulmonary disease: indacaterol versus tiotropium. Am J Respir Crit Care Med 2010;182(2):155–62.

71. Jenkins CR, Jones PW, Calverley PM, et al. Efficacy of salmeterol/fluticasone propionate by GOLD stage of chronic obstructive pulmonary disease: analysis from the randomised, placebo-controlled TORCH study. Respir Res 2009;10:59.
72. Aaron SD, Vandemheen KL, Fergusson D, et al. Tiotropium in combination with placebo, salmeterol, or fluticasone-salmeterol for treatment of chronic obstructive pulmonary disease: a randomized trial. Ann Intern Med 2007;146(8):545–55.
73. Vogelmeier C, Bateman ED, Pallante J, et al. Efficacy and safety of once-daily QVA149 compared with twice-daily salmeterol–fluticasone in patients with chronic obstructive pulmonary disease (ILLUMINATE): a randomised, double-blind, parallel group study. Lancet Respir Med 2013;1(1):51–60.
74. Wedzicha JA, Decramer M, Ficker JH, et al. Analysis of chronic obstructive pulmonary disease exacerbations with the dual bronchodilator QVA149 compared with glycopyrronium and tiotropium (SPARK): a randomised, double-blind, parallel-group study. Lancet Respir Med 2013;1(3):199–209.
75. Welte T, Miravitlles M, Hernandez P, et al. Efficacy and tolerability of budesonide/formoterol added to tiotropium in patients with chronic obstructive pulmonary disease. Am J Respir Crit Care Med 2009;180(8):741–50.
76. Calverley PM, Rabe KF, Goehring UM, et al. Roflumilast in symptomatic chronic obstructive pulmonary disease: two randomised clinical trials. Lancet 2009; 374(9691):685–94.
77. Rennard SI, Calverley PM, Goehring UM, et al. Reduction of exacerbations by the PDE4 inhibitor roflumilast–the importance of defining different subsets of patients with COPD. Respir Res 2011;12:18.
78. Bateman ED, Rabe KF, Calverley PM, et al. Roflumilast with long-acting beta2-agonists for COPD: influence of exacerbation history. Eur Respir J 2011;38(3): 553–60.
79. Calverley PM, Martinez FJ, Fabbri LM, et al. Does roflumilast decrease exacerbations in severe COPD patients not controlled by inhaled combination therapy? The REACT study protocol. Int J Chron Obstruct Pulmon Dis 2012;7:375–82. http://dx.doi.org/10.2147/COPD.S31100.
80. Albert P, Calverley P. A PEACE-ful solution to COPD exacerbations? Lancet 2008; 371(9629):1975–6.
81. Calverley PM, Anderson JA, Celli B, et al. Cardiovascular events in patients with COPD: TORCH study results. Thorax 2010;65(8):719–25.
82. Kesten S, Jara M, Wentworth C, et al. Pooled clinical trial analysis of tiotropium safety. Chest 2006;130(6):1695–703.
83. Stephenson A, Seitz D, Bell CM, et al. Inhaled anticholinergic drug therapy and the risk of acute urinary retention in chronic obstructive pulmonary disease: a population-based study. Arch Intern Med 2011;171(10):914–20.
84. Jones PW, Singh D, Bateman ED, et al. Efficacy and safety of twice-daily aclidinium bromide in COPD patients: the ATTAIN study. Eur Respir J 2012;40(4):830–6.
85. Celli B, Decramer M, Kesten S, et al. Mortality in the 4 year trial of tiotropium (UPLIFT) in patients with COPD. Am J Respir Crit Care Med 2009;180(10):948–55.
86. Singh S, Loke YK, Enright PL, et al. Mortality associated with tiotropium mist inhaler in patients with chronic obstructive pulmonary disease: systematic review and meta-analysis of randomised controlled trials. BMJ 2011;342:d3215. http://dx.doi.org/10.1136/bmj.d3215.:d3215.
87. Dong YH, Lin HH, Shau WY, et al. Comparative safety of inhaled medications in patients with chronic obstructive pulmonary disease: systematic review and mixed treatment comparison meta-analysis of randomised controlled trials. Thorax 2013;68(1):48–56.

88. Wise RA, Anzueto A, Calverley P, et al. The Tiotropium Safety and Performance in Respimat(R) Trial (TIOSPIR(R)), a large scale, randomized, controlled, parallel-group trial-design and rationale. Respir Res 2013;14:40. http://dx.doi.org/10.1186/1465-9921-14-40.

89. Calverley PM, Rennard S, Nelson HS, et al. One-year treatment with mometasone furoate in chronic obstructive pulmonary disease. Respir Res 2008;9:73.

90. Martinez FJ, Boscia J, Feldman G, et al. Fluticasone furoate/vilanterol (100/25; 200/25 mug) improves lung function in COPD: a randomised trial. Respir Med 2013;107(4):550–9.

Pulmonary Issues in the Older Adult

Delia E. Frederick, MSN, RN

KEYWORDS

- Older adults • Pulmonary issues • Effects of aging • Pneumonia
- Chronic obstructive pulmonary disease

KEY POINTS

- Overall body changes in muscular strength, skeletal structure, and mobility, in addition to cardiovascular function, result in changes in pulmonary function.
- Decreased thirst response, and less moisture within the mucous membranes of the upper and lower respiratory tract contribute to thickened mucus.
- Community-acquired pneumonia and chronic obstructive pulmonary disease are typical respiratory diseases in older adults.

INTRODUCTION

Pulmonary diseases are not the highest ranked reasons for admission to hospital, nor are they the principal reason for death in the United States. Pulmonary complications are of concern for all individuals admitted to an intensive care unit (ICU). Chronic lower respiratory diseases result in the deaths of only 6.2% of adults older than 65 years, and deaths attributable to influenza and pneumonia occur in of 2.6% of adults older than 65. Morbidity for chronic lower respiratory diseases is 6.4%.[1]

Nevertheless, older adults do have anatomic and physiologic changes that adversely affect the protective mechanisms for the pulmonary system.[2] Some of the changes nurses see in older adults are due to normal aging processes, but others are related to disease processes. It is imperative that nurses should not assume that alterations in pulmonary status are due to aging, and thus fail to intervene to correct the pulmonary issue. The purpose of this article is to review the changes that occur with aging and elucidate their effects on the pulmonary system. Interventions to deter complications and recognize respiratory distress are also provided.

This article originally appeared in Critical Care Nursing Clinics, Volume 26, Issue 1, March 2014.
The author has nothing to disclose.
School of Nursing, The University of North Carolina at Greensboro, Unit #9, 44 White Oak Street, Franklin, NC 28734, USA
E-mail address: defreder@uncg.edu

Clinics Collections 6 (2015) 351–357
http://dx.doi.org/10.1016/j.ccol.2015.05.047

ANATOMY OF THE PULMONARY SYSTEM

The anatomy of the pulmonary system begins with the upper airway. The nose and mouth are entrances for air into the lungs. Atmospheric air is warmed and moistened as it courses through the nares. Adequate moisture of breathed air depends on a well-hydrated individual.[3]

The upper respiratory tract has 2 protective mechanisms to prevent foreign matter from entering the lower respiratory tract. The sneeze is a reflexive action that clears the upper airway when the presence of foreign matter enters the nose. This reflex is in place from the neonatal period until well into old age. The second protective mechanism is cilia within the posterior portion of the nares. Cilia are fine hairs that trap large foreign matter to prevent its entry into the lower respiratory tract. The cilia propel matter into the pharynx to be coughed out or swallowed. In a healthy older adult there is no decrease in the cough reflex.[3-5]

The pharynx has protective mechanisms in place to prevent aspiration of foreign matter into the lower respiratory tract. At the entrance to the lower respiratory tract, the tracheal opening, the glottis, is covered by the epiglottis during swallowing or at any time foreign matter makes contact with the glottis. This closure is a reflexive response that depends on cranial nerves IX (glossopharyngeal), X (vagus), and XII (hypoglossal). Effective swallowing is the result of coordination of these cranial nerves as well as many muscles, the cerebral cortex, the brainstem, and the cerebellum.[3,6]

The lower respiratory tract is enclosed in the thoracic cavity. The pulmonary system shares space with the heart and its structures. The skeletal structures of the thoracic cavity consist of an anterior sternum and a posterior vertebral column joined together by 12 pairs of curved ribs. Intercostal muscles allow for the movement of the skeletal structure necessary for inhalation and exhalation. In aging, reduced muscular strength or skeletal changes in the thorax can affect breathing even in the presence of healthy lung tissue.[2,4]

The trachea branches into 2 bronchi, then into the right and left lung fields. The right bronchus is straighter and more in line with the trachea, thus the risk of foreign-matter aspiration is more likely to occur in the right lung. The lungs are divided into lobes, of which there are 3 on the right and 2 on the left. The major lung fields are best auscultated on the back. It is important to assess lung sounds in all lung fields. Macrophages within the alveolar clusters consume foreign matter and bacteria that reach the terminal structures of the lungs. Gas exchange occurs at the alveolar-capillary membrane. The overall purpose of the pulmonary system is to deliver oxygen to the alveoli for diffusion into the bloodstream.[3,4]

ASSESSMENT OF THE PULMONARY SYSTEM

Respiratory rate provides a primary tool for determining homeostasis in individuals. The rate and effort of respirations in the older adult should be monitored, in addition to meticulous auscultation of lung sounds for abnormality. Tachypnea is an indication of hypercarbia, chemical irritation of the airways, or edema within the alveolar-capillary membrane tissue.[6] A full set of vital signs, including level of consciousness, is indicated to ensure stable oxygenation. Confusion, agitation, or both can indicate hypoxia. Tachycardia can be a sign of hypoxia.

Laboratory values are useful for evaluating pulmonary status.[7] Admission laboratory values may alert the nurse to potential risks of respiratory complications for an individual. Venous CO_2 can be referenced for metabolic processes in the absence of arterial blood gas. Fasting hyperglycemia on admission laboratory data has been found to be associated with higher rates of mortality in the presence of pneumonia.[8] An arterial blood gas indicates acid-base balance within the individual. Respiratory failure is indicated by a Pao_2 of less than 50 mm Hg and a $Paco_2$ of greater than 50 mm Hg. Brain natriuretic peptide (BNP) is a hormone secreted in response to elevated blood volume. Values of BNP higher than 100 µg/L indicate heart failure (**Table 1**).[6]

AGE-RELATED CHANGES THAT AFFECT THE PULMONARY SYSTEM

Older adults have a decreased thirst response, and thus may have less moisture within the mucous membranes of the upper and lower respiratory tracts. Poor hydration contributes to thickened mucus and increases the risk of the older adult being unable to clear sputum from the nose or lungs.[3] Older adults' intake and output, as well as blood urea nitrogen (BUN) and creatinine, indicate homeostasis of fluid volume. Excessive fluid volume impairs gas exchange at the alveolar-capillary interface.[6]

In older adults who have aspiration risk resulting from neurologic deficits, the cough response may be reduced. One small study of healthy older adults in a comparison with young healthy adults found a lower frequency of cough reflex in the older adults by a factor of one-third.[5] Speech volume and number of words spoken are affected by the volume of air within the lungs and the strength of the thoracic structures. The slow pace and length of idea delivery may suggest decreased cognition or may be attributed solely to the respiratory effort required to speak. Close attention to speech is needed to identify the effort of breathing in relation to decreased thinking in the older adult. Acute cognitive deficits may be related to hypoxia.[9]

Dysphagia in older adults can increase the incidence of foreign-matter aspiration. Impaired swallowing results in coughing or choking on thin liquids. Hoarse, gurgling sounds of the voice may indicate poor oropharynx clearance. Further investigation of airway sounds by auscultation starting at the trachea may aid in the assessment of ineffective swallowing. Dysphagic individuals require meticulous oral care to reduce the risk of aspiration pneumonia.[10]

As individuals lie in bed resting on their back, secretions can collect within the posterior lobes. Static secretions increase the risk of pneumonia development. Even

Table 1
Laboratory values related to the pulmonary system

	Arterial Blood Gases		
	Acidosis	Normal Value	Alkalosis
pH	<7.35	7.35–7.45	>7.45
CO_2, mm Hg	>45	35–45	<35
HCO_3, mEq/L	<22	22–26	>26
O_2, mm Hg	—	80–100	—
Vco_2, mmol/L	Metabolic	24–30	Metabolic
Brain natriuretic peptide (BNP), µg/L			<100
Serum glucose level, mg/dL			70–110
Sodium, mg/dL			135–145
Potassium, mg/dL			3.5–5.0
Chloride, mg/dL			100–106
Blood urea nitrogen, mg/dL			8–25
Creatinine, mg/dL			0.6–1.6

Data from Venes D, editor. Tabor's cyclopedic medical dictionary. 19th edition. Philadelphia: F.A. Davis; 2001. p. 2448–50; with permission.

healthy older adults' epithelial lining has been found to have an increase in neutrophils and a decrease in macrophages when compared with that of younger adults. Macrophages are effective in eliminating foreign matter and bacteria that reach the lower respiratory tract regions. The decrease in macrophage numbers may place older adults at greater risk for infection within the lungs.[4,11]

Changes in ventilation-perfusion matching and shunting occur with age. This widened alveolar-arterial oxygen gradient does not seem to change the arterial pressures of O_2 or CO_2. Despite this, the older adult may not perceive hypoxic or hypercapnic events in the same way younger adults do, and thus may fail to alert health care personnel. Even though the lack of O_2 or excess CO_2 may cause no apparent distress, abnormal O_2 and CO_2 values are always a cause for concern.[3,4]

Tachypnea is the best indicator of respiratory compromise in the older adult. Febrile presentation cannot be relied on for evidence of infection; only 50% of older adults have a fever with infection.[9,10] Tachypnea with or without activity may not be accompanied with the complaint of dyspnea by the older adult. In fact, older adults experiencing bronchoconstriction may not perceive the symptom even with the occurrence of significant constriction. Tachycardia from any cause can result in hypoxia from poor tissue perfusion.[3,4]

Overall body changes in muscular strength, skeletal structure, and mobility lead to changes in pulmonary function. Musculoskeletal changes alter thoracic mobility. These restrictions have a negative effect on respiration. All older adults have some decrease in thoracic muscular strength and skeletal movement, but some older adults have the added complication of comorbid diseases that increase the effort of breathing. Osteoporosis, spinal column changes such as kyphosis or scoliosis, and traumas to the chest require the individual to exert more effort to breathe in comparison with those unaffected by musculoskeletal disease. Positional support is needed to improve effective respiration. Older adults have improved lung aeration if the head of the bed is elevated at least 15° and as much as 90°. Individuals with chronic obstructive pulmonary disease (COPD) may prefer the orthopnic position.[2,4,12]

Typical Respiratory Diseases in Older Adults

Older adults are at greater risk for pneumonia related to heightened inflammatory activity within the alveoli and bronchiolar spaces. Boyd and Orihuela[13] found increases in inflammatory cells within the lungs and blood of healthy older adults. Although these cells are present, they do not have the effectiveness of fighting infection that occurs in younger adults. It is therefore possible that this contributes to their increased risk of community-acquired pneumonia (CAP). Individuals with COPD have even greater numbers of inflammatory cells than healthy older adults, and their risk of CAP is even greater than that of healthy older adults. Alterations in the pulmonary environment make it clear that pneumonia vaccines are protective in the older adult population.[1]

Individuals who present to the hospital with CAP have signs of acute respiratory infection that include cough, dyspnea, and, possibly, fever. A chest radiograph will indicate an acute infiltrate. Older adults are typically infected with *Streptococcus pneumoniae*, *Haemophilus influenzae*, or *Klebsiella pneumoniae*. Individuals who are admitted to the ICU for CAP have comorbidities. These patients also have fever, tachypnea, tachycardia, and hypotension. A presentation of abnormal chemistries includes arterial pH lower than 7.35, BUN level higher than 64 mg/dL, sodium level less than 130 mEq/L, glucose level greater than 250 mg/dL, Pao_2 less than 60 mm Hg, and Sao_2 less than 90%, as well as a pleural effusion on radiographs. Confusion caused by the altered homeostasis is common.[14]

The nurse should anticipate the treatment of CAP within the ICU to include a macrolide, a fluroquinolone, and a β-lactam. These antibiotics are administered intravenously for 1 week to 10 days. Individuals need to be afebrile and clinically stable before antibiotics are discontinued.[14]

Early signs of COPD are identified as a chronic cough with mucus production, although a cough may occur without noticeable mucus. Forced expiratory volume (FEV) at this time may fall within normal limits. The progression of COPD is apparent with further symptoms of dyspnea and diminishing FEV values. In the elderly, the diagnosis is confounded by the changes of aging that produce decreased FEV and dyspnea. Nonetheless, older adults who have smoked have greater challenges with breathing than do older adults who have quit smoking or have never smoked. Nurses should implement smoking-cessation education for all smokers regardless of the level of disease.[15]

Simple questions designed by the Global Initiative for Chronic Obstructive Lung Disease (GOLD) reveal the toll COPD takes on individuals diagnosed with the disease. Activity levels are graded from 0 to 4, with 0 being breathlessness with strenuous activity and 4 being too breathless to participate in activities of daily living without becoming breathless (**Box 1**). COPD is also quantified from mild to very severe by evaluating FEV after bronchodilator administration. Mild COPD, called GOLD 1, occurs with a FEV of greater than or equal to 80% of the predicted value of expired air for the same age, gender, height, and weight in persons without pulmonary compromise. Very severe COPD trends to such poor FEV that the expired air is less than 30% of the anticipated volume for similar persons without COPD (**Box 2**).[15]

Pulmonary support of individuals with COPD may require the administration of bronchodilators and, at times, corticosteroids. Airways normally dilate with inhalation and constrict with expiration. In the presence of bronchoconstriction and inflammation of COPD, airways become too narrow for effective expiration. β-Agonist bronchodilators exert an effect on β-receptors of the sympathetic nervous system, keeping airways open on expiration. Anticholinergic bronchodilators interfere with the parasympathetic nervous system's stimulus to constrict airways, also keeping airways open with expiration. The β-agonist albuterol and the anticholinergic ipratropium are often combined for the reduction of acute symptoms. Long-acting β-agonists and anticholinergics are prescribed for maintenance care.[15]

Box 1
Modified Medical Research Council (mMRC) questionnaire for assessing the severity of breathlessness

mMRC Grade 0: I only get breathless with strenuous exercise

mMRC Grade 1: I get short of breath when hurrying on the level or walking up a slight hill

mMRC Grade 2: I walk slower than people of the same age on the level because of breathlessness, or I have to stop for breath when walking on my own pace on the level

mMRC Grade 3: I stop for breath after walking about 100 m or after a few minutes on the level

mMRC Grade 4: I am too breathless to leave the house or I am breathless when dressing or undressing

Adapted from Fletcher CM, Elmes PC, Fairbairn MB, et al. The significance of respiratory symptoms and the diagnosis of chronic bronchitis in a working population. Br Med J 1959;2:257–66.

Box 2
Classification of severity of airflow limitation in COPD (based on postbronchodilator FEV$_1$)

In patients with FEV$_1$/FVC <0.70
GOLD 1: mild   FEV$_1$ $\geq$80% predicted
GOLD 2: moderate   50% $\leq$FEV$_1$ <80% predicted
GOLD 3: severe   30% $\leq$FEV$_1$ <50% predicted
GOLD 4: very severe   FEV$_1$ <30% predicted

Abbreviations: COPD, chronic obstructive pulmonary disease; FVC, forced vital capacity; FEV$_1$, forced expiratory volume in 1 second.

Pulmonary Interventions

Oxygen is useful to deter hypoxia in older adults with pulmonary issues. The use of oxygen must be balanced with consideration of the individual's drive to breathe. An older adult with healthy lungs will have a hypercarbic drive to breathe, whereas an older individual with COPD develops a hypoxic drive to breathe. Close observation of respiratory rate and effort on all older adults with oxygen therapy is necessary. Long-term use of oxygen is recommended for those individuals who have a Pao$_2$ less than 55 mm Hg as evaluated over a 3-week period.[15]

Noninvasive ventilation support has been shown to improve the quality of life for individuals with sleep apnea and COPD. Bilevel positive end-expiratory pressures for inspiration and expiration offer a way to regain adequate oxygenation and relieve hypercarbia in individuals with respiratory failure. The use of noninvasive ventilation requires an individual who is alert, with minimal mucus production, and who is calm enough for application of the facemask.[16] Noninvasive ventilation is as effective for respiratory failure in older adults as endotracheal intubation, but with shorter intensive care and in-hospital stays.[17]

Critical care nurses should encourage teeth brushing and flossing after each meal and bedtime in awake patients. Total-care patients need to have oral care provided at least 4 times a day. Water should be offered to maintain hydration in older adults.[9]

DISCUSSION

Nursing care for older adults requires the knowledge of the physiologic changes in the pulmonary system that result from aging. Bedside nursing care activities that assess and intervene in pulmonary alterations or age-related changes can reduce the number of complications in older adults. Oral care, water supplementation, and body positioning to ease breathing and release musculoskeletal structures may aid older adults in preventing complications attributable to normal aging.[2,3,9]

Further interventions are required for older adults with pulmonary diseases. Nurses can identify individual needs by attending to respiratory rate and effort. Changes in level of consciousness, confusion, agitation, or anxiety should alert the nurse to assess oxygen saturation as well.[17] Nurses should encourage smoking cessation in those older adults who continue to smoke. Even individuals within critical care settings will benefit from ambulation and positional passive exercises to release chest-wall tension.[11,15]

Nurses will continue to care for the older adult in critical settings for the foreseeable future. The population of older adults is increasing. It is important that nurses recognize the difference in expected pulmonary system changes during the aging process, and the pulmonary complications arising from pulmonary disease.

REFERENCES

1. Center for Disease Control and Prevention. Available at: http://www.cdc.gov. Accessed February 28, 2013.
2. Watsford ML, Murphy AJ, Pine MJ. The effects of ageing on respiratory muscle function and performance in older adults. J Sci Med Sport 2006;10:36–44.
3. Martini FH, Nath JL. The respiratory system, fundamentals of anatomy & physiology. 8th edition. San Francisco (CA): Pearson-Benjamin Cummings; 2009. p. 825–73.
4. Zeleznik J. Normative aging of the respiratory system. Clin Geriatr Med 2003;19: 1–18.
5. Chang AB, Widdiconbe JG. Cough throughout life: children, adults, and the senile. Pulm Pharmacol Ther 2007;20:371–82.
6. Parkes R. Rate of respiration: the forgotten vital sign. Emerg Nurse 2011;19(2): 12–8.
7. Venes D, editor. Taber's cyclopedic medical dictionary. 19th edition. Philadelphia: F.A. Davis Co; 2001. p. 2448–50.
8. Castellanos MR, Szerszen A, Saifan C, et al. Fasting hyperglycemia upon hospital admissions associated with higher pneumonia complication rates among the elderly. Int Arch Med 2010;3(16):1–7.
9. Huber J. Effects of utterance length and vocal loudness on speech breathing. Respir Physiol Neurobiol 2008;164:323–30.
10. Eisenstadt ES. Dysphagia and aspiration pneumonia in older adults. J Am Acad Nurse Pract 2010;22:17–22.
11. Takeshita T, Tomioka M, Shimazaki Y, et al. Microfloral characterization of the tongue coating and associated risk for pneumonia-related health problems in institutionalized older adults. J Am Geriatr Soc 2010;58:1050–7.
12. Ekstrum JA, Black LL, Paschal KA. Effects of a thoracic mobility and respiratory exercise program on pulmonary function and functional capacity in older adults. Phys Occup Ther Geriatr 2009;27(4):310–27.
13. Boyd AR, Orihuela CJ. Dysregulated inflammation as a risk factor for pneumonia in the elderly. Aging Dis 2011;2(6):487–500.
14. Hull CE. Community-acquired pneumonia management guidelines. Clinician Reviews 2007;17(9):28–34.
15. Global Initiative for Chronic Obstructive Lung Disease. Global strategy for the diagnosis, management, and prevention of chronic obstructive pulmonary disease (updated 2013). Available at: www.goldcopd.org. Accessed February 20, 2013.
16. Gursel G, Aydogdu M, Tasyurek S, et al. Factors associated with noninvasive ventilation response in the first day of therapy in patients with hypercapnic respiratory failure. Ann Thorac Med 2012;7(2):92–7.
17. Ramadan FH, El Sohl AA. Comment: respiratory failure in older adults. Respiratory Medicine. 2006; (13616706). pdf 20483752.

Printed and bound by CPI Group (UK) Ltd, Croydon, CR0 4YY

03/10/2024

01040398-0014